CONTROVERSIES
ABOUT
STUTTERING THERAPY

CONTROVERSIES ABOUT STUTTERING THERAPY

Edited by
Hugo H. Gregory, Ph.D.
Professor of Speech and Language Pathology
Director of Stuttering Programs
Northwestern University

University Park Press
Baltimore

UNIVERSITY PARK PRESS
International Publishers in Science, Medicine, and Education
233 East Redwood Street
Baltimore, Maryland 21202

Copyright © 1979 by University Park Press
Composed by University Park Press, Typesetting Division.
Manufactured in the United States of America by
The Maple Press Company.
Second printing, September 1980

Library of Congress Cataloging in Publication Data

Main entry under title:

Controversies about stuttering therapy.

Includes index.
1. Stuttering. 2. Speech therapy. I. Gregory, Hugo H. [DNLM:
1. Stuttering. 2. Stuttering — Therapy. WM475.3 C764]
RC424.C57   616.8'554'06   78-9923
ISBN 0-8391-1257-2

Contents

v

Contributors

Eugene B. Cooper, Ph.D., Professor and Chairman, Communicative Disorders, University of Alabama, University, Alabama 35486

Hugo H. Gregory, Ph.D., Professor of Speech and Language Pathology, Director of Stuttering Programs, Northwestern University, Evanston, Illinois 60201

William H. Perkins, Ph.D., Professor, Graduate Program in Communicative Disorders, University of Southern California, Los Angeles, California 90008

Bruce P. Ryan, Ph.D., Chairman, Communicative Disorders Department, California State University, Long Beach, California 90840

Joseph G. Sheehan, Ph.D., Professor of Psychology, University of California (UCLA), Los Angeles, California 90024

Ronald L. Webster, Ph.D., Professor of Psychology, Director of the Communications Research Institute, Hollins College, Roanoke, Virginia 24020

Dean E. Williams, Ph.D., Professor of Speech Pathology, University of Iowa, Iowa City, Iowa 52242

Preface

There has always been considerable controversy about the problem of stuttering and stuttering therapy. The purpose of this book is to clarify existing confusion about differing points of view by first stating controversial issues in the evaluation and treatment of stuttering and reviewing the literature pertaining to each; by second, presenting a specific discussion of these issues by recognized contemporary authorities who are active clinicians and researchers; and finally, by making a comparative analysis of the similarities and differences among the approaches described by the authors.

The contributors have responded to the issues in terms of their ideas, clinical experience, and research. They have referred to their most recent work and shown how this experience influences their thinking. In the comparative analysis, I have attempted to bring into focus the decisions clinicians have to make in therapy, as related to the issues discussed, and how the controversies, to some extent, may be resolved.

It is recommended that the book will be of greatest value if the review in Chapter One is studied before reading the six chapters by Cooper, Perkins, Ryan, Sheehan, Webster, and Williams responding to the issues. It should be understood clearly that the final chapter is not a summary. In this last chapter, "The Controversies: Analysis and Current Status," I have attempted to be very concise and review briefly what has come before only when it is essential to the logic of the discussion or when it appears necessary to prevent misinterpretation. Therefore, maximum comprehension of the analysis and conclusions in the final chapter depends upon a careful reading of each author's contribution.

Comparative analysis demands objectivity, and I have tried to be equal to the task. But, since I, too, am a practicing clinician with an evolving point of view, I am sure the reader will detect points in my analysis that could be viewed differently or explored more thoroughly. After all, a major thrust of this book is to stimulate students and practicing clinicians to continue the process of reflecting on these issues as they make decisions about evaluation and therapy.

Many people made this book possible. My mother and father, who very early helped me to form attitudes of appreciation for different points of view, have profoundly influenced my professional behavior and goals over the years.

For the last sixteen years my colleagues at Northwestern University have encouraged and supported my work in stuttering. I have learned much from them. When I conceived the idea of this book, Roy V. Wood, Dean of the School of Speech, and Roy Koenigsknecht, Head of the Program in Speech and Language Pathology (now Chairman of the Department of Communicative Disorders), offered tremendous support and arranged leave time for me to work specifically on this task.

Richard Schiefelbusch, University Professor and Director of the Bureau of Child Research at the University of Kansas, listened to my ideas about the book and made a number of useful suggestions.

I am indebted to my wife, Carolyn (who has now been with me for more than one-half of my life), for her encouragement and professional commentary.

Gratitude is also expressed to Professor Stephen McFarlane at the University of Nevada for his reactions to parts of the manuscript and his helpful suggestions.

Last, but certainly not least, I want to express my appreciation to the authors who joined with me in generating what we hope will be a unique and valuable book. Perhaps the reader can imagine the excitement with which I received the chapters, interested to see just how each contributor had responded to the controversial issues. Their work with me had a significant influence on my thinking about stuttering and its treatment and, for me at least, has enriched our friendships.

chapter ONE

Controversial Issues: Statement and Review of the Literature

Hugo H. Gregory, Ph.D.

It is appropriate to begin this book by stating and developing controversial issues related to the evaluation and treatment of stutterers. In doing so, reference will be made to the specific work of contemporary clinicians and researchers and to earlier contributors to provide a historical perspective. The following major issues will be discussed:

1. Teaching the stutterer to "stutter more fluently" versus teaching the stutterer to "speak more fluently"
2. Attitude change: what is it, and is it needed?
3. Psychotherapy for stutterers: what is it, and is it needed?
4. The appropriate management of stuttering in children
5. Planning the transfer of changes to the natural environment and dealing with the problem of relapse
6. Criteria for assessing the results of stuttering therapy; reports on the results of therapy

Before writing their chapters, the contributors read this review and discussion and considered the questions at the end of each section. The first chapter therefore should provide a frame of reference for reading the ones to follow, and like all of this book should serve as a focus for further discussion.

TEACHING THE STUTTERER TO "STUTTER MORE FLUENTLY" VS. TEACHING THE STUTTERER TO "SPEAK MORE FLUENTLY"

Stutter More Fluently Approach

Teaching the stutterer to stutter more fluently is the first of two general approaches to working with confirmed or secondary stutterers.[1] This approach is emphasized by Sheehan and Van Riper and is based on the ideas that the stutterer should make his[2] speech behavior the object of study, become familiar with it, and then gradually modify his stuttering by first thinking of and seeing how he can stutter more easily. Clinicians who adhere to this method believe this is an effective way to modify the stutterer's speech and to reduce avoidance behavior. It is said that the stutterer is not avoiding or inhibiting stuttering as much because he is letting it occur, then studying and modifying the behavior.

Van Riper — Identification, Desensitization, Modification Van Riper (1973) describes a sequence of therapeutic activities in which the stutterer identifies the overt behaviors and covert reactions associated with stuttering, and then learns to vary his general behavior first, before proceeding to variations in the stuttering behavior directed toward more fluent speech. Finally, activities are included that are intended to stabilize and generalize the changes made.

Van Riper emphasizes the stutterer's learning to vary the behaviors involved, beginning with those avoidance and postponement behaviors such as "Ah, Ah, Ah," which he sees as more under the stutterer's voluntary control than escape behaviors such as a prolonged fixation of the tongue for an alveolar sound, which are more closely related to core stuttering behaviors. He refers to the desensitizing effect, as well as the counterconditioning effect, of

---

[1]Discussion in this section focuses on confirmed or secondary stuttering, in most cases beyond elementary school age. The section on the appropriate management of children will deal with this issue as involved in therapy for children.

[2]Masculine pronouns are used throughout the book for the sake of grammatical uniformity and simplicity. They are not meant to be preferential or discriminatory.

these identification and modification activities. In discussing "modification: teaching a fluent form of stuttering," he says:

> The basic goal in this stage is to modify and shape the form of his stuttering so that it may occur without impairing the stutterer's communication or contributing to the maintenance of the disorder . . . *The sequential ordering* of the sounds he produces when stuttering should come as close as possible to that which characterizes normal utterances. Whatever the stutterer is doing that is inappropriate to the normal production of the sound, syllable, word or utterance should become a vivid error signal so that it can be altered in the direction of the normal utterance. (1973, pp. 311–312)

In the latter portion of the modification stage the enhancement of proprioceptive monitoring is emphasized utilizing auditory masking, delayed auditory feedback, and pantomiming. Then follow the procedures of cancellation, pull-out, and the use of motor planning and preparatory sets. Van Riper (1973) sums up by saying that the stutterer learns to stutter fluently and without the old struggle and avoidance. Historically, and up to the present, Van Riper (1963, 1971b, 1973) appears to believe that the stutterer's willingness to stutter, albeit in a modified way, is a very powerful psychological aspect of therapy that will lead to the most lasting and satisfying change in fluency.[3]

Sheehan — Avoidance Reduction, Role Acceptance, Role Taking
Sheehan (1968, 1970a, 1975) advocates the stutterer's acceptance of self in the dual roles of stutterer and normal speaker, that he accept stuttering as something he does, and that he take initiative to monitor and change the behavior. Perhaps a few quotations are the best way to introduce a brief review of his role theory and therapy.

> The acquisition of fluency in stuttering should come about indirectly, through the reduction of avoidance, through being open, through accepting the role of a stutterer. Anything that the stutterer has to do in a special or direct way to "achieve fluency" is probably wrong. (1970a, p. 25)

> For adults, a paradoxical feature of the problem is that role acceptance as a stutterer leads to being able to perform the role of a normal speaker, and the attempt to become a completely normal speaker leads back to the role of a stutterer. (1970a, p. 30)

---

[3]Starkweather (1973) provides an interesting behavioral analysis of Van Riper's therapy.

Since Sheehan believes, as does Sarbin (1964), that role enhancement with self-involvement is the best way to bring about changes in self-concept (he mentions the motto, "you are changed by what you do"), his avoidance reduction therapy consists of role assignments (Sheehan, 1975). For example, the clinician and client can explore the stutterer's stuttering; the stutterer can learn to monitor his speech; or the stutterer can learn to succeed by stuttering openly and easily, resisting time pressures, pausing and phrasing (use of silence), and voluntary stuttering. Increased fluency is seen as a by-product of these activities, which, with the exception of learning to pause and phrase, do not focus on improving the flow of speech. Sheehan reminds us that he does not use instruction in phrasing to help the stutterer avoid stuttering. Rather, he uses the procedure to teach a tolerance of silence, a confidence in being able to stop talking and to start again.

Bloodstein — Altering Tension and Fragmentation Another prominent contributor to stuttering therapy, Bloodstein (1958, 1975a) appears to adhere to the stutter more fluently point of view in his work with confirmed stutterers, those he refers to as being in Phase IV of four general phases of development he describes. He states:

> The central problem of treatment is not the difficulty of bringing about fluency, but the high probability of relapse; few quick cures are likely to be durable; and, in general, the most reliable way to achieve a lasting reduction of stuttering is to do it slowly and gradually through a process that enlists stutterers' comprehension of what they do when they stutter, why they do it, and how and why they are capable of altering their behavior. (1975a, p. 79)

Bloodstein describes procedures for analyzing the tension and fragmentation characterizing the stutterer's speech in order to help the stutterer see how he prevents himself from speaking more fluently by "pinching" and constricting the speech mechanism in various ways. As an aid to the stutterer's understanding of these unadaptive behaviors, Bloodstein suggests giving a description of the vocal apparatus. Thereafter, the objective is to achieve a pattern of stuttering "that is milder, simpler, less conspicuous, and less impeding to speech" (1975a, p. 82). Like Sheehan, Bloodstein recommends acceptance of the role of stutterer as he speaks, a role that can change as speech changes. Bloodstein's approaches to speech modification seem to be similar to those described by Van Riper.

Speak More Fluently Approach

Replacing stuttering speech behavior with fluent speech has been studied and advocated by several contributors during the last 15 years. Various approaches to instating fluency, as described below, are used, and features of the initially obtained fluency are usually modified to accomplish speech that is perceived as normal.

Goldiamond — *Instating a New Speech Pattern*   Goldiamond (1965) used delayed auditory feedback (DAF) in a negative reinforcement procedure to *instate fluency* beginning with oral reading and then attempted to transfer the fluency into other speaking situations. My office was approximately 50 yards from Goldiamond's laboratory at Southern Illinois University, where the work began in the late 1950s; therefore, it has been especially interesting for me to follow this development. Growing out of some basic experiments with disfluency and stuttering as operant behaviors, Goldiamond (1965) instructed subjects to use a prolonged speech pattern in reading while experiencing 250-msec DAF. The 250-msec delay served to negatively reinforce the prolonged pattern, for if the subjects tried to read faster the delay would have a disruptive effect. In other words, to avoid the aversive effect of DAF, a prolonged pattern was maintained. Once the new slowed speech pattern was established, the delay was faded out in 50-msec steps. In shaping the response pattern to normal speech, the reading rate was increased by presenting the material on a screen in front of the subject at faster rates. If previous patterns reappeared, the conditioning procedures as described were reinstated. More recently, Goldiamond (1977) has discontinued the use of DAF; instead, the technician or clinician models a new junctured speech pattern for the client. The junctured speech pattern can be learned in approximately 20 1-hour sessions. Goldiamond states that he tells prospective clients that he will teach them a new speech pattern that they can choose to use or not to use, "like a new coat that can be worn or left hanging in a closet."

Cherry and Sayers; Brady — *The Use of Masking and Rhythm*
Since Lee's 1951 article, "Artificial Stutter," there has been considerable interest in the integrity of auditory processes in stutterers and the effects that various forms of auditory and other sensory stimulation have on stuttering. In 1950, I attended my first American Speech and Hearing Association Convention at which

John Black and Grant Fairbanks demonstrated delayed auditory feedback equipment. As I, a stutterer who had been lucky enough to have therapy, talked under the influence of delayed sidetone, Black and Fairbanks noted that it was easier for me to control the DAF effects because I concentrated on tactile-kinesthetic feedback, something I had learned to do in therapy. Subsequently, in the last 25 years, a number of clinicians have used various forms of auditory stimulation including DAF, but also white noise and the rhythmic beat of a metronome. Cherry, Sayers, and Marland (1955) and Cherry and Sayers (1956) wrote about the total inhibition or the complete suppression of stammering (sic) using white noise at a high intensity level. Brady's study (1968) in which he used a metronome to instate fluency in severe, chronic stutterers was widely publicized as a successful approach. Initially, using a table model metronome, speech was paced one syllable to each beat. Metronome speed was changed gradually from 60 beats per minute to 100–120 beats per minute to attain a normal speaking rate. Later, a behind-the-ear type of metronome was introduced and gradually used outside the clinician's office. The loudness of the metronome could be gradually faded. When the subject encountered difficulty, a number of options including slowing the beat of the metronome were available.

In Poland, Adamczyk (1959, 1965) and Adamczyk, Sadowska, and Kuniszyk-Jozkowiak (1975) have used DAF (the echo and reverberation methods) to train stutterers in the production of fluency by having subjects time the production of syllables spoken. At the 1965 meeting of the International Logopedic and Phoniatric Society, Adamczyk described a telephone-echo system in which stutterers in Lublin, Poland, could telephone a number and practice speaking under DAF, either with their clinician present or while they were alone (Adamczyk, 1965).

There is much controversy about the use of these auditory stimulation procedures in therapy and about how the resulting fluency is produced. However, Beech and Fransella (1969) assert, based on studies comparing the effect of rhythmical metronome beats with arrhythmical beats and other tasks defined as distracting, that we should not dismiss the possibility of a valid therapeutic process involved. The reading of Bloodstein's (1975b) review and his comment that there may be a programming effect in the rhythmic stimulation of a metronome suggests that Bloodstein believes the increased fluency produced by a metronome could have legitimate therapeutic effects. Van Riper (1973) completes his assessment of syllable-timed speech and metronomic methods by saying:

> From all we have read and from all we have seen and personally ex-perienced, we would conclude that, at least in its present form, the use of this kind of speech training for the confirmed stutterer is inad-visable. (p. 70)

Ingham and Andrews (1973) sum up their review by stating, "All that one can conclude from the data is that stuttering is reduced in some 'rhythm therapies' and may carry over in some subjects" (p. 414). Ryan (1974) states the possibility that, like DAF, auditory stimulation procedures such as white noise and beats from a metronome are "stimulus support or stimulus control devices" (p. 78) and may be useful in establishing fluent speech.[4]

Perkins — Replacement of Stuttering with Normal Speech   In three reports on the replacement of stuttering with normal speech, Perkins (1973a, b) and Perkins et al. (1974) have delineated the ra-tionale for an approach, described the procedures, and commented on the effectiveness of therapeutic activities aimed toward the establishment of fluent speech, normal breath flow, normal prosody, and normal rate. The goal of establishing fluent speech is ac-complished by using DAF in very much the same manner as described by Goldiamond, although like Goldiamond he states that the clinician's modeling of a prolonged syllable pattern is also effec-tive. Perkins et al. (1974) stress that normal rate and prosody are essential to the acceptance of increased fluency by the stutterer. Thus they conclude that perhaps the primary need for rate control procedures is to serve as a "scaffold for perfecting the breath management skills of normal speech" (1974, p. 416). Breath management skills include adjusting the length of the phrase ap-propriately in terms of rate, initiating a phrase with an easy vocal attack, maintaining continuous airflow from the beginning to the end of the phrase, and blending syllables smoothly in a phrase. The following statement is an example of the type of analysis of the behavioral dimensions of speech that Perkins' clients learn:

> They know...that easy repetitions indicate a rate that is too fast, whereas pressure characteristics of repetitions, prolongations, or hesitations are signs of mismanagement of the breath stream, usually in conjunction with excessive rate. (Perkins, 1973a, pp. 290–291)

---

[4]Mysak (1960, 1966) presents a theory of stuttering and an interesting rationale for therapy with reference to auditory feedback and servo mechanisms.

A reader recognizes in Perkins' approach to the replacement of stuttering with normal speech that he utilizes his training and experience related to the normal speaking process, and all of the pathologies of speech including voice problems, to analyze the behaviors involved in the flow of speech and to modify the stutterer's speech. He recognizes that stutterers can speak normally under certain circumstances and, therefore, emphasizes that he is teaching them what they can do when they encounter difficulty. Apparently, learning to speak normally when difficulty is anticipated has to be a very highly conscious process, at least in the beginning.

Webster — Precision Fluency Shaping   Webster has been working with stutterers for several years developing a behavioral treatment now designated as the Precision Fluency Shaping Program. He states that "stutterers make the sounds of speech incorrectly" (1974, p. 35). To help the stutterer be able to initiate the characteristics of fluent speech with increasing efficiency, Webster is concerned directly with the teaching of target behaviors that generate fluent speech, e.g., gentle onset of voicing, and correct position, force, velocity, and duration of articulation. To reconstruct voice onsets, said by Webster to be "the single most important target in the program" (1975a, p. 4), a small instrument, the Voice Monitor, is used to measure voice onset characteristics.[5]

Webster (1974, 1975a) considers two aspects of the Precision Fluency Shaping Program of crucial importance: 1) breaking instruction down into the smallest units of phonation and articulation beginning with sounds and syllables and progressing to one-syllable words, two-syllable words, etc., and 2) providing for intensive practice resulting in overlearning the target responses. The latter is said to be crucial for transfer, a topic discussed later in this chapter. Although Webster does not say it, perhaps this overlearning is necessary if the stutterer is going to modify his speech, when as Perkins said, he expects difficulty or, as some other clinicians might say, when the speaker is in a more stressful situation. Webster makes no mention of emotional arousal or stress, probably because these variables cannot be specified as can be the phonatory and articulatory gestures involved. For the purpose of this discussion, the following quote should help the reader sense the essence of Webster's approach:

---

[5]Agnello (1975) has also developed an instrument designed to assist stutterers with voice onset skills.

The duration of the one-syllable word was greatly exaggerated at the outset. With increased proficiency in attaining the gentle onset and duration speech targets, the amount of prolongation was reduced until, by the time the subjects were working with three-syllable words, they were producing words of a duration that would be associated with the speech rate of 100 to 130 words per minute. At the next stage of the program the subjects constructed short sentences. After that longer sentences were constructed . . .

Subjects began to transfer practice on single words into their home environment early in the program, to practice some limited conversation at home using an exaggerated slow speech pattern, and then as the progression through the program continued, they transferred longer and more comprehensive fluent speech behavior into their everyday lives. (Webster, 1974, p. 36)

In his lecturing and writing, Webster (1974) has been critical of those speech-language pathologists who, he says, have not "attempted to apply systematic, direct, manipulative techniques to stuttering" (1974, p. 28). He implies that this is because psychotherapy is "perhaps the most pervasive treatment devised for stuttering . . ." (1974, p. 24). He seems to see a parallel between the lack of a behavioral approach in psychotherapy and the same in speech-language pathology and speech therapy for stutterers, a parallel that some speech-language pathologists probably would not agree exists to the degree perceived by Webster. Although speech-language pathologists and psychologists (Sheehan, 1970b; Van Riper, 1973; Bloodstein, 1975a), describing behavior modification approaches to stuttering therapy, have spoken of fear and anxiety reduction as a crucial aspect of the rationale for what they do, nevertheless, they have taught the stutterer how to modify his behavior in ways that were well structured and systematic. However, it is true that the structure has not usually been as specific as that evolved by Webster or that involved in Ryan's programmed learning procedures.

Finally, Webster has encouraged those who have a tendency to criticize fluency-producing therapies (e.g., the use of a metronome) as only distractions, to be more open to empirical observation of what appears to have beneficial effects. Accordingly, these observations should lead to much thought and study.

Ryan — Systematic Programmed Instruction   The main thrust of Ryan's 1974 book, *Programmed Therapy for Stuttering in Children and Adults,* is the systematic programming of therapy in a series of steps, each defined in terms of stimulus, response, consequence, and criteria. The target of these programs is fluent speech.

Ryan says this may not be the only goal that therapy should achieve, but that it certainly should be one of them! He describes the establishment, transfer, and maintenance of fluency in children and adults in four programs designated as operant: 1) Traditional, 2) DAF, 3) Punishment, and 4) Gradual Increase in Length and Complexity of Utterance (GILCU). Interestingly, with reference to the controversy being discussed, the Traditional Program is an adaptation of Van Riper's method of analyzing and modifying stuttering behavior employing identification procedures, cancellations, pull-outs, and, finally, fluent productions. The DAF Program relies on procedures stimilar to Goldiamond's. In describing the Punishment Program, Ryan reminds us that Shames (1970) believes that much stuttering therapy as practiced in the last 25 years is composed of punishing events, e.g., cancellation (interrupting speech or communication after a stuttered word). Thus, Ryan (1974) looks at the use of punishing consequences in a program from a broad perspective but points to verbal contingencies and time-out as especially useful procedures. The GILCU Program is "concerned with the development of fluent speech through the careful control of the evoking stimuli" (Ryan, 1974, p. 87). The subject is instructed to read one word fluently, then two, then three to six, followed by one sentence, two sentences, etc., and finally in later program steps, 5 minutes of reading fluently. As in all of Ryan's work, the program is continued from reading to monologue and conversational modes. Of the four programs, the GILCU has been used with the younger subjects and is even mentioned as appropriate for preschoolers if, as one assumes, appropriate materials are substituted for reading.

Ryan has had the greater amount of experience with the Traditional Program and the DAF Program. In comparing the four, he recommends that the clinician adopt the one "which best can be accomplished in his or her individual setting with the equipment and skills available to him or her" (1974, p. 90). In other words, his view is that fluency can be produced in several different programs. With reference again to the controversy of "stuttering more fluently" or "speaking more fluently," Ryan appears agreeable to using an adaptation of Van Riper's technique even though he does not share Van Riper's conviction that to deal effectively with stuttering the stutterer should learn to stutter more fluently.

Others such as Haroldson, Martin, and Starr (1968), Leach (1969), and Shaw and Shrum (1972) have presented operant conditioning procedures to reduce stuttering and increase fluency.

Wingate — Improved Vocal Modulation in the Production of Stressed Syllables and the Forward Flow of Speech   During the last decade, Wingate (1966, 1967a, b, 1971) has studied prosodic and linguistic factors related to stuttering and has analyzed the relationship between these factors and conditions resulting in the reduction of stuttering (Wingate, 1969, 1976). Recently, Wingate (1976, 1978) has described a broad therapeutic program for stutterers that includes counseling (giving information and dealing with feelings and attitudes) and that focuses on the modification of the person's speech by "generating the experience of fluency and helping the patient understand the basis for how fluency is achieved" (1976, p. 329). The understanding referred to stems from Wingate's analysis: 1) that stuttering occurs almost exclusively on stressed syllables,[6] when the subject cannot manage the phonatory changes related to the production of stressed vowels in the flow of connected speech, and 2) that procedures such as singing, choral speaking, shadowing, rhythmic speech, and DAF ameliorate stuttering because they produce prosodic changes, increased duration of phonation, reduced rate, reduction of stress contrasts between syllables, etc., that make it easier to actualize stress increases and keep speech flowing.

In Wingate's method, the above mentioned procedures that ameliorate stuttering are used to demonstrate that increased fluency can be obtained by making certain prosodic modifications. The melody aspect of speech is illustated; one of the procedures, called "sounding," is used as follows:

> Sounding is to ordinary speech as humming is to a song; it consists of producing the melody without the words...A good point to begin is with the use of a single rhyme. Nursery rhymes are good; so are very lyric kinds of poems such as 'The Village Blacksmith.' This should be followed by examples from less metered poetry and then some prose, including bits of ordinary conversation. (Wingate, 1976, p. 337)

Techniques that follow are aimed toward showing that speech melody is the expression of linguistic stress, that certain syllables are stressed and others are unstressed, and that speech is ballistic, i.e., it involves smooth and continuous motion in a temporal pattern

---

[6]Wingate (1976, p. 262) comments: "Occasionally stuttering will be observed to involve an unstressed vowel immediately preceding a syllable bearing stress prominence...It seems reasonable to hypothesize that in such cases coarticulatory planning for the adjustments necessary to express stress is slightly premature."

that involves changes in phonation (volume, duration, and pitch) as the underlying, basic process. Again, reading poetry is used for practice. Exaggeration of melody patterns at slower rates is used for emphasis. When the stutterer anticipates difficulty, he is advised to focus on moving into the vowel sound of the stressed syllable, a skill he has been practicing. Wingate offers a number of suggestions for implementing his approach and developing skill in natural speaking situations. He states that effective results require earnest effort.

Wingate's therapy is classified as a speak more fluently approach because stuttering and associated behaviors are only examined briefly to illustrate the nature of the problem; learning the melody of fluent speech is the focus of treatment. In fact, Wingate considers the analysis of stuttering behavior as recommended by Cooper, Gregory, Sheehan, Van Riper, and others as inefficient. In passing, one final point of considerable interest about Wingate's point of view is revealed in the following quotation:

> It is more realistic to understand this defect, in its observable occurrence, as something that *happens*. It is not meaningfully understood as essentially something one *does* — unless we are willing to speak in the same manner about such other actions as stumbling, yawning, hiccoughing, trembling, and the like. (Wingate, 1976, pp. 326–327)

In other words, stuttering is a phonatory dysfunction, but apparently the person can either adjust to the dysfunction and experience a remission of stuttering or receive treatment that helps in dealing with the dysfunction.

Schwartz — Airflow Technique Schwartz (1974, 1976) hypothesizes that stuttering is related to the lack of normal inhibition of what he designates as the airway dilation reflex. According to him, this reflex acts at the level of the nostrils, tongue, pharynx, and larynx to widen the breathing passage when there is a sudden need for a substantial amount of air. If the neurophysiological inhibition is not normally established, stress ordinarily associated with speech and increased air pressure involved in speech production brings about the reflex: "the vocal cords open wide, and the child becomes temporarily speechless" (Schwartz, 1976, p. 33). To compensate for this possibility, Schwartz believes that a child anticipating such an occurrence learns to close the vocal folds tightly, producing what is called a "laryngospasm." This, he says, is the heart of the stuttering problem, and the struggling observed in stuttering is a reaction to the laryngospasm.

In describing therapy, Schwartz observes that former stutterers he interviewed exhibited "tiny airflows" just before they spoke. He hypothesized that these observed, but not verified by research, airflows were used to ". . .ensure an opening of the vocal cords prior to speaking" (1976, p. 84). From this he formulated his treatment described as follows:

> I now began to experiment with airflow technique. I started by asking a stutterer to produce a long, audible, and relaxed sigh. I then asked him to sigh once again, and when halfway through it, to say a one-syllable word. The stuttering aborted immediately. I increased the number of one-syllable words spoken on a breath. Again, there was no stuttering. (Schwartz, 1976, pp. 84–85)

Schwartz's therapy is based on the passive airflow technique. He views therapy as needing to be intensive during the early stages, as involving changes in self-concept as well as fluency, and as being long-term, although changes in fluency can be rather immediate. In his book, *Stuttering Solved,* in which there are no references to the literature, Schwartz does not mention that Gifford (1956) described a similar approach to therapy. In listing steps in the training process for stutterers, Gifford describes "Learning how to release the voice on the outgoing breath stream, using the 'sigh principle' with the breathy tone quality" (p. 53).

The pretentious title of Schwartz's book, *Stuttering Solved,* the informal, "after dinner speech" style of writing, the omission of references and bibliography, and the apparent premature generalization from a proposed "model of the core of the stuttering block" (Schwartz, 1974, p. 169) to the claim that he has explained stuttering have made the book a very controversial one (see Gregory, 1977).

Summary and Discussion

Whereas contributors such as Bloodstein (1975a), Sheehan (1970a, 1975), and Van Riper (1973) seem to place the objective of studying and monitoring speech behavior ahead of the accomplishment of increased fluency in working with confirmed stutterers, Brady (1968, 1969), Cherry and Sayers (1956), Goldiamond (1965), Perkins (1973a, b), Ryan (1974), and Webster (1974) seem more interested in bringing about an efficient (rapid) increase in fluency and an efficient (rapid) decrease in stuttering.

Realizing the possibility of some misrepresentation by categorizing clinicians' beliefs, we have seen that, in general, the first group thinks that by learning to monitor and gradually change the stuttering behavior the stutterer is reducing his sensitivity to stuttering (desensitization), and simultaneously this prepares the way for the most effective modification (counterconditioning) of stuttering to take place. Step by step, avoidance behavior is reduced and approach tendencies are increased. The stutterer sees himself in the realistic role of a person who is changing, a person who stutters but who is stuttering more and more fluently. Voluntary stuttering is used for the additional desensitization derived (Van Riper, 1973; Sheehan, 1975) from emitting such disfluent behaviors as simple repetitions and prolongations purposefully (see also Damste, 1970). Through these procedures, the stutterer can move toward increased fluency with more confidence that he can cope with avoidance and inhibitory tendencies. Bloodstein (1975a), Sheehan (1970a, 1975), and Van Riper (1973) acknowledge that there are easier ways to increased fluency, but that their general approach is the most effective way to prevent serious recurrence and relapse. The dichotomy between fluency and stuttering is reduced.

Brady (1968, 1969), Cherry and Sayers (1956), Goldiamond (1965), Perkins (1973a, b), Ryan (1974), Webster (1974), and Wingate (1976) countercondition the stutterers' inappropriate unadaptive speech behavior by using the procedures discussed to instate or increase fluent speech. With the exception of the identification procedure used in Ryan's Traditional and DAF Programs, the transition is from speech containing occurrences of stuttering to some form of fluent speech flow with minimal, if any, attention to the monitoring of stuttering. Oftentimes, the fluency obtained initially is shaped (Ryan, 1974; Webster, 1974; Goldiamond, 1965). This group has been more devoted to operant conditioning and systematic programming than has the stutter more fluently group, and the proponents imply that this systematic approach is significant in the rationale for what they do and the eventual outcome of their therapy.

Ryan (1974), in answering the charge that these procedures, e.g., the DAF shaping programs, are merely distractions, points out that most therapy procedures for stuttering have suffered from an inability to condition long-term fluency. We will see later in this chapter that some of these clinical investigators emphasize additional components (e.g., Brady uses systematic desensitization) in a therapy program. Ryan acknowledges the anxiety factor in stuttering and the stutterer's fear of stuttering. Apparently, his opinion is that building speech fluency is one of the best ways known at present to diminish anxiety about stuttering, increase approach behavior, and decrease avoidance behavior. This exemplifies the attitude of many operant conditioners that the best way to deal with obscurely defined emotion is by changing overt behavior. Proponents of the stutter more fluently approach say these speak more fluently approaches do not desensitize the person to stuttering and disfluency and, in fact, may increase sensitivity to disfluency.

Other Contributors

Several other contributors to contemporary ideas about stuttering therapy are judged, based on their publications, not to be associated closely with either of the two schools of thought being analyzed, or appear to combine some aspects of both in the methods they advocate for helping confirmed stutterers accomplish normally fluent speech.

Shames — The Accommodating Nature of Operant Conditioning Shames and his students (Shames, Egolf, and Rhodes, 1969; Shames, 1975) have demonstrated ways in which adaptations of therapeutic procedures advocated by Van Riper (1963), Sheehan (1958b), and others for reducing stuttering can be implemented utilizing operant conditioning principles. Actually, Ryan's work on his Traditional Program (Ryan, 1964), begun in his doctoral dissertation directed by Shames, was such a demonstration. However, the objective of these demonstrations has not been to have the stutterer stutter more easily or fluently, but rather to reinforce modifications of speech aimed more directly toward increasing the operant behavior of fluency. On the other hand, a rapid, efficient increase in some form of fluency does not seem to be the objective as much as it is in the case of Goldiamond's, Perkins', or Webster's approaches using DAF or the clinician's modeling to establish such fluency. Shames and Egolf in their book, *Operant Conditioning and the Management of Stuttering* (1976), have emphasized that operant conditioning procedures can accommodate stuttering therapy procedures arising from various theories about the disorder and its treatment. In my opinion, this emphasis has been helpful to speech-language pathologists striving to integrate new developments into their clinical practice. Shames and Egolf view operant behaviors broadly (covert attitudinal responses included), and we will, therefore, return to their work in the following section dealing with attitudes.

Williams — Speech Exploration, Increasing Easy Normal Speech Williams (1971), with reference to therapy for school-age children, describes his approach in which there is an analysis of the person's total talking behavior, how he talks, and how he interferes with talking, "talking easy" and "talking hard." According to Williams, a person learns that when he makes a "mistake" while talking he can make the mistake easily. Williams cautions not to focus on stuttering, but on the overall way of talking. Thus, he seems to attempt to prevent the person from attending to stuttering or striving for fluency; he directs the person to a way of talking in which the person senses and changes disruptive tension that interferes with the forward movement of speech.

Brutten and Shoemaker — Extinction of Emotional Responses and Adjustive Behaviors   Brutten and Shoemaker (1967) and Brutten (1975) view stuttering therapy as involving the deconditioning of negative emotion that through learning has come to disorganize speech and cause stuttering (defined as repetitions and prolongations of parts of words) and the counterconditioning of instrumental behaviors that the stutterer learns as he copes with negative emotion. Earlier, Brutten and Shoemaker (1967) recommended a careful analysis of instrumental coping behaviors (secondary behaviors) and massed repetitions, similar to negative practice, to extinguish these responses. Recently, Brutten (1975), commenting on the behavioral mixtures in stuttering, has said:

> The stock use of a particular tactic or combination of procedures independent of the behaviors involved is questionable. Awareness of the behaviors involved, the tactics available, and the individual's responsivity needs to replace slavish devotion to inflexible clinical procedures. (p. 255)

Cooper — Reducing Associated Behavior, Fluency Initiating Gestures, Feeling of Control   Cooper (1965, 1968) differentiates between the moment of stuttering, the act of "getting stuck," and the behaviors that have been conditioned as reactions to the core behaviors. The early stages of therapy include identification and analysis of these behaviors. Then the stutterer is taught to modify those behaviors that are said to be reactions to the stuttering. In this way, Cooper seems to be instructing the client to accept the stuttering but reduce the associated behaviors. Cooper implies that this acceptance of stuttering reduces avoidance tendencies while the person gradually strives, under the clinician's direction, to reduce learned avoidance and inhibitory behaviors such as head shaking, accessory sounds, and tense articulatory contacts. Most recently, Cooper (1976) has described helping the stutterer use certain fluency-initiating gestures (slow speech, easy speech, smooth speech, etc.) that result in his having increased feelings of fluency control.

Gregory — Analysis and Modification of Stuttering, Building New Psychomotor Speech Patterns Gregory (1968, 1973a) adopts a position that specifies that in most cases the unadaptive stuttering behavior needs to be monitored and changed in such a way that the person becomes acquainted with the topography of his stuttering. But he also advocates that the stutterer practice new psychomotor speech patterns. Thus, the beginning stages of therapy are more like those of Van Riper and Sheehan and the later stages utilize methods like those used by Perkins, Ryan, and Webster. Gregory presents a sequence of activities aimed toward simultaneous desensitization (reduction of fear-arousing stimuli including the occurrence of stuttering) and counterconditioning of stuttering responses. The sequence includes analysis of stuttering and the use of negative practice, cancellations, pull-outs, and altered preparatory sets, voluntary disfluency, delayed responses, building up new psychomotor speech patterns,[7] and other individualized and appropriate modifications of speech.

Building up new psychomotor speech patterns, the part of therapy that stresses normal speech fluency, begins later in therapy. Gregory (1968) says:

> At that time in therapy when avoidance tendencies are diminishing and approach tendencies are increasing, improvement of speech skills is stressed by teaching appropriate rate control (through the use of phrasing and the proper duration of vowel sounds), better vocal inflection, and an increased awareness of the variations in articulatory pressure which can be used in producing sounds . . . The significance of this activity is that it increases even further the stutterer's positive expectations, feelings of hope, and approach tendencies, as contrasted to his negative expectations and avoidance tendencies. (p. 124)

The ability to be more flexible in speech (as opposed to the stutterer's usual rigidity) and to learn more flexibility including increased fluency is in part a product of the earlier clinical work directed toward analysis and modification, but also the work on the improvement of speech skills. Influenced by programmed instruction developments such as Ryan's work, Gregory and Mordecai (1977) have written programs specifying stimuli, responses, consequences, and criteria in employing identification, monitoring, modification, and transfer procedures.

---

[7]In a similar vein, Frick (1965) has described the use of motor-planning procedures for the treatment of stutterers.

Questions for Contributors

1. Should we have as our goal the changing of the secondary stutterer's speech to more fluent speech utilizing procedures *from the beginning of therapy* that modify the behaviors involved with reference to the physical production of normal speech and with minimal or no reference to the individual's behaviors associated with what we label as stuttering?
2. Should we have as our goal the changing of the secondary stutterer's speech to more fluent speech by helping the stutterer learn to monitor his physical speech behavior, including behavior labeled as stuttering, and then gradually modify his speech?
3. Just as the fluency shaper may overemphasize fluency, is it possible that clinicians who adhere to the more fluent stuttering approach get overly focused on stuttering and do not focus sufficiently on the varying characteristics of normal speech?
4. Can work on monitoring and observation of stuttering behavior early in therapy be combined with more direct work on normal speech flow as therapy continues?
5. Is it possible that different stutterers need different approaches, depending on the type of behavior emitted, the severity of their speech difficulty, and their reaction to their speech?
6. Is the controversy between the two groups diminished when advocates of both approaches include a carefully planned desensitization-generalization program recognizing the stress component or the conditioned emotional arousal (Brutten and Shoemaker, 1967) involved in stuttering?
7. Although clinicians' stated objectives may differ, are clients learning some of the same things in a therapy program? Sheehan (1970a) notes that he does not use phrasing to avoid stuttering. Rather, he uses this procedure to teach the tolerance of silence, a confidence in being able to stop talking and start again. Is the same tolerance learned in Perkins' or Webster's therapy when stutterers practice the same general behavior? To be beneficial, does it need to be pointed out to the client what he is learning?

ATTITUDE CHANGE: WHAT IS IT? IS IT NEEDED?

Gregory (1968), with reference to Allport (1935) and Mowrer (1960a, b), suggests that attitudes be viewed as mediating responses, dispositions to respond in certain ways based on emotional conditioning and a person's beliefs. Defined in this way, attitudes include affective and cognitive responses to stimuli. We gauge attitudes by verbal statements, nonverbal behavior, and perhaps some physiological measure (e.g., galvanic skin response) of affective responding.[8] Awareness of attitudes varies; consequently, it may or may not be possible to verbalize an attitude at a certain point in time.

We recognize that changing the stutterer's speech by teaching the person to "stutter more fluently," "speak more fluently," or however it is done, results in cognitive and affective changes. Thus, attitude change is occurring. This has been recognized by speech-language pathologists but has received added emphasis from speech-language pathologists and psychologists such as Ryan (1974) and Webster (1974), who have created precise speech change programs. However, Sheehan (1970a, 1975), who, as we have described, is associated with a different philosophy from that of Ryan or Webster, also stresses that behavior change (role enactment, as he sees it) brings about attitudinal or self-concept changes.

Therefore, the focus of controversy about attitude change in stuttering therapy is not whether behavior change produces attitude change. Instead, it is related to the extensiveness of procedures used *directly* to change beliefs and affective responses. For purposes of discussion, procedures in which cognitive attitudinal change is the major objective are considered first, followed by those in which affective attitudinal change is emphasized. It is realized that cognitive or belief-oriented approaches involve an affective component and vice versa. Mowrer (1960a, b) states that cognitive, affective, and motor aspects of behavior are conditioned one to the other by classical conditioning.

Cognitive Attitudinal Change

In behavioral psychology there is considerable evidence that awareness of intended target behaviors, what is being reinforced, and under what conditions, has an influence on learning (Bandura, 1969). Imagery and symbolic cues represent the principle cognitive means for this awareness. Wischner (1969), in commenting on

---

[8]Because these three responses can be viewed and studied as operants, some operant conditioners recommend analyzing attitudinal behavior in the same way as other behavior, i.e., in terms of stimulus consequences and associated discriminating stimuli (see Bandura, 1969, pp. 599–624, for a review of attitude change theories and strategies).

behavior therapy and stuttering therapy, questions the relationship between what a person says to himself and what he will actually do; in other words, the effects of self-verbalization on conditioning. Speech-language pathologists' treatment of stutterers has a long history of using interview-type counseling approaches, in an individual and group therapy setting, to explore the beliefs of stutterers or the parents of stutterers and to impart needed information. Just as these verbal interaction, thought-oriented approaches have been criticized in psychotherapy as less effective, current stuttering therapists with a behavior analysis/behavior modification point of view have questioned the value of attitude-oriented verbalizations between clinician and client. I suspect that this criticism has often been sharp to emphasize a point. In other words, the intended message may be: "Talking about the problem may be needed but don't talk to the extent that you do not focus adequately on the modification of the stutterer's speech." We all know of situations in which conversations between clinicians and clients that are not goal oriented are probably wasteful. However, practically speaking, all clinicians influence the client's beliefs about the problem, about himself as a stutterer, and about therapy by comments they make and by information and instructions they give (Williams, 1968). Verbal interaction is such an accepted and expected part of our society that it is hard to imagine a situation in which the clinician does not influence the client through this process.

Many clinicians, including myself (Gregory, 1968, 1973a), have stressed the evaluation of beliefs and attitude change. As pointed out (Gregory, 1968), in modifying attitudinal responses the clinician is essentially an operator in the field of language going about his work in the following ways:

1. He searches out with the client certain attitudes as revealed by the client's verbal report.
2. He helps the client acquire new verbal labels, in other words, new terminology that helps him to extend his understanding of his attitudinal and overt behavioral reponses.
3. He selectively rewards certain statements made by the client that he considers as indicating a change of thinking in the desired direction.
4. He makes certain interpretations that are appropriately timed. (Gregory, 1968, p. 112)

Johnson (1961b, 1967) and Williams (1957, 1968, 1969) have discussed the role of evaluations and beliefs in the development of stuttering and the need for work on the examination of these beliefs in therapy. In 1950, while an undergraduate student, I heard Johnson describe the influence of general semantics upon his ideas about stuttering. Johnson believed that the way the person came to think about his speech, stemming from the meanings of words and the influence these had on his thinking and behavior, were very important. For example, the label "stutterer" was misleading. A person could be both a stutterer and a nonstutterer at the same time. Furthermore, a person must not overgeneralize by saying "I stutter," but he must observe the specific things he does when he talks. Perceptual and evaluative reorientation, accomplished in a dialogue between client and clinician or in group sessions, became a significant part of Johnson's program of therapy. Williams (1957) extended this development and has most recently suggested ways to talk with children that bring about clarification of beliefs and a congruence between beliefs and behavior monitoring and change (Williams, 1971).

Sheehan (1970a, 1975) describes stuttering therapy as involving both motoric and attitudinal aspects. We see in Sheehan's therapy the teaching of an attitude about therapy, and he lists ideas that have been found supportive for any stutterer. For example, as related to the controversy about speech modification discussed earlier, he says, "You have a choice — you can exercise a choice to stutter openly and smoothly" (1970a, p. 277). Sheehan (1970a) also stresses work with the attitude of important listeners in the stutterer's environment. Perkins et al. (1974) observe that since stuttering begins at an early age the person's whole mode of living is influenced by the experience he has as a speaker. They imply that a needed psychotherapeutic aspect of therapy should relate to this; they also recommend exploring attitudes of family and friends. Van Riper (1973) advocates an exploration of attitude change analogous to an exploration of speech change.

Some discussions of attitudes appear to be, to some degree, a commentary on what these writers observe resulting from the contemporary emphasis of operant conditioning on overt observable behavior and a de-emphasis on cognitive and emotional variables that are not readily observed. Cooper (1965, 1968, 1976) continues to show considerable interest in the stutterer's immediate and private interpretations of experiences. In his descriptions of Interpersonal Communication Therapy (IPC) (Cooper, 1968) and Personalized Fluency Control (PFC) (Cooper, 1976), he includes steps for modifying perceptions, feelings, and attitudes during the clinician-client relationship. The affective component of this relationship, stressed by Cooper, is discussed in the next section. Cooper concludes that behaviorism applied to modifying the stutterer's speaking should be combined with phenomenological approaches to self-awareness. He quotes Combs and Snygg (1959):

> People do not behave according to the facts as others see them. They behave according to the facts as they see them. What governs behavior from the point of view of the individual himself are his unique perceptions of himself and the world in which he lives, the meanings things have for him. (Combs and Snygg, 1959, p. 17)

Murphy and Fitzsimons (1960) advocate therapy that emphasizes the individuality of every stutterer and the impact of attitudinal shifts. More recently, Murphy (1970), in commenting on conditioning in stuttering therapy, has said:

> The clinician's job must be more than simply describing and shaping stutterers; it should be to experience and understand them, and to help them chart the course of their own becoming. (p. 109)

Many contemporary behavior analysts and modifiers are perplexed by such a recommendation. They ask: What does the clinician do? What are the therapeutic operations? To Murphy, the existing subjectivity in the client-clinician relationship is crucial; for in reality, life is personal and subjective. Murphy is concerned that the dynamic interaction of interpersonal relations and intrapersonal reactions are not given attention by some therapists who center upon overt, more observable behavior.

Ryan (1974) refers to attitude as an operant aspect of stuttering defined by verbal statements. He goes on to suggest that it is stuttering that produces attitude problems. Finally, Ryan suggests the possibility of a combined therapy program including fluency training and attitude change such as that reported by Blind, Shames, and Egolf (1971) and Shames and Egolf (1976), in which the thematic content of the client's verbalization is shaped. In modifying thematic content, the clinician reacts with verbal approval to statements of the client defined as positive and with verbal disapproval to negative statements. For example, if the client says, "I sometimes change words when I think I am going to stutter," the clinician recognizes this as a positive response because the client is describing an avoidance behavior and using language that implies he is taking responsibility for the behavior. Thus, the clinician repeats or paraphrases the client's response and adds what Shames and Egolf (1976) call a positive tag line, such as, "good description,

I understand." Shames and Egolf's data show that the content of stutterers' verbalizations can be modified using this procedure, and they conclude that operant principles can be applied to modify the content of a stutterer's thinking. Perkins (1973b) recommends the incorporation of these content modification procedures in therapy to increase positive language responses. He, like Shames, Egolf, and Rhodes (1969), implies that an increase in positive language responses represents a change in a person's assumptions.

Affective Attitudinal Change

Certain procedures are a direct attempt to countercondition-desensitize a person's disposition to respond with negative affect to certain stimulus conditions. Others are more general and involve affective responses of a client to the clinical situation in which the clinician states that he is being accepting, empathic, genuine, etc.

Brutten and Shoemaker (1967) and Gray and England (1972) have applied Wolpe's systematic desensitization-counterconditioning approach in a direct effort to reduce the affective reaction of negative emotion associated with certain speech cues. Relaxation is commonly used to reciprocally inhibit or countercondition negative emotion. Based on an extensive interview, the clinician helps the client construct a hierarchy of feared speaking situations. The client then imagines a situation, or perhaps an aspect of the total situation in the beginning, and strives to stay relatively relaxed. When the relaxed criteria are reached at one point in the hierarchy, the same procedure is repeated at the next level. Clinicians using this procedure believe that the reduction of negative emotion results in 1) reducing the core stuttering behaviors elicited by negative emotion, and 2) making it easier to deal with coping or secondary behaviors motivated by higher levels of negative emotions. In passing, we recognize the cognitive elements involved in this approach. As described, there is imagery, but no doubt there is self-verbalization, too.

I use relaxation procedures to enable stutterers to be more calm in stressful speaking situations (Gregory, 1968). In this case the goal is to reduce negative emotion in a hierarchy of speaking situations beginning with the least stressful. Relaxation work is an integral part of an overall therapy program. Both Brutten and Shoemaker (1967) and myself (1968, 1973a) report the use of role playing in the clinical environment to prepare the client for the transfer of reduced responding with negative emotion to real life situations.

Biofeedback procedures, providing the subject with some observable indications of what is going on internally, are being explored as direct approaches to modifying emotional responses.[9] These techniques may be used in the counterconditioning and desensitization procedures just mentioned by measuring electromyographic (muscle) responses, galvanic skin resistances, heart rates, and blood pressure. Usually, these responses are transduced into visual or auditory feedback signals for monitoring purposes.

Those who use specific procedures aimed toward the modification of beliefs, assumptions, evaluations, etc., often describe differing types of client-clinician relationships that are appropriate at various times in therapy. The personal nature of this relationship is emphasized. For one thing, as the client and clinician work together they need to be able to trust each other. The clinician becomes a unique person in the experience of the client. Likewise, as mentioned by Ainsworth (1977) and Murphy (1970, 1974), the clinician responds in such a way that the client recognizes that the clinician is interested in him as a unique human being. Sometimes, this is referred to as a humanistic emphasis.

The relationship between the client and the clinician relates to the clinician emitting certain verbal responses designated as warm, interested, empathic, supportive, accepting, congruent, confronting, etc. (Rogers, 1957; Murphy and Fitzsimons, 1960; Cooper, 1965, 1968, 1976; Gregory, 1968; Sheehan, 1970a; Van Riper, 1973, 1975; and Murphy, 1974, 1977). The important element is the affective response of the client to the clinician's behavior. If the relationship between client and clinician is not characterized by some significant emotional responding, then it is said to be more intellectual and less significant to the client in terms of understanding and potential for growth and long-term change. Viewing therapy this way, the clinician can have general goals that may become more specific as the clinical relationship develops, but the clinician is described as being open to the unique experience of the client. The clinician, therefore, does not program therapy as specifically as some clinicians oriented to operant conditioning or programmed instruction may wish.[10]

---

[9]For an extensive review of biofeedback procedures, see Shapiro and Surwit (1976), and for a review of studies in stuttering, see Shames and Egolf (1976). Also, see Guitar (1975).

[10]A number of clinicians are exploring ways to combine elements of differing approaches. For example, some emphasize the affective nature of client-clinician rela-

Empathic responding is one type of response that many writers in psychotherapy and stuttering therapy have described as representing a display of affect by the clinician that influences the client's exploration and understanding of feelings. In responding empathically, the clinician is identifying as best he can with the feeling or affective reaction the client is experiencing and communicating this understanding to the client.[11] If the clinical relationship is one in which the client appreciates the nature of his personal relationship with the clinician, then the clinician's empathy is reinforcing and should increase the client's willingness to continue expressions of feeling. One of the principal objectives of this is to increase the client's self-understanding and willingness to accept the experiencing of affect. The clinician is saying, "Accept your emotional reactions more and begin to explore." Clinicians who work with stutterers are reminded of the similarity between this and the exploration of stuttering behavior as recommended by some authorities. The clinician's status and the clinical atmosphere are probably important in that the clinician's interest and acceptance are rewarding to the client. With reference to the modeling of behavior, it may be that the clinician is modeling an attitude toward the client (e.g., less punitive) that he wants the client to adopt as a self-attitude.

Just as with most clinical procedures, there are many possible outcomes of such methods as these. The labeling and discussing of feelings, it is hoped, lead to decreased negative emotion and the client's increased ability to be more accepting of himself and to plan more realistically for the future. In stuttering therapy, this type of activity sometimes leads to decreases in stuttering, but it is also thought to enable the person to cope better with the modification of his speech. This interaction also may be preparation for the more direct desensitization of emotional responding described at the beginning of this section.

Cooper (1968, 1976) notes that the affect of a relationship between client and clinician changes during stuttering therapy. This

---

tionship but also use rather specific behavior modification techniques at times considered appropriate. See Gregory (1968), Sheehan (1970a), Van Riper (1973), Emerick and Hood (1974), and Cooper (1976).

[11]The clinician presumably recalls some past experience similar to the client's and to some degree re-experiences the event by using self-verbalized cues to evoke the feeling.

change appears analogous to the shifting role of the clinician during therapy described by Sheehan (1968, 1970a).

Questions for Contributors

1. Can we ignore dealing with the thoughts and ideas the stutterer has about himself as related to the speech behavior we wish to change, even though we cannot at present deal as precisely with the content as with the speech behavior itself?

2. Will it suffice in bringing about the desired change and stabilization of change to deal principally with the stutterer's speech and only incidentally with beliefs and/or affective responses?

3. Do some clinicians who make little or no reference to dealing with the client's beliefs actually do so by the way they orient the client to therapy or by instructions given? For example, if the operant paradigm $S_D\text{----}R_{consequence}$ is taught, is this teaching a certain orientation to the problem?

4. Should a therapy program include procedures aimed toward optimizing the assumed interreciprocating effects among changes in speech, affective responses, and beliefs by including specific techniques related to each?

5. Just as some clinicians may overemphasize speech analysis and modification per se, is it possible that some clinicians become too involved in attitudinal components and do not focus significantly on modifying speech behavior?

6. Just as it was asked whether stutterers need variations in approaches to speech modification related to individual differences in the problem, is it possible that some stutterers have more need than others for therapy aimed at clarifying and shifting beliefs or modifying affective responses? If the answer to this questions is "yes," how do we carry out the differential evaluation?

7. Can we increase the objectivity of the identification of attitudinal responses, the clinician's role in therapy, and measurement by such methods as Thematic Content Modification Programs (Shames, Egolf, and Rhodes, 1969) and anxiety-deconditioning procedures using electro-skin-conductance measures (Gray and England, 1969)? Will this lead to improvements in therapy, or will these attempts to be objective hamper the relationship between clinician and client and thereby impede therapy?

PSYCHOTHERAPY FOR STUTTERERS: WHAT IS IT, IS IT NEEDED, AND IF SO, HOW SHOULD IT BE DONE?

Psychotherapy

The current practice of psychotherapy involves broad philosophical differences. These differences are probably most clearly illustrated in the assumptions and procedures of psychoanalytic therapy as contrasted with behavior therapy patterned after operant conditioning. Freudian psychological theory regards maladaptive behavior as the outward manifestations of unconscious causes. Emotional re-education and insight resulting from free association, dream analysis, analysis of transference, etc., lead to improved adjustment as the person understands why he feels and behaves as he does. Behavior therapy patterned after operant conditioning emphasizes that we are dealing with learned maladaptive behavior. This behavior is not an outward manifestation of some unconscious conflict in the Freudian sense. Behavior can be understood and analyzed in terms of consequences of the behavior and associated stimuli (designated as discriminated stimuli). Consequently, behavior can be changed by analysis and re-education procedures involving instruction, reinforcement, generalization, etc.

Realizing the hazard of simplification, if we think of psychoanalytic therapy as stressing insight, and behavior therapy based on the operant paradigm as emphasizing action, most other psychotherapies are seen to be more like one or the other, or to combine elements of insight and action. For example, Rogers' (1951) client-centered therapy has developed in part as a reaction to interpretation by the clinician that is characteristic of psychoanalysis; yet, like psychoanalytic therapy, Rogers' approach relies on the development of insight and largely assumes that appropriate behavior change will follow. Ellis' (1962) rational-emotive therapy aims toward helping the client understand the relationship between his distorted thoughts and behavior. Ellis moves the client from insight to action, but the person's behavior change is not planned by client and clinician as specifically as it would be by a psychotherapist using the operant paradigm as the frame of reference.

Using psychological procedures, psychotherapists treat many different psychological problems related to thinking, emotional responding, and overt behavior. Medically trained psychiatrists doing psychotherapy may also utilize therapeutic drugs. Some behaviorally oriented psychotherapists, probably known as behavior therapists or behavior modifiers, deal with the modification of stuttering behavior.

Psychotherapy and Stuttering Therapy

Twenty-five years ago, when I first began to work with stutterers, many psychotherapists were critical of the speech pathologists' work with the stutterer's stuttering. During the 1940s and the 1950s, the psychoanalytic model of inner conflict resulting in symptoms had a great influence on psychotherapy. Psychotherapists usually viewed stuttering as a symptom of conflict. Therefore, psychotherapy for stuttering, like psychotherapy in general, was directed to the resolution of emotional conflict. Then, it was thought, the symptoms would be resolved.

The advent of more behavioral approaches in psychotherapy and contributions such as those of Sheehan, beginning in 1954 with his article on an integration of psychotherapy and speech therapy in stuttering therapy (Sheehan, 1954b), has alleviated this criticism of speech therapy for stutterers as being symptomatic and superficial. Sheehan (1954b) recommended a sequence of treatment in which speech therapy that focused on the stutterer's feelings as a stutterer and his attempts to handle word and situation cues was offered first. He stressed the type of speech therapy that did not suppress the stuttering behavior but that dealt with a reduction of avoidance and the modification of speech in a context of understanding associated conflicts, feelings, and attitudes. The psychotherapeutic portions of the treatment involved the releasing and expressing of feelings, developing more adequate interpersonal relationships, and preparing the stutterer for an adjustment to increased fluency. As a speech pathologist teaching about and specializing in stuttering therapy and as a psychologist teaching courses in psychopathology and psychotherapy, Sheehan currently advocates an action-oriented, behavior change approach to psychotherapy. In commenting on psychotherapy through action he says:

> Insight oriented psychotherapy may facilitate change when it is a supplement to action; insight retards change whenever it serves as a substitute for action. (1970a, p. 284)

Van Riper (1971b, 1973) views the stutter more fluently approach, reviewed earlier in this chapter, as a form of psychotherapy in which the stutterer's self is equated with his stuttering; thus, by modifying the stuttering and the avoidance and inhibition involved, the stutterer's self-concept is changed. Van Riper (1973) states that he has drawn upon his knowledge of many psychotherapeutic procedures in therapy for stutterers. Bloodstein (1975a) mentions the need for a psychotherapeutic relationship in stuttering therapy. Perkins (1977) concludes that, unless psychotherapy is included in stuttering therapy, it is more likely that the problem will resist permanent modification.

In this discussion, we have said that there are many different approaches, known as psychotherapy, for dealing with psychologically based problems. In addition, it has been shown that as psychotherapy became more behavioral in orientation, and that as psychologists and speech-language pathologists working with stutterers interpreted more of what they did as psychotherapeutic, psychotherapists became more accepting of speech modification activity in stuttering therapy.

An issue that concerns students in speech-language pathology preparing to work with stutterers, and professional speech-language pathologists as well, is: What are the differences between speech therapy and psychotherapy, and how much of a psychotherapist does the speech-language pathologist need to be to work with stutterers? I have discussed this with many professional speech-language pathologists, psychologists, and students in class. The following statements represent my present point of view:

1. Psychotherapists, counselors, and speech-language pathologists share techniques in common, but the problems they understand through training and experience are usually different. All three specialists may use procedures aimed toward insight, affective change, and behavior change. The speech-language pathologist's role is specific to speech and language problems. He understands these problems better than other specialists do. A counselor's process of understanding and advising a person is usually specified by designations such as vocational, rehabilitation, and educational. Ordinarily, a psychotherapist's role is to deal with emotional distress and unadaptive behavior that are less specifically focused (more pervasive) than those with which a speech-language pathologist or a counselor would work. Finally, all have to understand their qualifications and limitations resulting from training and experience. Some speech-language pathologists may specialize with stutterers, others may work

with them. Also, a few psychotherapists have specialized in
stuttering therapy.
2. Call the techniques psychotherapeutic or whatever you may, the
    competent clinician, in addition to sufficient knowledge about
    stuttering, has to know procedures for analyzing and dealing
    with stuttering behavior and the stutterer's thoughts (cognitive
    responses) and feelings (affective responses). Furthermore, if he
    does or does not use a procedure, he should be able to give a ra-
    tionale in terms of his belief about the problem of stuttering and
    such issues as those discussed in this book.

Referral of Stutterers for Psychotherapy

Diverse results have characterized research findings pertaining to
the personality and adjustment of stutterers, but most commentaries on the literature (Goodstein, 1958; Johnson, 1967; Sheehan,
1970a; Bloodstein, 1975b) conclude that stutterers, as a group, do
not show a particular personality pattern. Sheehan (1970a) states
that the slight differences between stutterers and control groups
shown in some studies are the type of differences that could be
related to difficulties in speaking situations. Although there is
disagreement about the effectiveness of different approaches to
therapy, stuttering therapy that results in reduced stuttering and
increased comfort in interpersonal relationships should meet the
needs of stutterers as revealed by these personality studies.
Sheehan (1970a) concludes, "To say that stutterers need psychotherapy or can profit from it is like saying people need psychotherapy or can profit from it" (p. 132).

Brady (1968), a psychiatrist who has used a metronome to instate more fluent speech in stutterers, employs Wolpe's desensitization therapy when needed and in addition reports that some stutterers require psychotherapy if they have a poor self-image, passive
behavior, and other maladaptive characteristics that may be
predicted from the social nature of a stuttering problem. With
reference to the last, all clinicians working with stutterers should be
able to deal with these attitudinal and behavioral characteristics
related to the social frustration of stuttering. Bloodstein (1975a)
states that some stutterers need "broader forms of personal
guidance" if their insecurity or inadequacy makes it difficult for
them to profit from stuttering therapy. Gregory (1973a) suggests
that a psychological consultation be part of the differential evalua-

tion of stutterers. In this way, individual adjustment patterns can be more thoroughly evaluated and additional consultation or referral, if needed, can be arranged before, during, or after stuttering therapy.

Questions for Contributors

1. Recognizing the many variations in practices that exist, is it appropriate to say: Speech-language pathologists, psychotherapists, and counselors share techniques in common, but the problems they understand as a result of their training and experience, and with which they are prepared to cope, are different?
2. If we define psychotherapy as dealing with more general problems of personal adjustment or personal adjustment not specific to the speech problem, are there stutterers who need this type of assistance before, during, or after stuttering therapy?
3. Should a psychological consultation to discover those who may need psychotherapy be included in the initial stages of evaluation and therapy?
4. When we as clinicians decide to refer to a psychotherapist, do we choose on the basis of the procedure he utilizes, i.e., insight directed, insight and action directed, behavior analysis/behavior modification directed, etc.?

STUTTERING THERAPY FOR CHILDREN

Contemporary issues pertaining to the prevention and/or treatment of stuttering in children include the following: 1) What is the nature of disfluent[12] speech in children, what are the normal variations in fluency, and how do we define and identify a fluency problem such as stuttering or cluttering? 2) What factors are considered in the evaluation of a child aimed toward the prevention of stuttering, the

---

[12]In this connection, there is disagreement about the spelling of the word *dis*fluency (*dys*fluency). Twenty years ago, nonfluency was often used. The Latin root "non" means absence. Today, *dis*fluency is preferred by many because the Latin root "dis" means apart, separated from. The ones who prefer disfluency object to dysfluency since the Greek word root "dys" refers to ill, bad, or hard. Not all disruptions in speech flow are bad. *Dis*fluency indicates not fluent. Then the designation of more normal to more abnormal is left to the use of other appropriate modifying words. Some, such as Brutten and Shoemaker (1967), prefer dysfluency to emphasize that the normal condition of speech flow is fluency. Accordingly, there is a reason for all disruptions.

management of early developmental stages, or the treatment of a more advanced or confined stuttering problem? 3) What are appropriate intervention strategies?

Fluency, Disfluency, and Stuttering

As language is acquired and as articulatory proficiency develops during the years of childhood, there are, at the same time, changes in the flow of speech, noted by the quality and quantity of speech disfluency. Speech-language pathologists' classifications of disfluency have been oriented to their interest in stuttering, and therefore have focused on the repetition of phrases, words, and parts of words (repetitious disfluencies) plus prolongations. Psycholinguists, with their initial interest in the influence of cognitive and emotional variables on language encoding, have given particular attention to pauses and revisions (nonrepetitious disfluencies).

As speech-language pathologists and psycholinguists broadened the objectives of their fluency research, classifications expanded to the point that we can now be hopeful that we are approaching agreement on a more universal system. Brownell (1973) formulated the following comprehensive classification system:

A. Repetitions
    1. Monosyllabic unit
       a. Sound
       b. Syllable
       c. Word
    2. Polysyllabic unit
       a. Word
       b. Phrase
B. Prolongations
C. Unfilled pauses
    1. Grammatical (pauses at grammatical junctures)
    2. Hesitations (pauses at nongrammatical points)
D. Filled pauses
    1. Interjections of sounds
    2. Interjections of words
E. Revisions
F. Incomplete phrases
G. Broken words
H. Unfinished words

I believe this is a useful classification system, considering the need to study the fluency of clinical cases more thoroughly and to continue investigations of fluency related to age, sex, communicative situations, the nature of a child's communicative message, etc.

What do we know about the age changes in the occurrence of these disfluency types and the quantity and quality of disfluency that is clinically significant? Davis' (1939) classical cross-sectional study of repetitions showed that there was a general trend toward less repetition of words and phrases between 24 and 62 months of age. Subsequently, studies by Branscom, Hughes, Johnson, and Oxtoby (e.g., Branscom, Hughes, and Oxtoby, 1955) confirmed this finding. In all of these studies, syllable repetition was very infrequent and did not change significantly between 2 and 5 years of age. Of importance, in terms of the information to be reviewed in this section, Davis (1939) reported that both the frequency of instances of syllable repetition and the number of repetitions involved (Ma Mama vs. Ma Ma Ma Mama) were the best indicators of marked deviation. DeJoy (1975) showed that there is a significant decrease in part-word repetitions, word repetitions, phrase repetitions, and prolongations between 3½ and 5 years of age. Interestingly, grammatical pauses increased. In general nonrepetitious disfluencies (revisions, interjections), the types of disfluencies that are more characteristic of adult speech, did not decrease significantly between ages 3½ and 5.

Listener reaction studies (Boehmler, 1958; Giolas and Williams, 1958; Williams and Kent, 1958), in which observers listened to disfluencies drawn from the speech samples of both nonstutterers and stutterers, have shown that there is greater agreement in classifying sound and syllable repetitions and disfluencies rated as more severe as stuttering. Revisions and interjections are judged infrequently as stuttering.

In another study that has a bearing on the quality and quantity of disfluency that is clinically significant, Emrick (1971) examined the speech behavior of typically disfluent and highly disfluent nonstuttering children. In comparing the rankings of the types of disfluencies in the two groups, word repetitions, part-word repetitions, and disrhythmic phonations (prolongations) showed a higher rank order in the highly disfluent group while interjections and revisions showed a higher rank order in the typically disfluent group. In other words, as total disfluency increased, word repetition, part-word repetition, and prolongations increased more than the other types.

Several studies have revealed that speakers who are considered to be stutterers demonstrate substantially greater amounts of sound and syllable repetitions and prolongations (Davis, 1939; Voelker, 1944). In the last of three studies of the onset and development of stuttering, Johnson et al. (1959) acknowledged that the parents of stuttering children reported the presence of sound and syllable repetition at the onset of stuttering significantly more often than was reported by parents of a matched group of nonstuttering children.

Wingate (1962, 1964a) and Van Riper (1971a) maintain that breaks in the fluency of individual words are less normal than the repetition of words and phrases, pauses, revisions, and interjections. The data briefly noted in this review — which indicate that this type of disfluency (sound and syllable repetition, prolongation) occurs very infrequently in most children, that there is a decrease in the frequency of these disfluencies between ages 3½ and 5, that listeners are much more likely to judge these disruptions at the word level as stuttering, and that stuttering children show a greater occurrence of this behavior — support an assumption that clinicians should be more concerned when there is an increase in the frequency of this type of disfluency. Of course, the next step is to be more definitive about the quantitative aspect, i.e., how many sound or syllable repetitions or prolongations should signal the clinician to be concerned? Van Riper (1971a), in listing guidelines for differentiating normal and abnormal disfluency, mentions numerous criteria, among which are the following: 1) syllable repetitions: more than two per 100 words; more than two repetitions per instance; irregular patterns; and 2) prolongations: more than one per 100 words; more than 1 second in duration. In my experience, these criteria are reasonable and useful guidelines. Prolongations ending in fixed postures and other signs of increased tension in the lips, jaws, and larynx are more obvious characteristics of stuttering.

Some stutterers' speech is characterized not only by the disfluency types mentioned heretofore and by accessory behaviors, but also by a rapid, slurred, and jerky pattern typified by the running together of words. This behavior has been termed "cluttering," and is referred to by some clinicians as "poorly organized speech" because that is the impression one gets when listening. We see children (nonstutterers, beginning stutterers, and confirmed stutterers) who have "cluttering components," as we express it, in their speech patterns. In terms of the objective of this section, to review current knowledge about variations in speech fluency and the identification of fluency problems, we have not made as good progress toward establishing specific criteria for making clinical judgments about cluttering as we have about stuttering.

Evaluation

This section surveys issues involved in the evaluation of children when the evaluation is aimed toward the prevention of stuttering, the correct management of early developmental stages, or the treatment of children with a more advanced stuttering problem. Evaluation procedures vary in scope from brief informal observation of a child and some discussion with the parents to a complete diagnostic evaluation including a case history, observation, and testing. The clinician's beliefs about the nature and development of fluency, the occurrence of disfluency, and conditions related to stuttering influence what he does.

Speech Analysis   Observation of the child's speech is a part of all evaluations. As described in the previous section, clinical reports and research in recent years have enabled clinicians to be more definitive in their judgments related to variations in the fluency of speech and what should be viewed as an emerging fluency problem or as stuttering. In brief, it was concluded, based on a survey of research, that we should be concerned about the fragmentation of a word by sound and syllable repetition or prolongations. Furthermore, it was stated that Van Riper's quantitative guidelines were reasonable: 1) two or more syllable repetitions (containing more than two repetitions per instance) per 100 words, and 2) one or more prolongations (1 second or more in duration) per 100 words (Van Riper, 1971a). Of course, the speech sample should be sufficient in length, at least 500 words, to be representative. Van Riper (1971a) lists several other qualitative guidelines for differentiating normal disfluency and stuttering. Cooper (1973) developed a Chronicity Predition Checklist for School Age Stutterers, in which one of the variables studied is behavioral characteristics during speech. After observing the child and interviewing the parents, the clinician records answers to questions about the child's speech. Several of Cooper's questions parallel observations included in Van Riper's guidelines previously mentioned. Examples of Cooper's other questions are:

1. Is the schwa vowel inappropriately inserted in the syllable repetition?
2. Is the airflow during the repetitions often interrupted?
3. Is vocal tension often apparent during the repetition?
4. Are there observable and/or distracting extraneous facial or body movements during the moment of disfluency? (1976, p. 48)

Riley (1972) has reported the use of a stuttering severity instrument based on three parameters: 1) frequency of repetition and prolongation of sounds and syllables, 2) duration of the longest blocks, and 3) observable physical concomitants. Procedures are delineated for obtaining a total frequency score, total duration score, total physical concomitant score, and total overall score for nonreaders and for children who read. For the latter, conversational samples are also included. Percentile and severity equivalents, based on 109 stuttering children, are given. This procedure is useful for determining the severity of a problem, but observations of fragmentation at the word level described above (Wingate, 1964a; Van Riper, 1971a; Cooper, 1973, 1976) are the most useful in determining the existence of an emerging behavior about which the evaluating clinician should be concerned. In the same vein, Bloodstein's (1975a, b) description of speaking behavior associated with his analysis of four phases of the development of stuttering is useful in establishing the severity of a child's stuttering. Johnson, Darley, and Spriestersbach (1963) describe several dimensions of the stutterer's behavior including the consistency of stuttering on certain sounds, words, and in certain situations that should be evaluated. This observation indicates the strength of cues associated with unusual disfluency or stuttering.

Other Factors Evaluated   When evaluating a child to determine if a problem exists or to decide the nature of an existing fluency problem, speech-language pathologists, regardless of the extensiveness of the evaluation, desire information about the parent or other informant's perception of the child's speech and to the extent possible, the child's attitude about talking. Johnson's contributions (Johnson et al., 1959; Johnson, 1967) highlighted the need to know the way in which the parents and others perceive the problem in comparison with the clinician's observation and even the evaluation of the child himself.

Williams (1969, 1971) has described "talking to a child about talking" as an approach to picking up clues about his enjoyment of speech and possible reactions to the way he talks. Williams has reported a study showing that all children have attitudes toward speaking that they can express in answer to questions such as: How do you like talking? What do you like most (least) about talking? In what situations do you like to talk most (least)? I have found this approach effective in evaluating the attitudes of beginning and more advanced stutterers.

Most authorities, regardless of specific point of view, have considered environmental influences to be important in the development of stuttering; thus, they have included procedures for obtaining information about communicative stress, the child's emotional climate in general, and interpersonal relations (Speech Foundation of America, 1962, 1964; Brutten and Shoemaker, 1967; Wyatt, 1969; Glasner, 1970; Sheehan, 1970a, 1975; Gregory, 1973a; Shames and Egolf, 1976).

In the last 15 years, speech-language pathologists have examined receptive-expressive language and articulation in beginning stutterers with increasing care. This is attributable to two circumstances: 1) increased interest in the effects of specific characteristics of the communicative message (idea, word selection, syntax) on fluency (Bloodstein and Gantwerk, 1967; Emrick, 1971; Muma, 1971; Brownell, 1973; Helmreich and Bloodstein, 1973; DeJoy, 1975), and 2) continuing reports that a notable number of stuttering children are delayed in language development, have specific language problems, or have articulation problems (Berry, 1938; Bloodstein, 1958; Andrews and Harris, 1964; Rutherford, 1977). Boehmler (1970) points out that instrumental coping behaviors in a child's speech can result from language formulation inadequacies and minimal problems of motor patterning for the production of speech. Information about general development and medical factors is considered by many speech-language pathologists to be important because delayed physical development and motor coordination or illness may be associated with delayed speech and language development or impaired motor control of the speech mechanism, which could contribute to disrupted fluency. In school-age children, Bloodstein (1958) notes the relationship between learning to read and the beginning of stuttering in a number of cases; thus, there is a need to evaluate the child's educational programs.

Evaluation Systems   The foregoing brief review of factors mentioned in current literature as contributing to the development of stuttering shows that the clinician chooses among numerous possibilities in organizing an evaluation. Luper and Mulder (1964), in their book on stuttering therapy for children, recommend an extensive case history and evaluation of the child, and throughout their discussion of therapy they show how various kinds of information are useful. However, the relationship between information from the evaluation and treatment is not specific. Bloodstein (1958, 1975a), in writing about stuttering as an anticipatory struggle reaction, implies the need to explore numerous provocations for stuttering (delayed speech, defective articulation, cluttering, oral reading difficulties, etc.) that, when combined with unusual sensitivity or excessive parental demands, may lead to the child viewing speech as a behavior he has to be very careful about. Glasner (1970), although he stresses emotional factors, believes in an extensive evaluation of developmental factors. He says:

> A careful examination of the child and the uncovering of any possible etiological factors should precede treatment. Stuttering in the young child, therefore, will not be approached as a single uniform problem of development, and the treatment will of necessity vary with the needs of the child. (1970, p. 252)

In 1973, Gregory authored a brief introductory book, *Stuttering: Differential Evaluation and Therapy,* in which he described a broad case history, clinical observation, and testing approach to differential evaluation. He gave the rationale for each procedure with reference to current theory and research information. In addition, Gregory attempted to be specific in describing how therapy is individualized, based on the findings of a differential evaluation. He stated:

> Differential evaluation results in decisions about therapy . . . The onset and development of stuttering is complex and the treatment must not be fragmented . . . The initial evaluation is just the beginning of an important, perhaps rather long, involvement which will produce new information, causing the clinician to modify his earlier opinions. (1973a, pp. 23–24)

Gregory (1973a) also mentioned the value of a psychological consultation to obtain information on intellectual functioning and more subtle attitudes in a child or his parents that may not be perceived by the speech-language pathologist.

Brutten (1975), with reference to his idea (Brutten and Shoemaker, 1967) that repetitions of syllables and prolongation are responses to conditioned negative emotion and that other behaviors commonly associated with stuttering (e.g., word substitutions) are adjustive instrumental responses, has created a battery of procedures for differentially assessing antecedent stimuli and resulting responses. Referring to what is fundamental about therapeutic decision making, Brutten says:

> For therapy to have a firm practical base, it is necessary to know the particular adjustive responses used to cope with specific situational and word difficulties and the stimulus circumstances that set the occasion for their occurrence. (1975, p. 254)

In describing a case selection procedure to be used in a school situation, Cooper (1976) discusses seven steps necessary in reaching a therapy enrollment decision:

1. Initial contact
2. Speech-language pathologist's evaluation
3. Teacher interview
4. Parental interview and testing
5. Chronicity assessment
6. Parental follow-up
7. Enrollment decision

This system includes an elaborate guide to observation, testing, and the scaling of behavior.

Van Riper's (1954, 1963) multiple etiology concepts about stuttering have always implied the necessity of a broad differential evaluation. His most recent discussion (Van Riper, 1971a) of different tracks of development, based on a survey of 300 case folders, shows how the speech behavior in the beginning stages differs among children and how different conditions (emotional trauma, word finding, etc.) are possibly associated with these speech characteristics.

Intervention Strategies for Children

During recent years the findings from retrospective research that from 50% to 80% of those who once stuttered for a significant time period recover spontaneously (Andrews and Harris, 1964; Sheehan and Martyn, 1966, 1970; Dickson, 1971; Cooper, 1972) have highlighted the possibility that conditions contributing to more deviant disfluency do change or can be changed. Just as speech in a child is in the process of development, Williams (1971) points out that stuttering is always a problem in the process of developing. We can all agree that the management of the child's development in such a way that normally fluent speech is facilitated and the early developmental stages of stuttering are handled wisely is our most important task.

We have referred to individual differences in children beginning to stutter. Obviously, in young children 3–8 years of age, each year of age is a very significant variable in and of itself in making decisions about the treatment of the child. Therefore, the speech-language pathologist must have a sufficient understanding of child development including knowledge about speech and language development, cognitive maturity, and social development. The reader may think this is a rather obvious statement; nevertheless, authorities such as Williams (1971) and Van Riper (1973) have pointed to the need to think even more carefully than we have about specific procedures for working with children. Williams warns that we have sometimes generalized our approaches with adults to children. Gregory (1973a) says that therapy with preschool children is developmental in orientation, not corrective. A more corrective approach may be used if unadaptive behavior becomes more severe.

Developmental Intervention   When parents express concern about the fluency of a child's speech, the clinician is invited to enter into the ongoing process of events in a child's life. He hopes that by joining the child, his parents, and others, the direction of the developing process toward stuttering or more serious stuttering can be changed.

Those, such as Glasner (1970) and Sheehan (1970a), who emphasize the interpersonal aspects of the development of stuttering, advocate family-centered therapy. Glasner believes that the prognosis of treatment for the preschool child is good if the treatment is not limited to the symptomatic level but deals with the child's sensitivity, social adaptation, and the parent's adjustment. Sheehan states: "With a young child still in the family circle, direct speech therapy should more often be a last resort rather than a starting point" (1970a, p. 303). Just as Sheehan believes in action-oriented therapy for adult stutterers in which they gain insight into feelings and attitudes, he recommends that the *parents* of young children explore their behavior and associated feelings by carrying out behavioral assignments. Both Sheehan and Glasner place great importance on the clinician's relationship with the child, the affect-oriented behavior discussed in the section on attitudes. As expected, both discuss the nature of effective parent counseling.

Procedures derived from an orientation similar to Glasner's and Sheehan's, but involving behavioral observations and changes that are described more specifically, are those of Shames and Egolf (1976). The clinician observes the child's interaction with his parents to discover disequilibriums in the relationship assumed to occasion increased disfluency or stuttering. An example given is a mother who was demanding and authoritative, asking her child questions with little time for replies. The therapeutic strategy, in this example, was for the clinician to assume a role opposite to that of the mother, one in which the initiation of conversational topics by the child was reinforced and time for lengthy utterances was provided.

An approach, also focusing on parent-child interaction as a crucial variable, yet relying to a greater extent on observations by the parents, has been described by Zwitman (1978). His program is intended to be used by clinicians in counseling parents who are concerned about the fluency of their preschool child's speech. The use of certain of the seven sections in the program is based on observation of features of the child's disfluency and characteristics of the home environment. Each section, e.g., the one "How to Deal With Your Child's Speech," includes a questionnaire for parents, a checklist for parents to use in assessing their behavior, and directions for clinicians to follow. Zwitman's work is predicated on the concept that response contingencies by the parents can be used to modify the child's behavior and that, in turn, changes in the child's speech and other behavior will reinforce the parents for carrying out the clinician's program. The specificity of this child management program is emphasized.

Wahler et al. (1970) reported a study in which stuttering in two children (ages 4 and 9) was reduced when contingencies were applied to secondary problems such as oppositional behavior and frequent shifts of attention. Based on observation, the researchers were satisfied that the stuttering behavior was not reduced because the secondary behavior and stuttering shared common stimulus control variables or because differential attention was given fluent and stuttered speech. It was concluded that "control of the stuttering was most clearly related to specific aspects of the child's own behavior — namely, changes in their secondary problems" (p. 427). Experienced clinicians are probably not surprised by the finding of this study, but research aimed toward a better understanding of these results needs to be done.

Other clinicians such as Bloodstein (1975a), Luper and Mulder (1964), and Van Riper (1973) also focus on the interpersonal aspect of therapy and providing parents information about speech development, but in addition, their therapy includes procedures for facilitating the child's fluency. Bar (1971, 1973) describes an approach to the treatment of children as young as 2 years of age in which therapy concentrates on helping the child become aware of his natural fluencies and his ability to speak fluently. Historically, some clinicians seem to have developed the attitude that a clinician cannot see a beginning stutterer for therapy, that he can only see the parents. The Speech Foundation of America's publications (1962, 1977) and films[13] on the prevention of stuttering, as well as the author just mentioned, emphasize that we can work with a child to increase and reinforce fluency without working with disfluency or stuttering in a way that calls the child's attention to his speech in a counterproductive way. To the contrary, the procedures suggested for increasing the child's positive feelings about talking should countercondition minimal negative reactions that may be developing. To make the point, here are two suggestions made by Van Riper (1973): 1) a play situation between adult and child that progresses from solo to cooperative play, with little talking at first, and then with more verbal interaction in which the clinician models sentence structure and fluency that are, as Van Riper says, "within the child's reach," and 2) speaking accompanied by a rhythmic timing device such as a metronome or the clinician's finger tapping. Bloodstein (1975a) makes similar suggestions and joins Van Riper in commenting that fluency-producing procedures that would be deceptive if used with an adult can be used effectively with a child to increase his approach feelings, i.e., his confidence about speaking. They remind us to keep in mind the plastic nature of the child's developing speech. Johnson (1946, 1967) discussed the importance of not reacting differentially to the child's disfluency. In parental counseling, he focuses on reducing fluency disrupters.

Bloodstein (1975a), in his anticipatory struggle hypothesis, emphasizes the role of environmental pressure in the development of stuttering. Therefore, he recommends that the following points be considered in counseling parents:

---

[13](1) Prevention of Stuttering: (Part I) Identifying the Danger Signs. (2) Prevention of Stuttering: (Part II) Family Counseling and the Elimination of the Problem. (3) Stuttering and Your Child: Is it Me? Is it You? Available from Seven Oaks Productions, 8811 Colesville Road, Silver Spring, Maryland 20910.

1. Any effort to change some of the parents' behavior must start with the removal of guilt about the child's stuttering. (p. 58)
2. We must insist on the removal of all speech pressures. (p. 59)
3. When necessary, the parents should be helped to understand in what respects they might be less restrictive and demanding in their attitudes toward the child's behavior as a whole. (p. 60)
4. In a certain number of cases psychotherapy may offer the only practical hope of reducing parental pressures. (p. 61)

These four points are illustrative of statements made about parent counseling in the literature on stuttering (Luper and Mulder, 1964; Johnson, 1967; Glasner, 1970; Sheehan, 1970a; Gregory, 1973a; Van Riper, 1973). One realizes the knowledge, and skill derived from practical experience, required to deal with this aspect of therapy.

Before desensitization as a concept was considered in detail in the literature on stuttering therapy, Egland and Van Riper (Van Riper, 1954) described a procedure, called desensitization therapy, in which stress-producing stimuli are introduced gradually after the child has been brought under the influence of fluency-producing stimuli. When the child's behavior indicates that the threshold of occurrence of particular disfluency types is being approached, the clinician returns to the production of fluency-producing stimuli. In this way, the child is helped to become less sensitive to communicative stress that disrupts fluency or increases stuttering.

As previously noted, Wyatt (1969) and Van Riper (1973) have provided suggestions for the use of modeling procedures. Hill and Gregory (1975) have described work with preschool children in which the child is rewarded for imitating the clinician's more easy, relaxed speech in a play school atmosphere. The clinician's utterances (stimuli to the child) vary along a continuum from shorter to longer (increasing syntactic complexity) and from less to more meaningful (e.g., naming, description, interpretation). These procedures are carried out in the context of a language activity program. Desensitization is utilized as it is judged to be appropriate and productive. Gregory (1973a) discusses variations in therapeutic strategy based on a continuing differential evaluation.

The foregoing discussion of developmental intervention has mentioned the emphasis on different factors by certain writers. It seems that parent counseling, including the providing of information and steps to alter the interaction between parent and child, is deemed necessary by most clinicians. Most advocate working with the child. Some see this work focusing mostly on interpersonal relations (between clinician and child, between parent and child). Others include language- and fluency-facilitating activities. Contributors such as Ryan (1974), Webster (1974), and Brutten (1975) offer minimal comment on therapy for preschool children.

Intervention with More Confirmed Stutterers My training in general semantics (Lee, 1941; Johnson, 1946) leads me to use the word "more" in this heading to tell the reader of my awareness of the matter of degree. To construct language to represent the facts is difficult in talking about stuttering therapy, and it is particularly so at this point. In most instances in this section, I am writing about the child who is elementary school age and who displays varying degrees of awareness that speech is difficult. When we observe the youngster we see fragmentation at the word level and perhaps some struggle behavior. Again, it is emphasized that each year of age is an important variable and each child is unique.

Williams (1971), Van Riper (1973), and others have described the way in which we have sometimes generalized our clinical attitude about adults to these children. Some have talked to them as though they were much more mature and have used speech analysis and modification procedures similar to those used with adults. On the other hand, I have also observed clinicians treating these children in ways similar to those discussed in the previous section on the preschool beginning stutterer, perhaps with parent counseling and indirect or no work with the child. In the last 10 years a number of clinicians have presented specific procedures for working with more advanced stuttering in children. As I review this work, the issues discussed will relate to those raised in the discussion of "stuttering more fluently" vs. "speaking more fluently" and the section on attitudes.

With the publication of his chapter, "Stuttering Therapy for Children" (Williams, 1971), and with his many lectures on the topic, Williams' ideas on the appropriate way to intervene with children have become widely known. On the subject of the child's attitude, Williams stresses that faulty beliefs and associated affective reaction patterns are just beginning to develop, and therefore the clinician's objective is to keep these attitudes from progressing to a level at which the child feels he cannot cope. Williams describes a concrete therapy program, called a positive approach to learning, that deals simultaneously with attitudes about talking and an exploration of the motor act of speaking. Here are a few sample topics: 1) how we learn to say words, 2) how we talk words into sentences, 3) how we observe what we do, and 4) how feelings of being scared or embarrassed can interfere with doing the things we want to do. With the clinician's guidance, the child explores what he does to interfere with talking and makes a comparison of "talking hard" and "talking easy." One thing Williams says a child can learn is that when he makes a mistake while talking he can make the mistake "easily." He cautions the clinician to focus not on stuttering but on the overall way of talking. As we interpret Williams' objectives, the child does not strive for fluency but rather for a way of talking in which he learns to sense and change disruptive tension that interferes with the forward movement of speech. Parent and teacher counseling is also deemed important. Finally, drawing on experience from a project in which he studied therapy for stuttering in a school system, Williams analyzed the problems involved and made suggestions for implementing a stuttering therapy program in the schools. Since so much stuttering therapy is done in the schools, Williams' comments help us to see that additional special attention must be given to the improvement of therapy in this setting.

Van Riper (1973) and Bloodstein (1975a) seem to agree that with elementary-school age children the clinician should first attempt fluency-increasing procedures since the learned cues associated with stuttering and the child's self-image as a person having speech difficulty may both be relatively weak. Bloodstein (1975a), with reference to what he classifies as a Phase II stutterer, recommends the use of suggestion by giving these children techniques, presumably such as slowing down, phrasing, following a metronome, etc., about which the clinician professes confidence. His clinical experience indicates that these approaches often supply just the confidence the child needs. Of course, parent counseling, developing of the child's personal qualities, etc., are also a part of therapy. In a similar vein, Van Riper (1973) says:

> As we have advocated for the beginning stutterer, when we work with younger children with advanced stuttering, we again may occasionally use various forms of timing devices, unison speech and other fluency increasing techniques so that they can know again some freedom in speaking. (p. 434)

In the opinion of Bloodstein and Van Riper, the clinician should not reject techniques such as these, which, with reference to their points of view, would not be the most appropriate for an adult. The clinician should not generalize from adult to child.

In connection with the use of these fluency-producing techniques as an initial approach with children in whom it is difficult to evaluate their habit strength of the problem, Bloodstein (1975b) states that operant conditioning procedures may prove to be quite appropriate. I use this speculative comment by Bloodstein to introduce reports by Ryan (1971, 1974) on operant procedures applied to stuttering therapy for children. Ryan (1971), utilizing some of the same programmed instructional approaches described in the first section of this chapter, reported successful results with five children ranging from 6 to 9 years of age. Furthermore, he stated:

> Spontaneous transfer of fluent speech was demonstrated by at least four of the five children . . . (p. 278)

> Operant procedures, that is systematic therapy programs with small steps and appropriate reinforcement, were demonstrated to be an effective strategy for helping children with stuttering problems. (p. 280)

> Some speech clinicians may wish to view these programs as only one part of the total treatment process. They may be used in conjunction with other forms of therapy for stuttering. (p. 280)

Again, it seems that Ryan believes that the use of programming is very effective, and although he has studied several methods he is accepting of the idea that there may be a number of ways to obtain normally fluent speech. I speculate that Ryan would be accepting of Williams' (1971) concept of the "easy speech" aspect if Williams' work were programmed in terms of stimulus, response, reinforcement, and criterion.

Regarding the previous discussion of "stutter more fluently" vs. "speak more fluently" as philosophies of therapy, in reference to young children as compared to adults, there seems to be less difference of opinion between clinicians such as Bloodstein or Van Riper as opposed to Ryan. Goldiamond and Webster, whom we associated with the "speak more fluently" approach, have reported little or no experience with children. Gregory (1973a), in commenting that secondary stutterers of elementary-school age need a concrete and organized approach to the modification of speech, indicates that careful programming and reinforcement, as emphasized in the operant conditioning literature, can be applied beneficially in working with this age group.

If it becomes necessary to work with escape and struggle behaviors, Van Riper (1973) utilizes an approach more similar to that of working with an adult in which the child is helped to differentiate between easy stuttering and hard stuttering. But, he states there is very little identification of the specific sound and word cues involved because, to the child, the cues are ordinarily more general, e.g., more associated with "getting started" at the beginning of a statement. Emerick (1965) describes a similar approach for children 7-12 years of age who are struggling noticeably and attempt to avoid or disguise their difficulty.

Another prominent contributor of special techniques for children, Cooper (1965, 1976), describes procedures for helping the child conceptualize the problem at his cognitive level and for modifying his speech. A graphic representation of the child's stuttering, "the stuttering apple," is worked out by the clinician and the child. The "core" of the apple is "getting stuck on words." Circles drawn around the core represent "things I do when I stutter," such as struggle behaviors and attitudes. From this frame of reference, therapy consists of modifying the behavior that has been conditional to the core behavior and then teaching fluency-initiating gestures such as easy onset, easy contact, and slow speech. As we found in discussing attitudes in stuttering therapy, Cooper places considerable importance on the client's cognitive and affective changes in therapy, and this is true of his work with children. He says there has to be a real emotional involvement on the part of the child. The clinician, at the appropriate time, confronts the child when he says, e.g., that he did not do an assignment because he was embarrassed. The clinician, in a kind, sensitive manner, asks "What do you mean 'embarrassed'?"

Gregory (1968, 1973a, b), and Gregory and Haerle (1976) in some unreported work, have described a step-by-step system of stuttering therapy that is concrete, i.e., related directly to the child's speaking experience, and that emphasizes the role of the clinician as a model. A less specific approach is used at first in which the clinician, beginning with short one-word utterances and working up to longer, more complex ones, models "more easy relaxed speech with smooth movements." Pausing and the resistance of time pressure in talking is an aspect of the program. "More easy relaxed speech with smooth movements" is transferred eventually to conversation and social speaking situations. If the cues associated with stuttering on particular sounds or words are of the strength that stuttering still occurs, then a more specific analysis using identification of tension, negative practice, and work on modification of preparatory sets, etc., is used. Of importance, more specific analysis is used only to the extent necessary. In summary, if the less specific approach of modifying speech in a general way is effective, then that is all that is needed. Otherwise, more specific analysis and modification can be used.

Parent counseling has been mentioned throughout this discussion of therapy for more confirmed stutterers. Most writers, like Sheehan (1975), point to the importance of counseling the parents to change the parent-child relationship and of informing parents about the child's therapy so that they may be supportive. Gregory and Haerle (1976) model specific behavior changes for the parents and then reinforce the parents for appropriate responding. DeFeo (1975) has used videotapes to teach parents how to identify and respond to both adaptive and unadaptive behaviors in the child.

Questions for Contributors

1. Do we have adequate information about the fluency dimension of speech, disfluency, and stuttering to accurately identify a fluency problem?

2. How are decisions made about what factors are considered in the evaluation of a child aimed toward the prevention of stuttering, the management of early developmental stages, and the treatment of children with a stuttering problem?

3. Does the case history provide information that, although not as reliable as direct observation, may help in understanding a problem better by directing observation and testing of a child and his parents?

4. Do we need to strive for greater objectivity in our evaluation by generating procedures that are more quantifiable? Just as some refer to the need for a positive affective relationship in certain stages of therapy, is this also important in evaluation and is there a chance that being more objective will impair this?

5. Should therapy for children focus first on the child's environment while time for observation is taken in making a decision about work with the child?

6. Should therapy for the beginning stutterer of preschool age include only parent counseling and therapy with the child aimed toward a release of feelings and an improvement of interpersonal relations?

7. In addition to a parent counseling program and therapy to facilitate interpersonal adjustment, is it appropriate to include activities for the beginning stutterer that build fluency?

8. When and how do we modify the speech flow of a more confirmed stutterer? How does the approach differ depending on age, consistency of cues associated with stuttering, and severity of struggle behavior?

9. Can we through our work with the child's speech modify his attitudes about talking? Can we also utilize some discussion type approaches, aimed toward attitude change, that are concrete and related to the child's direct experience?

10. How broad in scope does our treatment of children need to be? Are there contributing factors that require the participation of other professionals?

TRANSFER OF CHANGES TO THE NATURAL ENVIRONMENT AND THE PROBLEM OF RELAPSE

With most stutterers, regardless of age, the modification of stuttering or the production of increased fluency is not particularly difficult. This generally recognized fact is a favorable factor for therapeutic change, but at the same time the history of stuttering therapy reveals that both clients and clinicians have been sometimes deceived by this. Procedures utilized in the modification stages of therapy and during the transfer and maintenance period must be based on an understanding that the stutterer will have to cope with varying degrees of relapse and that continued improvement will involve stabilizing changes and generalizing new responses to more difficult speaking situations.

Advocates (Sheehan, 1970a, b; Van Riper, 1973; Bloodstein, 1975a) of the stutter more fluently approach to the modification of stuttering emphasize that their methods are the most effective way to prevent recurrence and relapse because avoidance tendencies and behaviors are confronted and dealt with in a more systematic way than in fluency-instatement programs. In addition, the stutterer is said to view himself more realistically as a person who is changing, a person who is stuttering more and more fluently. He becomes increasingly less sensitive about stuttering. Those who recommend procedures aimed directly, from the beginning of therapy, toward instating more fluent speech emphasize that their systematic teaching of modified speech production results in much more effective learning by the stutterer and consequently a better ability to respond successfully when difficulty is anticipated. Webster (1974, 1975a) in particular maintains that intensive practice of target behaviors, resulting in overlearning these responses, is crucial to the person's ability to perform in the natural environment. Perhaps two examples can summarize the matter. If one of his clients regresses, Sheehan (1970a) may say that such occurrences may be expected and that the stutterer must strive even more to reduce avoidance tendencies. If one of Webster's clients has increased difficulty, he may say it is because the client has not been conscientious in practicing the target behaviors that generate fluent speech (Webster, 1974).

Clinicians using reinforcement contingencies on either a less formal or a more formal programmed basis have pointed to the effect of reinforcement schedule on the stability of modified speech behavior. In modifying the stutterer's speech, there should be a gradual shift from continuous to intermittent reinforcement. Intermittent reinforcement is more characteristic of the natural environment; therefore, the clinician should thin out the schedule within the clinical setting as a particular aspect of change is being stabilized. It is also likely that intermittent reinforcement encourages the development of self-reinforcement, a topic that has been given significant consideration recently.

External reinforcement in learning must generalize to internal or self-reinforcement if behavior is to be maintained. This phenomenon has been subsumed in recent literature into a broader discussion of self-control or self-regulation procedures. Speech-language pathologists, like psychologists and educators, have known that self-control had to occur in the learning or therapy process, and they have seen the importance of self-monitoring in learning self-control (Sheehan, 1970a; Van Riper, 1973). I teach self-evaluation from the beginning of therapy, as the stutterer analyzes his speech, and this is emphasized throughout therapy. Even though self-regulation has been considered in stuttering therapy, much more needs to be done along the lines of current work in clinical psychology (Kanfer and Phillips, 1966, 1970; Goldfried and Merbaum, 1973).[14] Interestingly,

---

[14]Bandura (1969), Kanfer and Phillips (1970), and Goldfried and Merbaum (1973) provide excellent reviews of theory and research in this area. Watson and Tharp (1972) have authored a useful self-modification manual. Hanna and Owen (1977) describe specific self-control procedures for facilitating transfer and maintenance in stuttering therapy.

although Skinner has been thought of as an uncompromising environmentalist, in *Science and Human Behavior*, he said:

> The individual "chooses" between alternative courses of action, "thinks through" a problem while isolated from the relevant environment, and guards his health or his position in society through the exercise of self-control. (1953, p. 228)

Apparently, Skinner regards self-control as behavior like any other behavior. Thus, self-control is learned in varying degrees depending on our personal histories and can be improved in therapy.

Kanfer and Phillips (1970) describe a group of procedures for improving self-regulation under the term "instigation therapy." Three stages are involved: 1) attending to and monitoring behavior, 2) evaluation of behavior using predesignated behavioral criteria, and 3) consequating the behavior, i.e., self-reinforcement or punishment. My observation is that speech-language pathologists functioning clinically have not formalized self-consequation procedures as well as they have monitoring and evaluation. Furthermore, much more attention should be given to planning monitoring, self-evaluation, and self-consequation in the natural environment. If these behaviors are taught precisely during the modification stages of treatment, they can be more readily incorporated and extended during carryover and after formal therapy ends.[15]

In addition to the influence that procedures used earlier in therapy have on the outcome of stuttering therapy, clinicians recognize the need to utilize specific procedures aimed toward generalization or transfer of changes to the natural environment. Traditionally, clinicians have accompanied stutterers on "field trips" and given them assignments of practicing new behavior in "nucleus" situations outside the clinic. Gregory (1968) describes facilitating change outside the clinic by bringing the stutterer's family, friends, and other interested persons into the clinic to participate in role playing and other activities of a group. To determine the situations that will be worked on during the role playing, the stutterer is asked to list speaking situations in a descending order of difficulty. Easier situations are worked on first. Group experience has many benefits including the practice of new behavior; and,

---

[15]A therapy program incorporating tape-recorded instructions of the language learning type as described by Peins, McGough, and Lee (1972) is a model that should be explored more extensively. It offers advantages during modification, as well as transfer stages of therapy.

related to self-control, it is possible that self-monitoring, evaluation, and reinforcement can be increased through vicarious learning. Sheehan (1970a) points to the advantages of group support during carryover. In recent years, I have provided a continuation program, meeting approximately twice a month, that the stutterer can attend as long as he wishes. If relapse requiring individual therapy occurs, the person cannot attend this program until he is able to continue transfer and maintenance procedures.

Sheehan (1970a), Perkins (1973b), and Shames (1975) agree that changes in speech behavior may need to be related to other more general changes in attitude and behavior if the stutterer is going to cope effectively with life situations. These observations are related to the earlier discussion of cognitive and affective attitude changes in stuttering therapy and the possible benefits of psychotherapy.

Perkins (1973b) describes the use of a normal speech generalization record in which the stutterer rates his ability to execute dimensions of normal speech (fluency, rate, etc.) in speaking situations of gradually increasing difficulty. He stresses planning situations in a sequence that the stutterer believes will permit him to succeed.

Ryan makes this interesting statement: "...there may be a danger in overtraining in the clinic setting in that such overtraining might interfere with transfer" (1974, p. 95). Therefore, as early as possible, physical setting, audience size, familiarity of audience, etc., should be varied. Ryan's maintenance programs involve the counting of stuttered words each day, clinic contact in which speech is sampled and progress is discussed, and home practice.

Williams (1971) describes conferences with parents, teachers, and friends to give instruction in the proper way to encourage and reinforce a child in carryover. Recently, DeFeo (1975), working with Gregory, has created videotape materials to train parents and teachers to recognize and reinforce appropriate speech responses in elementary-school age children.

Finally, like other aspects of stuttering therapy, generalization procedures probably have been influenced by the setting in which therapy is done and by the length of the clinician's program. If the therapy is in a residential setting, the clinician may stress overlearning as the way to enhance transfer. This is necessary since the client will be leaving to return home, perhaps several hundred miles away. If the therapy is scheduled on a longer-term basis, and the client lives nearby, transfer activities may be planned that involve a hierarchical analysis of speaking situations and a gradual extension of stimulus control.

This consideration of transfer to the natural environment has been shorter than previous sections of this chapter because so much information basic to this discussion has been covered earlier. However, this is probably the most important topic in the contemporary study of stuttering therapy!

Questions for Contributors

1. How can we improve procedures used through therapy, during the initial stages of conditioning and counterconditioning as well as the carryover phase of treatment, to improve performance of modified speech behavior in the natural environment?
2. Is the stability of change in speech related to changes in personal adjustment or, put another way, to changes in other behavior patterns besides speech?
3. What constitutes a realistic understanding on the part of the client of the difficulties of transferring modified behavior that involves a stress or emotional component to the variable circumstances of real life?
4. How can we improve the role of the client's social environment in the transfer and maintenance of specific behavior? For example, how can we utilize parents, teachers, and peers or friends more effectively as carryover observers and reward agents?
5. How careful should we be to remain involved in the therapy process until changes are firmly conditioned and generalized? How should we manage this if the client resides several hundred miles away from the center at which a concentrated course of therapy is received?

CRITERIA FOR THE SUCCESS OF
STUTTERING THERAPY: THE RESULTS OF THERAPY

The controversy about criteria of improvement is related in part to the clinician's basic beliefs about the nature of the problem and how to analyze and change behavior. For example, some clinicians who consider themselves strict operant conditioners focus almost exclusively on measuring occurrences of stuttering. Behavior therapists, who speak of the need to countercondition anxiety, attempt to evaluate this variable as well as changes in fluency. If the clinician considers cognitive attitudes important, then some evaluation of this, perhaps an attitude scale, is included in the outcome assessment. The following is a brief commentary on the problems involved in assessing results.

Measuring Stuttered Speech and Speech Improvement

There has always been agreement that the overt aspects of stuttering behavior are very accessible to observation and that change in speech should be measured. Much progress has been made in evaluating speech behavior beginning with the scaling of the severity of stuttering (Sherman, 1952, 1955; Young, 1961) and leading up to recent procedures for counting the number and various types of stutterings per 100 words or per 100 syllables emitted. Still, there is some question about what should be counted as a stuttered unit and the related aspects of speech that should be assessed.

What Should Be Measured   In the section of this chapter on the evaluation of children, it was concluded that fragmentation of a word by sound and syllable repetitions or prolongations is a more atypical form of disfluency. Studies (Davis, 1939; Voelker, 1944) have revealed that stutterers demonstrate substantially greater amounts of these disfluencies than do nonstutterers. Prolongations ending in fixed postures and other signs of increased tension in the lips, jaw, and larynx are more obvious characteristics of stuttering. If, based on our evaluation, we have concluded that there is a speech problem and if the individual is in therapy, it seems we are safe in counting these behaviors as stuttering and using these data as a frame of reference for change in fluency. In addition to the part-word repetitions, prolongations, and struggle behaviors just mentioned, some clinicians, including Ryan (1974), count whole word repetitions as stuttered words. Ryan says:

> After observing many people who stuttered we have decided to routinely count whole word repetitions as stuttered words. We believe it was better to err in the direction of over defining rather than under defining. (1974, p. 15)

By "over defining," Ryan seems to mean that if disruptions within words and struggle behavior were minimal, the counting of word repetitions would not be as significant in deciding the severity of a problem. Perkins et al. (1974), following the recommendations of Andrews and Ingham (1971, 1972a, b), believe that percentage of syllables stuttered is the most definitive measure. Although words are the basic units of meaning, syllables are the basic units of speech production.

In strict behavioral terms, we have to realize that there is some overlap between the disfluencies of stutterers and nonstutterers, and that an absolutely definitive description of stuttering is not possible. Moreover, in making judgments about the occurrence of stuttering we are confronted with the subtle way in which some stutterers substitute words and use circumlocutions to avoid anticipated stuttering. In large part, we have to rely on the person's report of these stuttering tactics.

Assessing the rate of a stutterer's speech is also necessary since particularly slow or rapid rates have been found to be associated with some individuals' stuttering patterns. In addition, a cluttering element may involve a more rapid rate. Therefore, rate is likely to change in therapy and is a dimension that should be measured. In fact, as we have seen, rate control is often involved in some therapies (e.g., Perkins, 1973a, b; Perkins et al., 1974; Webster, 1974). Ryan (1974) measures rate of talking and provides rules to follow in doing so. Perkins (1973b), in keeping with his emphasis on analyzing and modifying multiple dimensions of the speech process, recommends rating fluency, rate, breath and voice flow (phrasing), and prosody.

Stuttering Rate   There appears to be controversy about the most appropriate way to compute the rate of stuttering. As mentioned, Perkins et al. (1974) follow Andrews and Ingham's (1971) suggestion to calculate percentage of syllables stuttered. On the other hand, Ryan in his programmed therapy has reported number of stuttered words per minute. Ingham and Andrews (1973) criticize this measure, "because although appearing to use time as a parameter, it may not accurately reflect information on rate and sample size" (p. 419). Ryan and Van Kirk (1971) provide information on words spoken per minute along with words stuttered per minute, and this would appear to allay this criticism to a great extent, and especially so if sample size is also reported. However, I prefer percentage of stuttered words or syllables combined with measures of syllables or words spoken per minute as the most accurate measure of stuttering. The reliability of these various counts of disfluencies has proved satisfactory when the clinician has been appropriately trained (Johnson, Darley, and Spriestersbach, 1963).

More clinicians are charting progress in clinical treatment using speech measures like those just cited. Clinical reports in journals reflect this, and it is hoped that this development will lead to the publication of more meaningful case reports.

Valid Measures of Speech Behavior in the Natural Environment
The validity of measures of carryover made in the natural environ-

ment seems to be a greater problem in stuttering therapy than it is in therapy for other speech problems. No doubt this is a reflection of the complex and varying nature of stuttering behavior, a vital reality often cited in the literature (Van Riper, 1971a, 1973; Bloodstein, 1975b; Wingate, 1976). The stimulus conditions of the clinic can come to control or signify the occurrence of changes in speech. The stutterer's behavior will be influenced when a fragment of this control is present, e.g., a clinician or fellow client is nearby or the stutterer knows that the speaker on the telephone line knows about his therapy. "Reactive measurement effect" is the term now used to refer to the influence of these stimulus conditions on the assessment of a behavioral response (Rosenthal, 1966). If a tape recorder within the stutterer's view is used to make a posttreatment assessment, the tape recorder is said to have a reactive measurement effect that results in the stutterer's speech response being less representative of his usual behavior.

Andrews and Ingham (1972a) and Ryan (1974) have suggested the use of telemetry and other covert (concealed) recording systems. More research is needed, but Ingham (1975) concluded from a comparison of overt and covert measures, that "for some subjects, fluency attained under overtly recorded conditions may be illusory . . . and give a false impression of the efficacy of therapy" (p. 346). Covert recordings of results in realistic, complex situations are difficult and even involve an ethical question. Considering this, Perkins et al. (1974) settled for overt recordings and have attempted to arrive at clinical procedures that are predictive of measurements taken in real life with the client's permission. The connection between these issues and the earlier discussion of transfer to the natural environment can be seen. In reporting clinical work in professional journals and books, as well as in news releases to the popular press, newspapers, magazines, radio, and television, we should include information about the status of our knowledge of transfer and the problems involved in accurately determining success.

Other Improvement Measures

Gregory (1969), Sheehan (1970a), Van Riper (1973), Perkins et al. (1974), and Webster (1974) state that self-report data are important in assessing the person's subjective evaluation of improvement. Gregory (1969) found that adult stutterers, particularly less severe ones, tended to evaluate their own progress in therapy as more beneficial than a more objective procedure such as ratings of tape recordings may show. Perkins et al. (1974) have used a modification of the Iowa Stutterer's Self-Ratings of Reactions to Speaking Situations to tap self-evaluations. They reported that clients' attitudes toward speaking improved most during the generalization phase as compared to the earlier modification stages. Webster (1974) reported that the Perceptions of Stuttering Inventory (Woolf, 1967) is valuable in assessing the stutterer's change in feelings of struggle, avoidance, and expectancy. Using Erickson's scale of communication attitude (Erickson, 1969), Andrews and Cutler (1974) reported that attitude change was only partial after a course of behavior modification, but that when the stutterers completed a transfer program their attitudes became similar to those of nonstutterers.

While no current authorities view personality and anxiety change data alone as criteria for success, several do gather this information and compare it to speech change results and self-report information mentioned above. Perkins et al. (1974), using the 16 PF Test, the S-O Rorschach, and the Guilford-Zimmerman Temperament Survey, did not find any meaningful relationships between changes on these instruments and speech modification. They noted that their sample was too small to permit a firm conclusion that no relationship existed. Gregory (1969), using the MMPI, observed that certain positive changes in personality, such as decreased depression, phobic behavior, worry, and social withdrawal, began at the beginning of a waiting (control) period, when the stutterers began to anticipate help, and continued throughout therapy. In terms of the point of view held by some that stuttering is a symptom of personal maladjustment (Travis, 1957; Glauber, 1958), it is interesting to note that there were no instances in which stuttering therapy produced a group change toward poorer adjustment. Earlier, Sheehan (1954a) found Rorschach factors useful in predicting personality changes in stutterers but of no value in predicting speech improvement. As for anxiety, studies of this variable and stuttering have revealed an inconsistent relationship (Gray and England, 1972; see reviews by Perkins (1970), Van Riper (1971a), and Bloodstein (1975b)). Using palmar sweat prints as an operational definition of speech-associated anxiety (Mowrer, 1953; Brutten and Shoemaker, 1967), Gregory (1969) found that significant decreases in stuttering during therapy were not associated with decreases in palmar sweating.

Results of Stuttering Therapy

Ingham and Andrews (1973) and Bloodstein (1975b) have provided valuable reviews and commentaries on the results of stuttering therapy. This section examines the main points made in these two reviews and refers to several recent reports.

Ingham and Andrews (1973) began their analysis with a review of reports of the results of therapy based on the contributions of Bryngelson, Johnson, Sheehan, and Van Riper. They pointed to Gregory's study (1969, 1972) in which he demonstrated the effectiveness of procedures based on these authorities' concepts. Specifically, Gregory reported on a comparison of objectively rated speech changes in adults occurring 9 months before therapy, during 9 months of therapy, and 9 months following therapy. The 16 stutterers, as a group, showed a statistically significant decrease in stuttering during therapy and a nonsignificant regression during the 9-month follow-up period. These clients were not followed beyond this point. Both Gregory (1969, 1972) and Prins (1970) have suggested that procedures based on the work of Bryngelson, Johnson, Sheehan, and Van Riper need to be structured or programmed more precisely. Ingham and Andrews (1973) then proceeded with a critical evaluation of behavior therapies for stuttering. The reader is urged to examine this article since, for the purposes of this chapter, the following summary statements are brief:

1. Rhythmic speech — "All that one can conclude from the data is that stuttering is reduced . . . and may carry over in some subjects. But the similarity between reduced stuttered speech resulting from rhythmic speech and fluent normal speech . . . remains ambiguous." (p. 414)
2. Shadowing — " . . . the reported studies tend to imply that shadowing needs to be combined with other procedures . . . in therapy." (p. 416)
3. DAF/prolonged speech — " . . . some features of stuttered speech can be dramatically reduced in the laboratory, but little information is available on carry-over . . . beyond the laboratory . . ." (p. 418). However, it is noted that Curlee and Perkins (1969) report that subjects estimated a 75–90% decrease in outside situations. Speech is said to need to be more than fluent; it must also sound natural and spontaneous.
4. Masking — As long as the stimulus support of the masking noise is present, stuttering is greatly diminished.

5. Negative practice — Does not hold much therapeutic promise. Seems to have a differential effect on those stutterers who have blocks as compared to "repetition stutterers." "Blockers" become worse.

6. Anxiety reduction — "An overview of stuttering therapies using anxiety reduction suggests some evidence of reduced stuttering" (p. 426). Independent measures of anxiety need to be used more often.

7. Operant conditioning — It appears quite clear that stuttering can be reduced by contingent procedures. Transfer and maintenance programs (e.g., Ryan) are reported to be successful, but the reactive effect of clinical measurements is a problem. Some of these studies indicate degrees of relapse following treatment.

Ingham and Andrews stress the need in studies of therapy to establish the reliability of measurements, to measure rate of speaking as well as number of stutterings, and to assess transfer to the natural environment.

Bloodstein (1975b) presented a summary table of reports of treatment results covering speech pattern and behavior therapies, parent counseling and child guidance approaches, drug therapies, and other therapies. Based on his analysis, Bloodstein said:

> It is unmistakable that a very great variety of methods are indeed capable of bringing about what clinicians may regard in good faith as a successful outcome of therapy in a large proportion of cases . . . one would be inclined to infer that substantial improvement, as it was defined in these studies, typically occurs as a result of almost any kind of therapy in about 60 to 80 percent of cases. (1975b, p. 355)

To improve statements about results, Bloodstein urges greater use of objective tabulation of stuttering frequency and severity and evaluations of the stutterer's progress outside the clinic. Again, follow-up studies after the end of treatment are declared essential.

Several recent studies have attempted to deal with some of the issues raised in these reviews. Webster (1974) has carefully defined the dependent variable, disfluent words, and has established that the reliability of disfluent words counts ranges from 90% to 100%. In one study, results from what he describes as Program V, he reports:

> In the posttreatment oral reading tasks, 13 out of 20 subjects had disfluent word frequencies at or below 1 percent. In the posttreatment conversation measure, 9 out of 20 subjects scored at or below 1 percent disfluencies . . . The pretreatment and posttreatment differences for

both conversation and reading are significantly different at or beyond the .005 level when tested with the Wilcoxon signed-ranks test. (1974, pp. 37–39)

In addition, Webster stated that self-reports were consistent with the objective data. He noted an increase in verbal output but did not give data on speech rate.

Perkins et al. (1974) reported interjudge reliabilities of 0.92 for the frequency of stuttered syllables and 0.92 for syllable rate per minute. They compared two forms of behavior management: 1) control of rate to maintain fluency, and 2) control of rate to facilitate normal management of breath stream, phrasing, and prosody, as well as fluency. Stutterers treated with both methods showed significant ($p < 0.01$) reductions in the percentage of syllables stuttered during treatment and also to 6 months after treatment. When fluency and rate were combined as criteria of normal speech, only 44% of those receiving method 1 achieved normal speech as compared to 65% of those treated by method 2. Perkins et al. included data on judgments of normalcy by students not related to the program and on self-evaluations by the clients.

In a 1974 report, Ryan and Van Kirk (1974a) selected, for a detailed analysis, 50 clients from more than 200 seen in the preceding 4 years in a DAF operant program providing for establishment, transfer, and maintenance of normal, fluent speech. Stuttering was defined explicitly and no clinician was allowed to serve as an observer who did not attain, with training, a 90% criterion of agreement with another skilled observer. Two measures, stuttered words/minute (SW/M) and words spoken/minute (WS/M), were said to provide a two-dimensional description of the client's fluency. Mean total number of words stuttered per minute in reading, monologue, and conversation combined dropped from 8.4 before establishment program to 0.3 after establishment and 0.1 after the transfer program. As expected in this type of therapy, words spoken per minute went down during establishment, e.g., in conversation from 128.0 to 83.7, but returned to a slow normal rate of 135.3 after transfer. About maintenance, Ryan and Van Kirk (1974a) say:

> Thirty clients have been on maintenance. During maintenance checks they have demonstrated 0.1 SW/M (one stuttered word per 10 minutes of talking)...Their speech sounds normal...Additional casual observation of clients in their environments and reports of their friends or relatives indicate that they are continuing to speak fluently in a wide variety of settings. (p. 9)

This report meets the requirements of reliable measurements and the continued measurement of speech during therapy including transfer; however, objective data on speech in extratherapeutic settings are not available. In his 1974 book, Ryan admits the great difficulty of obtaining transfer measures not influenced by stimulus control factors associated with the clinic.

The report by Prins (1976) illustrates the way in which assessment of the results of ongoing therapy programs lead to modifications in approach. Prins describes his objective:

> In an attempt to improve its effectiveness, a traditional symptomatic stuttering therapy program for school-age children was modified to (1) focus more upon self-therapy activities while reducing group work emphasis; (2) specify more precisely the target responses used to replace stuttering; (3) establish clearer the criteria for client progress; and (4) to provide well-defined activities for the transfer of speech change. (1976, p. 452)

Results from an initial program and the modified program were compared using the Riley Stuttering Severity Index (SSI)[16] and a follow-up self-report questionnaire based on Van Riper's formula PFAGH+CS (Van Riper, 1963). Prins showed, based on the SSI, that both programs reduced stuttering about equally as well, but that the modified program resulted in continued improvement during the follow-up period as compared to some relapse during follow-up in the initial program. Overall, the self-report questionnaire confirmed that the changes made in the second approach improved therapy. Reliability coefficients on the SSI for frequency, duration, and physical concomitant observations were 0.96, 0.99, and 0.98, respectively. Prins concluded that the changes made had resulted in more effective maintenance of improved speech and a more positive perception of speech improvement.

Guitar (1976) pointed to the need for additional information about pretreatment factors associated with the long-term outcome of stuttering therapy (1 year after treatment). In a well designed study, he found that pretreatment attitudes were most highly related to outcome, followed by pretreatment severity of stuttering and personality measures. With reference to the often mentioned reactive measures problem, Guitar's subjects were contacted 12–18 months after treatment by "a management consultant...and a meeting was arranged in his office in a different part of the city from

---

[16]The Riley Index is described on page 36. See also Riley (1972).

the place of treatment" (p. 593). A 5-minute speech sample was obtained in this situation.

It is concluded that considerable progress is being made in the assessment of the process and outcome of stuttering therapy. Specific information about the identification of stuttering is usually reported and information is provided about the circumstances and the reliability of measurements. Since an unusually slow or rapid rate is often associated with a stuttering problem, and since rate control is involved in therapy, measurements of rate are recognized as essential. Baseline and follow-up data are generally seen as indispensable to a discussion of therapy; in fact, they are necessary in order to know if anything positive is occurring. Many clinical researchers think that related self-report information is useful. Currently, it seems that the greatest problem involves the making of realistic measurements of speech behavior in the natural environment.

Questions for Contributors

1. What is the most valid and effective way of assessing the status of the stutterer's speech?
2. Will we have to settle for the client's subjective report of how well follow-up samples coincide with "usual speech" or how well improvement is holding up in situations where there is some expectation of difficulty?
3. Do both objective and subjective techniques provide valuable information?
4. How can we acquire better information about prognostic indicators?
5. With reference to ethical conduct, should we in our public statements exercise modesty and due caution for the limits of knowledge and be very careful not to imply unrealistic results? Furthermore, if publicity about our work is a misrepresentation or exaggeration, is it our responsibility to correct this information conveyed to the public by, for example, writing a letter to the editor?

chapter TWO

Intervention Procedures for the Young Stutterer

Eugene B. Cooper, Ph.D.

The chapter begins with a discussion of the assumptions this author holds with respect to the problem of stuttering in young children and the roles of parents and speech-language clinicians in assisting the abnormally disfluent child to gain and to maintain fluency. The problem of identifying the very young chronic stutterer is then considered, followed by a discussion of the significance of clinician and parent attitudes toward the young stutterer. The author then describes what appear to him to be the kinds of attitudinal sets that will facilitate parent and clinician involvement in an effective intervention program. Procedures for teaching the young stutterer fluency-initiating gestures are described, as is the therapy goal of developing the child's feeling of fluency control. This is followed by a discussion of the need to consider the young stutterer's feelings and attitudes in any type of intervention program initiated, the need for formal verbal psychotherapy, and the author's views of the efficacy of intensive short-term therapy and nonintensive long-term therapy. Finally, there is a consideration of how the results might be assessed.

ASSUMPTIONS

Although there continues to be a controversy as to exactly how many young stutterers "spontaneously" recover from stuttering, there appears to be a general agreement among investigators that a significant number of stutterers do recover without therapeutic intervention (Cooper, 1976; Wingate, 1976). Cooper (1973), after reviewing studies of recovery from stuttering, suggested that speech-language clinicians might expect that as many as two out of any three stutterers they observe in a school-age population will recover without professional help and that the spontaneous recovery rate in preschool-age disfluent children might even be greater.

Wingate (1976), after reviewing the literature concerning recovery from stuttering, concluded, as this author has (Cooper, 1976), that parents of young stutterers must be doing more "right-things" than "wrong-things" in the ways in which they are responding to their child's stuttering. A review of the recovery from stuttering studies indicates that parents of recovered stutterers frequently advised their children to "slow down" or "take a deep breath before speaking." It is of more than passing interest to note that variations of both of these techniques are used in current therapy systems (for example, Webster's (1975) 'Precision Fluency Shaping Program' and Cooper's (1976) 'Personalized Fluency Control Therapy'). Obviously, the old admonition that parents must not draw attention to the child's speech should be re-examined.

The results of the recovery-from-stuttering studies and even more recent investigations concerning parental and clinician attitudes toward stuttering (Cooper, 1975; Crowe and Cooper, 1977; McLelland and Cooper, 1977; Fowlie and Cooper, 1978) have led this author to the conclusion that too many speech clinicians for too long have held to the belief that parents are the primary causative factor in stuttering in children and that parents generally do all the wrong things as they react to their children's disfluencies. Because of the lack of research supporting the hypothesis that parents cause stuttering and because of the existence of data suggesting that generally parents react helpfully to disfluent children, it appears that speech-language clinicians might be more usefully biased if they believed that parents of stutterers were not responsible for their children's disfluencies and were the most natural and efficient change-agents available with respect to their child's disfluencies.

The recognition that parents, through their early and active intervention procedures with their abnormally disfluent children, may be the primary factor in the significant number of "spontaneous" recoveries from stuttering observed in young children also leads this author to the suggestion that early and active intervention by clinicians may also facilitate recovery from stuttering.

Following are four assumptions that this author currently holds regarding the problem of stuttering in young children and the roles of parents and speech clinicians in assisting abnormally disfluent children in maintaining fluency:

1. Most stuttering behavior is the result of multiple co-existing factors including both physiological and psychological variables.

2. Typical parental reactions in terms of drawing attention to and in suggesting means to alter disfluent behavior generally facilitate the development of fluent speech in stuttering children.

3. Very young stuttering children exhibiting tension in the speech musculature and/or articulatory or phonatory struggle behavior during moments of disfluency can be taught to use fluency-initiating gestures efficiently and effectively.

4. In addition to instructing the parents and the young stutterer in how fluency-initiating gestures can be developed, the speech clinician has the responsiblity of assisting the young stutterer in identifying, developing, and reinforcing fluency-enhancing attitudes and feelings.

IDENTIFYING THE YOUNG STUTTERER

The problem of differentiating between normally disfluent children needing no therapeutic assistance and disfluent children who could benefit from assistance most frequently exists as an academic rather than a real problem. Generally parents and speech-language clinicians can determine with confidence if and when a child is struggling with disfluencies or is experiencing feelings that might exacerbate the disfluency problem (both indicators that the child needs help). However, parents and clinicians may observe young children being markedly disfluent with no apparent accompanying struggle behavior and giving no indications of any emotional response to the disfluencies. While the child's frequent disfluencies attract the attention of the parent and the clinician, the clinician may need to undertake a comprehensive analysis of the child's disfluencies before being able to determine if the disfluencies are suggestive of a chronic stuttering problem.

After reviewing the data available in the literature with respect to differentiating between a "normally" disfluent child and a child whose disfluencies are predictive of chronic stuttering, this author developed a Chronicity Prediction Checklist (Cooper, 1973) for research purposes. The checklist consists of 27 questions that the speech-language clinician may answer with yes or no responses after consultation with the stutterer's parents and after observations of and interaction with the stutterer. Responses to the questions provide historical data (such as onset, family history of stuttering) and information concerning the parent and child attitudes toward the stuttering (for example, does the child perceive himself as a stutterer?) and the current behaviors associated with the stuttering (for example, do prolongations last longer than 1 second?) Yes responses may be interpreted as predictors of stuttering chronicity, but no individual question weighting for predictive value was attempted. Research is continuing to determine the significance each of the items on the checklist might have in predicting stuttering chronicity.

Without attempting to review all of the variables noted in the literature as being indicators of stuttering chronicity and thus clues as to whether or not a disfluent child should be included in an intervention program, a summary of probable key clues to stuttering chronicity is presented in Table 1. It would be ideal if we could measure precisely and then assign a weight to each of the above noted variables, enabling us to arrive at a score that would tell us which children need help and which children do not. Unfortunately we do not have such a system and it is doubtful if we will have such a system in our lifetimes. Consequently, each clinician must make the difficult intervention decision on the basis of imprecise measurements of variables whose significance to the chronicity of stuttering remains questionable.

INTERVENTIONISTS' ATTITUDES

As suggested by the assumptions noted previously regarding the problem of stuttering in very young children, this author is of the opinion that drawing attention to the child's disfluencies may be helpful. Obviously, the manner in which attention is drawn to the

Table 1. Probable key clues to stuttering chronicity

Variable	Indication for intervention
Severity	
Frequency	If the child's disfluencies have occurred consistently on 5% or more of the words spoken in most speaking situations for at least a period of 6 months, the frequency of disfluency might be interpreted as being indicative of a potentially chronic problem needing a professional's attention.
Duration	If the average duration of the child's disfluencies is 2 seconds or greater, the duration of disfluency might be indicative of a need for therapy.
Articulatory patterns	If the amount of disfluency is characterized by a variety of articulatory gesturings suggesting that the child is attempting to "struggle free" from the moment of disfluency (as opposed to relatively simple repetitive movements), the resulting complex articulatory pattern might be indicative of a need for therapy.
Concomitant extra-articulatory behaviors	If the child's disfluencies are accompanied by extraneous facial or body movements such as eye blinks and arm swinging and an observable general increase in body tension, the child might benefit from therapy.
Client affective cognitive responses	If the client indicates negative feelings regarding the disfluent behaviors and the reactions of others to the disfluent behavior, the child may benefit from therapy.
Parent affective cognitive responses	If the child's parents indicate negative feelings regarding their child's disfluencies and express feelings and attitudes which the clinician perceives to be potentially detrimental to the child, the child might benefit from a therapeutic intervention program that includes parental participation.

disfluencies is a critical factor in determining if such an intervention strategy is helpful or harmful. The manner in which clinicians and parents approach young stutterers will, of course, be determined by the attitudes they hold toward stuttering and stutterers.

Clinician Attitudes

Investigators of clinician attitudes toward stuttering suggest that speech-language clinicians generally hold attitudes toward stutterers that might be evaluated as being negative and predictive of therapeutic failure (Yairi and Williams, 1970; Woods and Williams, 1971; Cooper, 1975). Yairi and Williams (1970) studied speech-language clinicians' impressions of elementary-school age boys who stutter. They obtained 127 returns (from 32 men and 95 women) of a questionnaire that had been sent to all 174 speech-language clinicians in Iowa school systems. Their open-ended questionnaire asked the clinicians to "list all words, adjectives, or traits which in your opinion are needed to adequately describe elementary school age boys who stutter." From the adjectives reported, Yairi and Williams concluded that clinicians demonstrated considerable consensus in their stereotypes of elementary-school male stutterers and that the most frequently mentioned traits were personality characteristics rather than physical or mental characteristics. Also, they found that most of the traits speech-language clinicians used to describe boys who stutter were judged to be undesirable characteristics (for example, nervous, shy, withdrawn, tense, anxious).

Woods and Williams (1971) used questionnaires completed by 45 speech-language clinicians in Iowa to study the way in which these clinicians perceived boys and men who stutter. The open-ended questionnaire requested each clinician to write five or more adjectives that in his opinion best described the adult male stutterer. From this total list, each clinician chose the five most descriptively relevant adjectives and listed them separately. These five adjectives were then rated by the clinician according to their degree of relevance in describing the adult male stutterer. Degrees of relevance included "very much," "quite a bit," and "slightly." These three categories, and the unspecified adjectives remaining after the five most descriptive traits were removed, provided a basis for giving a clinician's responses various weights (from 1 to 4), depending upon the relevance the clinicians attached to the adjectives they listed. Weighing the responses in this manner allowed comparisons to be made on the basis of the relevance of each adjective to the clinicians who listed it, in addition to the general comparison of percentages of clinicians who mentioned any one adjective. These responses were compared with the same information obtained about elementary-school age boys who stutter (Yairi and Williams, 1970). Many of the same adjectives were listed for both boys and men, indicating a fairly well established stereotype of a "stutterer" regardless of age. Furthermore, Woods and Williams judged most of these adjectives to be descriptive of undesirable personality characteristics for males. When the adjectives were grouped together into broad behavior categories, approximately 75% of the clinicians listed adjectives that grouped within the category of "nervous or fearful," and 64% listed those that were included in the category of "shy and insecure." Only 31% of the clinicians listed adjectives that reflected "abnormalities of speech." In discussing their results, Woods and Williams suggested that one would expect to see inappropriate and perhaps detrimental therapy with a stuttering child if the clinician expects children and adults who stutter to have similar personality traits and concomitant problems. They noted:

> Constructive stuttering therapy is more likely to occur when the clinician compares the child's behavior and feelings, for example, with the broad range of normal children's behavior and feelings rather than with the narrow range of the stereotype of the stutterer. (1971, p. 283)

Speech-language clinician attitudes toward stuttering and stutterers in 119 practicing clinicians from Pennsylvania and 23 from Michigan using the Clinician Attitudes Toward Stuttering (CATS) Inventory were studied (Cooper, 1975). The CATS Inventory consists of 50 statements to which clinicians respond by circling the words on a five-point scale ranging from "strongly agree" to "strongly disagree" that indicate their reactions to each statement. The clinicians completing the CATS Inventory in this study were primarily working in public school situations. Ninety-nine of the clinicians held bachelors degrees, 42 held masters degrees, and one held a doctorate. In the Pennsylvania sample, the mean with respect to years of experience was 6 years; such data were not obtained in the Michigan sample. Clinician responses to each statement were recorded as falling within one of three categories: acceptance of the attitude expressed in the statement, rejection of the attitude expressed, or neither. Data were prepared in terms of the percentage of clinicians rejecting, accepting, or remaining neutral to the attitude expressed in each of the 50 statements. Inspection of these percentages revealed no significant differences between the Michigan and Pennsylvania groups and no observable differences between the responses of clinicians holding bachelors degrees and those holding masters degrees. Fifty-six percent of the total sample of clinicians accepted and 32% rejected the statement that most stutterers have psychological problems. Only 14% of the clinicians rejected the statement that "stutterers display a distorted perception of their own social relationships." Fifty-eight percent of the clinicians accepted and only 24% rejected the statement that most stutterers possess feelings of inferiority. Twenty-five percent (or one in four) of the clinicians rejected and 49% accepted the statement that there are some personality traits characteristic of stutterers. Only 25% of the clinicians rejected the statement that parents of stutterers tend to possess identifiably similar personality patterns. Twenty-eight percent of the clinicians accepted and only 32% rejected the statement that parents are the primary factor in causing stuttering in their children. Forty-five percent of the clinicians rejected the statement that stutterers "have to some extent an underlying physiological impairment." Eighty-two percent of the clinicians accepted the statement that stuttering is the most psychologically devastating speech disorder, and 51% accepted the statement that clinicians must be more understanding of the feelings of their stuttering clients than their nonstuttering clients. In a discussion of these results it was noted:

> . . . a bigot has been defined as one who holds blindly to opinions in the face of overwhelming contradictory evidence. In view of the extensive evidence in the literature that stutterers do not possess characteristic personality traits nor do they characteristically possess personality disorders; in view of the mounting speculations concerning the significance of physiological factors in the stuttering syndrome; and assuming the attitudes noted in this study are characteristic of even a small percentage of clinicians generally, speech clinicians might be practicing a form of bigotry the ramifications of which are intriguing to contemplate. (Cooper, 1975)

Most theorists concerned with personality development note that children tend to adopt perceptions of themselves that are held by individuals perceived by the children as being in positions of authority. Assuming that preschool children would tend to perceive speech-language clinicians as being individuals of authority at least with respect to speech problems, the significance of any negative and distorted perceptions the clinicians might hold toward stutterers with whom they interact becomes obvious. Not only might the clinician's misperceptions, if adopted by the very young disfluent child, impede the recovery from stuttering that has been observed by several investigators (for example, Sheehan and Martyn, 1966, 1970; Dickson, 1971; Cooper, 1972, 1973; Lankford and Cooper, 1974), but the clinician might inadvertently reinforce the very stuttering behavior the clinician is attempting to eliminate.

Parent Attitudes

Recently, Fowlie and Cooper (1978) studied traits attributed to stuttering male children by their mothers. The Woods and Williams (1976) Adjective Checklist, containing 50 adjectives on 25 bipolar seven-point scales, was completed by 34 mothers of male stutterers ranging in age from 6 to 11 years and by 34 mothers of nonstutterers whose children were matched to the stuttering children on the basis of age, sex, grade level, and race. A group mean scale value for each of the 25 seven-point bipolar scales was obtained for the mothers of the stuttering children and for the mothers of the nonstuttering children. Mothers of the stuttering children described their children as being more anxious, introverted, fearful, sensitive, withdrawn, and insecure than did the mothers of the fluent children. The authors concluded that their results appeared consistent with the widespread stereotype of stutterers that has been reported in previous studies (for example, Erickson, 1969; Yairi and Williams, 1970; Woods and Williams, 1976).

While one could assume that a stereotype of stutterers exists because most stutterers actually behave in a characteristic manner even though no research has indicated such is the case, Woods and Williams (1976) suggest that a more satisfactory explanation for the existence of stereotype is related to the concepts of "state anxiety" and "trait anxiety" (Spielberger, 1966). It may be that listeners react to the momentary high "state anxiety" the stutterer is perceived as experiencing during the moments of disfluency and infer that the stutterer typically has a high level of "trait anxiety." This suggests that disfluent children may be perceived as being different from others when speech factors are not under consideration. Parents of disfluent young children may inaccurately perceive their disfluent children as being anxious when they are not anxious and may proceed to anticipate reactive behavior patterns to nonexistent negative emotional stimuli. In such situations, parents would be expected to adopt perceptions of their disfluent children that would more accurately reflect widespread stereotypes of stuttering children's behavior than their child's actual behavior.

In addition, parents of disfluent children frequently appear to believe themselves primarily responsible for causing their children to be disfluent (and why not, in view of the significant number of speech-language clinicians who do believe parents to be the primary cause of stuttering?). Such perceptions of parental guilt with respect to the cause of stuttering are reinforced too frequently, in the opinion of this author, by literature and films prepared by professionals who suggest that stuttering could be prevented if parents would follow simple guidelines used for developing good mental health in their children. One who accepted such guidelines literally easily could conclude that stuttering in children could be prevented if parents would listen without interruption to what their children have to say or if they would simply provide their children with a good model for speech. It is not difficult to understand why many parents do develop unreasonable guilt feelings with respect to their children's disfluencies. Perhaps it is more difficult to understand, in view of how frequently popular magazines contain articles suggesting parental involvement in the onset of stuttering, why so many parents react to their children's disfluencies with helpful concern and a realistic sense of their role in helping the child gain more fluent speech.

ATTITUDINAL SETS FACILITATING INTERVENTION

In a convention paper concerning controversies in stuttering therapy, this author (Cooper, 1977), after discussing therapy for the very young stutterer, concluded that sufficient evidence exists that speech-language clinicians may be perpetuating destructive and self-fulfilling prophesies through the unsubstantiated biases they hold with respect to the etiology of stuttering and the role played by parents in the maintenance of stuttering. While such a dictum may appear rather abrupt and capricious when in print, the sentiment expressed reflects accurately the concern this author has for the perpetuation by speech-language clinicians of unjustified and potentially disfluency-reinforcing parental guilt. It is for this reason primarily that the present discussion on helping the very young stutterer was begun with a set of assumptions about stuttering and about the roles the clinician and parent might play in an intervention program. Assuming agreement with those assumptions, the clinician would most likely approach the disfluent child without preconceived ideas regarding the variables that elicit and maintain

disfluency. In addition, the clinician's nonjudgmental and commu-
nication-facilitating approach to the parent might assist parents
and clinicians in identifying fluency-initiating behaviors for the
child.

In attempting to establish intervention-facilitating parental attitudes, the clinician might begin the initial meetings with the
parents by assessing the parents' knowledge of and attitudes
toward fluency problems. Simple checklists to assist in identifying
parental attitudes and knowledge of stuttering have been described
and are available for clinician usage (Cooper, 1976; Crowe and
Cooper, 1977). Once the clinician has an understanding of the
parents' perceptions of their child's fluency problem, the clinician
may begin to inform the parent of what has been observed with
respect to their child's fluency problem and what is known about
the typical development of fluency problems of that nature. Knowing the attitudes and knowledge that the parents have of fluency
problems, the clinician can stress information that may correct any
inaccurate perceptions the parents hold in the hope that intervention-facilitating parental attitudes will result. It is hoped that
parents will not be frightened by words themselves and be fearful of
using terms like "stuttering" in front of their children. Obviously, if
the parents are fearful of the word itself, the child may adopt their
fear with the result that the child now has the additional problem of
fearing a word that might have helped the child and the parents talk
about the fluency problem. In addition to being comfortable in using words that describe fluency problems, it is hoped that parents
will feel comfortable in discussing fluency failures with their children and in offering suggestions to the children in how they might
use their vocal mechanisms in a fluency-facilitating manner. If the
parents are able to communicate to their children that their concern
and their suggestions for altering speech motor patterns are
positive expressions of assistance rather than punishments for
"bad" behavior, the young child may adopt the kinds of attitudes
and behaviors that lead to increased fluency. It is in regard to identifying, developing, and reinforcing these attitudes and behaviors in
parents that the clinician can be of most help to the parent and the
very young disfluent child.

If clinicians assume that one of the more important goals in intervention programs for the young disfluent child is to prevent the
child from becoming so anxious about the disfluencies that the anxiety itself leads to additional fluency failures, parents will want to

do all they can to keep their children from responding in an overly anxious fashion to their disfluencies. The term "defused stuttering" has been used with parents to communicate the importance of reinforcing fluency-enhancing perceptions and attitudes in the child such as:

1. Stuttering is caused by many things — no one is "to blame" for the stuttering and no one is "bad" or "at fault" because they are disfluent at times.
2. Some people are more disfluent than others.
3. Most people stutter at times.
4. People can learn speech behaviors that can reduce stuttering.

Obviously, if the parent elects to attempt to convey to the child the above noted stuttering-defusing perceptions and attitudes, the parent cannot be successful by ignoring the child's stuttering behavior or in not reacting to the disfluencies. The parent who considers the child's disfluencies to be of a nature and frequency that the child should begin to learn the speech behaviors that can reduce the stuttering will want to communicate this to the child. It is in assisting parents in making such an evaluation that the clinician may be of significant assistance. For example, parents may have adopted unrealistic fluency expectations for all of their children after having observed the speech and language development of a sibling whose fluency was exceptional or even average. Speech-language clinicians, having knowledge of normal speech and language development and of the probable key clues to stuttering chronicity, can assist parents in determining if the child's stuttering behaviors suggest that the child would benefit from training to develop fluency-initiating behaviors and attitudes. If the clinician and the parent agree that the child needs fluency help, the clinician generally assumes the responsibility of instructing the parents in reinforcing the fluency-enhancing perceptions and attitudes noted previously and in identifying, developing, and reinforcing the use of fluency-initiating gestures.

TEACHING FLUENCY-INITIATING GESTURES

Before fluency-initiating gestures are described it might be helpful to the reader for the present author to review the development of his own thinking with respect to the question of whether clinicians should teach the stutterer to stutter more fluently or to speak more fluently. For years the author was of the opinion that if clinicians could eliminate the extraneous and peripheral things a stutterer does *when* he blocks and the behavior patterns adopted *because* of the stuttering, the block would take care of itself. While the frequency and severity of the moments of stuttering were significantly reduced through this approach, it was observed that many stutterers were not satisfied with the resulting level of fluency.

For the next several years the author used the widely used technique of teaching the stutterer to modify moments of stuttering to achieve more fluent stuttering. Stutterers were asked to superimpose on the involuntary stuttering a voluntary motor act that would result in a modification of the stuttering block. These activities were most frequently called "controls" and are known primarily as Van Riper's (1972) cancellations, pull-outs, and preparatory sets. With that approach to fluency control the author believes that many stutterers were helped. However, a problem seemed to persist. It was observed that most stutterers were able to achieve the feeling of control and experience periods of fluency ranging from several days to several months. Unfortunately, success in this approach presented difficulties with respect to maintaining fluency.

Many stutterers, when they "went on controls" as it was termed, became fluent rapidly and with little effort. This was termed the client's "flight into fluency." Unfortunately, with fluent speech, the stutterer had little or no opportunity to reinforce the use of controls or to develop skill in the utilization of a specific control during an actual stuttering block. In addition, clinicians frequently found themselves to be increasing rather than decreasing the complexity of the client's struggle behavior when they asked the stutterer to increase struggle behavior during the moment of stuttering. Again, the clinician proceeded under the assumption that by doing so the stutterer would be able to superimpose voluntary behavior over involuntary behavior and thus gain control of the stuttering. This rationale and approach to teaching more fluent stuttering were reevaluated in view of the frequently noted observation that almost all stutterers are fluent most of the time and that most stutterers when instructed are able to increase their fluency in most situations. The thinking was that if the stutterer's efficient and effective fluency-initiating behaviors could be identified and reinforced, the clinician could avoid the problems noted in teaching stutterers to control moments of stuttering. A fluency analysis checklist (Cooper, 1976) was created to determine which behavioral variables associated with speaking (for example, slow articulatory rate or breathing pattern changes) elicited fluency in each stutterer. As would be expected, fluency-initiating behaviors were observed for all stutterers with the effectiveness and the efficiency of the fluency-initiating behaviors varying markedly between stutterers. For example, some stutterers could markedly increase their fluency in all situations by what appeared to the clinicians to be inefficient and ineffective (in terms of facilitating communication) manipulations of speech-related behaviors such as the insertion of extraneous words and sounds. Following the identification of what appeared to be efficient and effective fluency-initiating behaviors, the clinician would assist the client in becoming proficient in the utilization of that behavior. The author was aware that the clinicians were using therapy techniques that had been described over three-quarters of a century ago by several authorities. For example, Makuen, who at the turn of the century was Professor of Defects of Speech in the Polyclinic Hospital for Graduates in Medicine at the University of Pennsylvania, noted in his work on the treatment of stuttering:

> The aim should be, not the cure of stammering, but the development of correct speech. . . . Stammering in the great majority of instances is due primarily to faulty or delayed phonation, or to a lack of promptitude in the vocal mechanism. . . . Without graded exercises covering a long period of time, the stammerer cannot talk in a prescribed manner. (1930/31, p. 25)

> He must be taught to bring all the processes of speech within the domain of his own consciousness, and he must learn to control them by volitional effort in the manner of a musician learning to play upon a violin. (1930/31, p. 26)

Robbins (1930/31), also around the turn of the century, while serving as director of the Boston Stammerers' Institute reported the following exercises as being the most helpful (in the order named):

1. The easy start of the first word to be spoken on each breath
2. Keeping calm, relaxed, and unhurried in everything they do
3. Slow breathing
4. The relaxation pause on empty lungs
5. Never holding the breath between breathing and speaking
6. Joining all words smoothly and easily together
7. Getting the attention more on vowels and less on consonants

Being aware that the techniques we were now proposing as "fluency controls" were not new, we assumed that by using more sophisticated programming procedures we could use these fluency-eliciting gestures effectively and efficiently in a therapy process that incorporated an attention to the client's feelings and attitudes as well as to the client's disfluencies. The author also became aware of Webster's (1975b) therapy program in which several "target behaviors" that seem to be similar to those fluency-eliciting behaviors listed above are identified and reinforced in the client through a series of lessons increasing in complexity and in a variety of speaking situations. Among the target behaviors Webster identified are the following: stretched syllable target, slow change target, smooth transition target, full breath target, and a gentle onset target. Webster considers the efficient utilization of these target behaviors in life situations and with varying speech sounds also to be targets. In addition, Webster has developed therapy instruments to facilitate the clinical instruction and reinforcement of the gentle onset target and the stretched syllable target.

The present author, continuing the development of what is now labeled Personalized Fluency Control Therapy, came upon a slogan that succinctly indicates the author's current thinking in regard to whether the stutterer should be taught fluent stuttering or fluent speech. It is now suggested that the client be taught Fluency-Initiating Gestures (FIGs) and that the client should adopt the motto: "Don't Fight It; Fig it!"

It is interesting to speculate how these fluency-initiating gestures result in fluent speech and how they might relate to etiological factors in stuttering. For example, assuming that Schwartz (1974) is correct that stuttering is related to a phonatory disorder, one might hypothesize that focusing on the modification of the stutterer's phonatory behavior through the easy onset fluency-initiating gesture might assist the stutterer in making compensatory phonatory adjustments that permit normal phonation and thus fluency for the stutterer. Investigators will and should continue to attempt to identify and to describe such relationships. However, this author, continuing under the assumption that stuttering is the result of multiple co-existing factors, is of the opinion that sufficient clinical data exist to indicate the usefulness of focusing on these fluency-initiating behaviors in therapy even though we are unaware of the underlying dynamics of the resulting changes in fluency.

Perhaps the individual seeking a term in keeping with the current level of understanding to describe how these behaviors elicit fluency might use the term "vigilance." This term was suggested by Cross and Cooper (1976) to indicate that the individual's attention was focused on his fluency rate. As has been demonstrated repeatedly (for example, Wingate, 1959; Daly and Cooper, 1967; Cooper, Cady, and Robbins, 1970; Siegel and Hanson, 1972; Cross and Cooper, 1976; Kimbarow and Daly, 1977), fluency is enhanced under conditions in which any type of stimuli is made contingent upon stuttering responses. The use of fluency-initiating gestures may serve the stutterer as a response-contingent alerting device and thus enhance the stutterer's vigilance. The term "vigilance" also is suggested to avoid the utilization of operant learning model terminology that may limit our conceptualization as to what is occurring when fluency changes are observed in the stutterer. As Cooper (1971) has noted and Siegel (1970) has concluded, we are impelled to seek explanations other than learning for stuttering behavior.

The effectiveness of any one kind of fluency-initiating gesture in eliciting fluency will vary from client to client. In fact, it appears that the possible number of behaviors that could be labeled fluency-initiating gestures is limited only by how many stutterers increase their fluency by altering their speech behaviors in unique ways. It is possible that clinicians might inhibit clients in developing their own unique and efficient fluency-eliciting behaviors by providing the client with a description of the common fluency-initiating gestures. It is for this reason that the clinician might wish to attempt to identify with the client characteristics (other than fluency) of the client's stuttered speech that are altered when the client is being fluent. Such attempts can be made by observing the client's speech in conditions that typically produce fluent speech (for example, reading in unison, following a metronome, shadowing another speaker, noise conditions, under delayed auditory feedback, or self-imposed rhythm). The client and the clinician may be able to observe differences in the client's fluent speech under these conditions (for example, less precise pronunciation, slower rate, a lower pitch, or an exaggeration of articulatory movements) that the client might transfer to other situations as fluency-initiating gestures (FIGs).

Although the clinician should be encouraged to assist older clients in developing their own "personal" FIGs, the clinician may introduce what have come to be called the "universal FIGs" (Table 2) because they appear effective in eliciting fluency in most stutterers.

Table 2. The universal FIGs

FIG	Speech characteristic
Slow speech	Characterized by a reduction in the rate of speech typically involving the equalized prolongation of syllables
Easy onset	Characterized by the initiation of phonation with as little laryngeal area tension as possible
Deep breath	Characterized by a consciously controlled inhalation prior to the initiation of phonation and typically used in conjunction with the easy onset FIG
Loudness control	Characterized by a conscious and sustained increase or decrease in the volume of the client's speech
Smooth speech (easy contact)	Characterized by light articulatory contacts with plosive and affricate sounds typically being modified to resemble fricative sounds
Syllable stress	Characterized by conscious loudness and pitch variations

Fortunately for both parent and clinician, the concept of FIGs can be communicated relatively easily to very young stutterers. A drawing of a FIG tree (Cooper, 1976) with the outline of four or five large figs spaces among the leaves and branches might be used effectively even for the preschool nonreader. For the reading-age stutterer, the child might be asked to write in the empty figs the names of the fluency-initiating gestures that the child, parent, and clinician have observed to be effective and worthy of reinforcement. The drawing then becomes the child's personal "FIG tree." For nonreading children, simple symbols can be developed and drawn in the empty figs to represent fluency-initiating gestures.

The author has found that the FIG tree has been most useful in conveying to very young children a sense of direction in what they are attempting to change in their speech behavior. This graphic representation has been used with very young children in conjunction with the "stuttering apple" (Cooper, 1976). The stuttering apple is created in the following manner: the clinician suggests to the child that the "core" of the stuttering problem is "getting stuck on words," or another term or phrase appropriate for the child. A small circle is drawn on a paper and the term agreed upon, such as "getting stuck," is written inside the circle. Next, the clinician encourages the client to note "things I do *because* I stutter, and things I do *when* I stutter." As the child (assisted by the clinician when necessary) notes such behaviors as "I blink my eyes *when* I stutter," "my hand jerks *when* I get stuck," "I don't answer in class *because* I stutter," etc., the clinician draws small circles attached to and surrounding the "core," writing in each circle the behavior that the child has noted. This procedure is continued until the child, with the aid of the clinician, has put in the graphic display all those behaviors associated with the moment of stuttering. Clinicians and clients typically identify additional stuttering behaviorisms as therapy progresses and these are added to the graphic display. A circle is then drawn around the "core" and all the attached labeled circles, and a "stem" is added to produce the "stuttering apple." The completed stuttering apple represents the client's stuttering behaviorisms.

The use of the stuttering apple to aid the child in the identification of the behavioral dimensions of the problems offers several important advantages. The graphic representation provides the client and the clinician with a similar conceptualization of the stuttering problem, thereby facilitating communication between clinician and child. Because the "apple" consists of behavior, the child is not threatened by the clinician forcing his attention to attitudes and feelings. Although we may successfully approach some adults with the direct question of how they "feel" about something, we have all experienced the problem of having children continually (and to us — exasperatingly) reply, "I don't know." By defining the problem in terms of behavior — "what I do" — the child is not asked to introspect as to how he feels. Actually, however, the same goal is achieved by focusing the client's attention on his behavior. The child's attitudes and feelings are reflected in the behaviors which comprise the stuttering apple.

Another important advantage in the use of the stuttering apple as a means of conceptualizing and identifying the client's problem is that it avoids the use of meaningless labels. Terms such as "secondaries," "starters," "avoidance," "anxieties," etc., are frequently meaningless to a client. The stuttering apple provides the child with a concrete description of his problem in his own words. Although the stuttering apple can be used effectively with most chronic stutters, it remains an individualized presentation of the stuttering problem. Finally, the stuttering apple has provided the child with a concrete description of his problem and thus, perhaps, reduced the child's vague and general fear regarding the previously undefined problem.

After the stuttering behaviorisms have been identified for the client through the use of the stuttering apple, the clinician may use the graphic representation to structure the initial phase of therapy (Cooper, 1976). The clinician suggests that the apple represents those things that the client wants to "do away with." Therapy becomes a matter of "eating the apple to its core." The clinician then discusses with the child which "bite" to take out first. The child is led to choose a relatively uncomplicated behavior to eliminate, such as "I blink my eyes when I stutter." The child can see on the graphic representation the concrete behaviorisms with which therapy will deal. Consequently, the vagueness of the immediate therapeutic goal is kept at a minimum. Also, the clinician and the child have a concrete and readily available reference as to the behaviorisms with which therapy will initially deal. The child can *see* where he is "going" in therapy.

Clinicians may approach the utilization of FIGs with parents and children in a variety of ways. It has been found advantageous to structure their use with the very young stutterer in the following manner:

1. The clinician describes for the parent and the child the concept of fluency-initiating gestures.
2. The clinician has the child try out in the clinical session, generally in the presence of the parent, a variety of FIGs.
3. Using the graphic representation of the FIG tree, the clinician assists the parent and the child in selecting which FIGs appear to be most efficient and effective for the child by writing the FIGs' names in the empty figs on the drawing of the tree.
4. The clinician, parent, and child agree upon which FIG to begin working.

It is assumed that the clinician, knowing the child's feelings, attitudes, and skills in using fluency-initiating gestures, generally is the best judge of how and when the child should begin using fluency-initiating gestures in the various speech situations. The clinician might wish to create a hierarchy of speech situations on the basis of the amount of difficulty the child experiences in the situations and then direct the child to begin working his way up the hierarchy by using FIGs in each of the situations until the level of fluency is acceptable to the child and, more important, until the child experiences the feeling of fluency control.

THE FEELING OF FLUENCY CONTROL

There appear to be differences among individuals describing stuttering programs with respect to what should be the end goal of therapy. While this author is of the opinion that the end goal of therapy should be the development in the client of a feeling of fluency control, others have developed therapy programs so that arbitrarily established stuttering frequency counts during predetermined speech activities in prescribed situations appear to be the goals of therapy. Making frequency counts of disfluencies in controlled situations may be less difficult and demonstrably more precise than assessing a hypothetical construct such as "the feeling of fluency control." However, it is suggested that the latter is a key, if not *the* key, variable in determining if a stutterer will maintain an acceptable fluency level upon termination of formal therapy. In addition to questioning whether stuttering frequency counts in prescribed speech modes and situations are valid indicators of an individual's general stuttering behavior in life situations, clinicians are aware that such pre- and posttherapy assessments frequently have little validity in reflecting changes in the complexity of the stutterer's struggle behavior or in the stutterer's fluency-facilitating or fluency-impeding attitudes and feelings. Again, while the stutterer's feeling of fluency control may be more difficult to define and to assess than stuttering frequency counts, it is the opinion of this author that the feeling of fluency control is the most important single variable in determining how successful the client has been in obtaining and will be in maintaining a level of fluency acceptable to the client.

The term "feeling of control" is not meant to be abstract. Rather, it is meant to refer to a response-specific visceral reaction that everyone has experienced in some aspect of their behavior, whether it be in typing class, shooting baskets in basketball, or playing the guitar. It is the visceral response of knowing you are capable of controlling a complex motor act. Athletes perhaps experience and are aware of the feeling of control most frequently when they note they played well because they "felt" in control — "psyched up," or, as they might say, "Man, was I with it!" The feeling of control that stutterers are encouraged to develop should be perceived as a very concrete and real experience, not as a hypothetical construct never to be experienced. Manning and Shrum (1973) noted the difficulties in communicating the "feeling of control" to clinicians and clients. While they noted that such a feeling might appear to be abstract and vague, they concluded:

> . . . such a feeling can be extremely identifiable and specific to the stuttering client. The client is able to "know" whether he is completely "in charge" of his speech or whether "the block has assumed command." Certainly the stutterer could indicate to the clinician when such control has been achieved. In many instances, though, the experienced clinician is able to identify such control or the lack of it. It is recognized, of course, that identification of this type of control involves a good deal of subjective evaluation on the part of both client and clinician. Perhaps more objective methods such as measurement of the absence of slight reduction of tension and anticipation as suggested by Bloodstein and Shogan (1972) would also serve to indicate whether or not the client has achieved control. (1973, p. 33)

Regardless of which procedures are being used in the modification of the stuttering pattern, clinical observations suggest that they are of value only if the stutterer *feels* he has changed the original stuttering pattern. Fluency-initiating gestures appear to be of little value in themselves unless the stutterer is developing a "feeling of control" when he uses them. To avoid having the stutterer focus on the modification technique rather than on the feeling of control, it may be advantageous for the clinician to continue to demand behavioral descriptions of the fluency-facilitating behaviors the client is using rather than to attach a label to the behavior. Unfortunately, once a label has been attached to a modification technique, the stutterer may focus on doing a good job with the technique rather than developing an ability to modify the speech act itself. For example, the stutterer may focus on doing a "good deep breath" rather than on being able to modify the speech act. It appears more appropriate for the clinician to ask: "Do you *feel* you were able to change the speech pattern in any way?" than to ask: "Did you do an easy onset or a deep breath?" As the client continues to experiment with various fluency-initiating gestures in different speech situations, his feeling of control over the speech pattern is reinforced. The client may enter the therapy situation and announce dramatically that he has the feeling of control. When asked to express this feeling, the controlled stutterer might report, "No matter how tough a speaking situation I'm in, or no matter how much stuttering I might have initially, I *know* that I can use my FIGs until I feel in control."

Fluency is perceived as being the by-product of the feeling of fluency control. The term "control" as used in this context refers to the ability of the stutterer to use fluency-initiating gestures in any speaking situation. The term "control" and the term "fluency" as used here are not meant to be synonymous. An individual may be capable of using fluency controls and continue to be disfluent. However, it is assumed that an individual who has experienced the feeling of fluency control and has the ability to use fluency-facilitating behaviors in even the most difficult situations will be capable of decreasing the disruption in communication and, with the feeling of control, will experience fewer disfluencies.

This author's clinical observations and the controlled evaluations of therapy programs in which he has been involved has resulted in the perception that the feeling of fluency control is critical to the maintenance of fluency following termination of therapy. Recently, Daly (1977), in discussing the results of a follow-up study of stutterers who had been enrolled in an intensive therapy program at a summer camp, made the following observations regarding the feeling of fluency control and the maintenance of fluency:

> It is our contention that stutterers must *earn* this "feeling of control." What happens when our clients acquire fluency too fast or when they experience "false fluency" very early in therapy? The change in speech fluency occurs so suddenly that the client is not aware of the monitoring he or she must do in order to maintain fluency in difficult situations. (1977, p. 5)

> These clients do not replace stuttering with normal speech — fluency just happens. Happy with their new speech pattern, many clients are not motivated to learn the speech components or targets necessary to retain fluent speech. These clients have not achieved the "feeling of control." Fluent speech and disfluent speech are still superstitious behaviors that just occur. It is with these "quick to fluency" clients that we have considerable difficulty. (1977, p. 6)

These observations support this author's opinion that one of the most important fluency-intervention attitudes that clinicians might assist parents in developing is the attitude that reinforcing the feeling of fluency control in their child is more important than having the child maintain an arbitrarily determined level of fluency.

FEELINGS AND ATTITUDES CONSIDERED

While there does not appear to be much disagreement among stuttering specialists that stuttering may be the result of the interaction in time of both physiological and learned factors, there does appear to be controversies between specialists with respect to what constitutes a total therapy program. This author is of the opinion that any stuttering program is inadequate if it does not at some time assist the individual in identifying and clarifying his feelings and attitudes about stuttering and fluency control. Others believe the attention to "attitudes" and "feelings" are unnecessary. Ryan (1974), for example, in arguing for an "operant analysis" approach to the treatment of stuttering, noted:

> Although it may be argued that any really effective approach to stuttering must include modification of speech, anxiety and attitude, the data coming of the operant/clinic-laboratory seem to indicate that the production of fluent speech alone tends to bring about concurrent changes in anxiety and attitude. In other words, to modify the attitudes and anxiety of the person who stutters, the best procedure is to provide him or her with the capability of speaking fluently. An operant analysis appears to permit and encourage the achievement of this goal. (1974, p. 12)

With the advent of detailed and systematic behavior modification programs based on a specific learning model such as the program described by Ryan (1974), speech-language clinicians were made aware of the vulnerability of the abstract hypothetical constructs upon which "insight approaches" to stuttering therapy had been based. Clinicians found themselves defensive as they discussed "self-actualization," "acceptance," "objectivity," or "self-concept." In comparison with the rigorously defined and experimentally manipulatable behaviors that receive the focus in behavior therapy, these terms appear indefinable and have been presented as being irrelevant to the manipulation of behavior.

Unfortunately, behaviorally oriented therapy programs that have not attended to the feelings and attitudes of the stutterer have resulted in the belief by many that, with the proper control of contingencies, fluency can be shaped and maintained in stutterers without much effort on the stutterer's part. While there appears to be little doubt that stutterers can be conditioned to *temporary* fluency, there appears to be every indication that, if the stutterer wishes to maintain that fluency, he must spent an enormous amount of "psychic energy" to do so. It is apparent that stutterers must possess this largely internally derived energy if they wish to maintain the fluency that was elicited with the clinician's artificially imposed conditioning strategies. The amount of control many stutterers need to exert to sustain totally fluent speech requires such an outlay of energy that they are capable of accomplishing little else. This author assumes that it is the speech-language clinician's duty to assist each stutterer in assessing how much energy he wishes to expend on the maintenance of fluency control. By doing so, the clinician will avoid imposing unrealistic fluency standards on the individual. If this variable is neglected, the clinician may succeed in making the stutterer feel less than whole when he is unable to maintain the fluency that can be so easily elicited in the clinical situation. The speech-language clinician can assist each stutterer in assessing how much psychic energy the client is both capable of expending and willing to expend on the control of fluency. The stutterer may be belittled when a therapy program is imposed upon him with externally derived criteria for success. On that basis alone it would appear to this author that therapy programs should attend to the individual stutterer's feelings, beliefs, attitudes, goals, and dreams — those very real things that will still largely evade the behaviorist's well defined, measurable, and manipulatable reinforcers.

Proceeding under the assumption that stuttering is the result of multiple co-existing factors, this author has viewed resistances to fluency change as following into three major groups:

1. Resistances that result primarily from physiological factors (that at this time continue to evade precise identification by investigators)
2. Resistances that result primarily from the individual's perceptions of self, environment, and the interaction of the two (that would indicate that a stutterer's feelings and attitudes would affect therapeutic progress)
3. Resistances that result primarily from established motolinguistic patterns (that would indicate that the stutterer may have speech habit patterns requiring therapeutic attention)

Assuming that such resistances to fluency changes are real and that clinicians cannot at this time precisely identify the physiological factors that may impede fluency changes, one would appear justified in concluding that stuttering treatment programs should include activities leading to the modification or at least evaluation of perceptions and to the modification of fluency-related motoric behavior.

In a more detailed analysis of the need to attend to the feelings and attitudes of stutterers in the therapy process, this author made the following observations:

In order to deal with the innumerable variables present in the clinical situation, the clinician is forced to develop organizing conceptualizations of the therapy process. These conceptualizations will be more or less abstract depending on the scope of the variables being included. The degree to which these conceptualizations mirror reality determines the clinician's ability to manipulate and to predict behavior. It is doubtful if a single theoretical framework exists which the clinician can adopt to give order to the manipulation of the innumerable events occurring in a therapy session. In fact, it may be naive to assume that one day we will have a single theoretical framework with which we can accurately account for the variability in human behavior. Presently, it appears more realistic for the clinician to choose selectively those conceptualizations which appear to reflect most accurately the class of behaviors to be modified. This pragmatic approach does imply that a clinician may be operating from more than one conceptual framework during any one treatment process. Such pragmatism is hardly puristic and the danger of practicing under the aura of an emasculated eclecticism is ever present. However, it appears wiser to attempt to conceptualize the problem in its entirety than to focus only on that aspect of the problem which can be defined and manipulated behavioristically.

The assumption is made that no single conceptual framework is broad enough and specific enough to explain adequately and accurately the determinants of human behavior. The continuing challenge is to create a more generic frame of reference with minimal distortions of reality. Until such a framework is developed, clinicians may find that current behavior therapy models do not present a complete rationale for clinical behavior. (Cooper, 1976, p. 8)

Being convinced that the speech-language clinician should attend to the stutterer's feelings and attitudes in the therapy process, this author has attempted to describe a therapy process that incorporates procedures to facilitate the identification of the stutterer's feelings and attitudes. Although aware that the clinician may not need to change a client's attitudes and feelings to enhance fluency, the author is convinced that the clinician and the client must at least identify them if therapy is to proceed efficiently and effectively. It appears that one of the major responsibilities of the clinician particularly with the young stutterer is to provide the client with sufficient information about stuttering so as to facilitate the client's adoption of realistic and fluency-enhancing attitudes and feelings. Table 3 briefly summarizes the four stages of Personalized Fluency Control Therapy.

As noted previously (Cooper, 1977), this author is of the opinion that while there may be many controversies in the area of stuttering therapy, the issue of whether to attend or not to attend to the feelings and attitudes of stutterers is the most important. Any stutter-

Table 3.   The four stages of Personalized Fluency Control Therapy

Stage	Therapy
1. Identification and structuring	The clinician assists the stutterer in identifying behaviors that occur during moments of disfluency and behaviors adopted as a result of the disfluencies. The clinician informs the stutterer of the procedures that will be followed in the therapeutic process and the rationale for focusing on the client-clinician relationship to facilitate removal of disruptive cognitive processing and, through the resulting therapeutic involvement, to facilitate the client's acquisition of fluency-initiating gestures.
2. Examination and confrontation	The clinician directs the client to begin modifying behaviors identified in the first stage of therapy. The clinician observes client behavioral patterns indicating client resistance to change. Having identified the client's resistive behavioral patterns, the clinician makes the client aware of these behavioral patterns. The goal of the clinician's confrontative behavior is to lead the client into an emotionally significant therapeutic involvement. Thus, the clinician reinforces client expressions of affect in response to the clinician's confrontations. Through shaping of client affective responses the clinician creates an affectively open therapeutic relationship.
3. Cognition and behavior orientation	The clinician reinforces client expressions of affect to facilitate client self-evaluation activities and to maintain client commitment to change. The clinician reinforces accurate, self-appreciative, and productive verbalized client cognitions and reinforces client behavioral expressions of adequacy. The clinician instructs the client in establishing self-reinforcing procedures for the maintenance and continued enhancement of the individual. Concomitantly, as the clinician begins to perceive that the client is realistic with respect to his feelings and attitudes regarding himself, is capable of self-reinforcement, and is aware of the amount of energy he is willing to expend on modifying the speech behavior, the clinician begins instructing

	the client in manipulating speech behaviors to determine which fluency-initiating gestures (for example, speech rate change, the gentle onset of phonation, or breathing pattern changes) appear most appropriate for the client. The cognition and behavior orientation stage is brought to a close when both the clinician and the client mutually agree that the client's potential for gaining and feeling of fluency control is maximized.
4. Fluency control	The clinician assists the stutterer in planning and using fluency-initiating gestures in the kinds of speech situations that had previously resulted in fluency problems for the client. The primary goal in this final stage of therapy is the development within the stutterer of a *feeling* of fluency control. Therapy may be terminated when the stutterer *feels* that no matter how difficult the speaking situation may be, he is capable of employing fluency-initiating gestures to obtain a level of fluency acceptable to him for the particular speech situation involved.

ing program that does not at some time assist the individual in assessing and clarifying feelings and attitudes about stuttering and fluency control is, in the opinion of the author, inadequate and may in fact be detrimental to the client. The proliferation on the market of exclusively behavior-oriented stuttering therapy programs inadvertently may be reinforcing the training of technicians without the skills necessary to assist others in identifying and handling feelings and attitudes. With the popularization of behavior modification principles and procedures, some training programs were criticized for training amoeboid compassionates without technical skills. Now it is hoped that the complete clinician can be trained: a humanist who is both a behaviorist and a phenomenologist.

PSYCHOTHERAPY

Being aware of the many significant contributions made by many psychotherapists of all orientations to the treatment of stuttering and being convinced that treatment programs for stutterers should include the identification of the stutterer's feelings and attitudes that will facilitate or impede therapy, this author has appreciated the value particularly of psychodynamically oriented, verbal psy-

chotherapy in the treatment of stuttering. However, this appreciation is not based on the assumption that all stutterers or even many
stutterers need psychotherapy. Rather, this appreciation for psychotherapy is based on the assumption that psychotherapists may
assist us in helping our stuttering clients make maximum utilization of the fluency-enhancing procedures we provide them. Reality
dictates that most speech-language clinicians do not have an opportunity to work in conjunction with a psychotherapist with the same
client and it does not appear necessary that they do so with all but a
very few stutterers.

The incidence of psychopathology in stutterers (which apparently can only be estimated on the basis of clinical experience
because of a lack of substantive data) does not seem to indicate a
need routinely to refer all stutterers for a psychodynamically
oriented psychological evaluation. However, stuttering therapy programs conducted by speech-language clinicians should be structured sufficiently to enable the clinician to assess the need for
psychological consultation during any phase of the therapy program.

The Personalized Fluency Control Therapy program summarized in Table 3 was developed with evaluational instruments to be
described later in this chapter that assist the clinician in determining the need for psychological consultation. Several of the instruments were developed to assess the feelings and attitudes of the
stutterer and to provide the clinician with some indications as to the
psychological state of the client with whom he will be working.

INTENSIVE VERSUS NONINTENSIVE THERAPY

One might assume that an ideal situation would be for the client to
be enrolled in an intensive therapy situation where 100% of his time
could be in therapeutic endeavors under the immediate and continuing supervision of the clinician. Such intensive therapy programs do
exist throughout the country in settings ranging from residential
summer camp situations to year-round intensive rehabilitation programs most frequently associated with university speech and hearing centers and comprehensive rehabilitation centers. In the University of Alabama intensive therapy program, clients have been able
to complete the therapy process in 8 weeks, during which time they
spent approximately 5 hours, 5 days a week in group and individual
therapy activities. Comparisons are not available of the therapeutic

results obtained in intensive relatively short-term therapy programs with the results obtained in the more typical program consisting of 1 or 2 hours a week of therapy for 1 or 2 years. It is apparent, however, that clients can benefit from therapy in either the short-term intensive therapy situation or the long-term nonintensive therapy situation. At one time, this writer was convinced that the short-term intensive program definitely was preferable to the long-term nonintensive type of therapy program. That is no longer the case. Too frequently, significant relapses have been observed in clients who were able to gain an acceptable level of fluency in a short period of time in an intensive program away from the client's home environment. Although again there are no data available indicating which program is preferable, this writer perceives in the long-term nonintensive program an opportunity to assist the client in developing fluency control skills slowly and methodically without a dramatic disruption of the client's life. On the basis of that conclusion, this author is now of the opinion that most school-age stutterers can be enrolled in efficient and effective therapy programs in the typical school situation in which clients receive 1 or 2 hours of therapy weekly on a long-term basis. Such a conclusion does not suggest that a combination of a short-term intensive program, in which basic fluency skills are introduced, and a long-term nonintensive program, in which the fluency skills are maintained, could not be provided the client with the advantages of both therapy forms.

ASSESSING THE RESULTS OF THERAPY

Having stated that stuttering therapy should include considerations of the stutterer's feelings and attitudes as well as the stutterer's disfluencies, the author is of the opinion that therapeutic success or failure should be determined on the basis of both changes in the fluency rate and changes in attitudes and feelings. To facilitate the assessment of changes in both attitudes and fluency, the following instruments (Cooper, 1976) were constructed: the Stuttering Attitudes Checklist, the Situation Avoidance Checklist, the Concomitant Stuttering Behavior Checklist, the Stuttering Frequency and Duration Estimate Record, the Client and Clinician Perceptions of Stuttering Severity Ratings, the Parent Attitudes Toward Stuttering Checklist, and the Longitudinal Stuttering Assessment Summary Sheet.

Stuttering Attitudes Checklist

The Stuttering Attitudes Checklist contains 25 statements about the client's feelings and attitudes toward his own stuttering; the client is asked to indicate if he agrees or does not agree. The statements have been worded in such a fashion as to make them appropriate, in most instances, for both children and adults. The statements may be read to clients if the clinician believes for any reason that client responses would be facilitated by doing so. The statements also have been worded so that client agreement with each of the statements might be interpreted as indicating an "undesirable" attitude on the part of the stutterer independent of whether the attitude may be justified. For example, the stutterer may agree with the statement, "My stuttering is my biggest problem." In reality, it may very well be the client's biggest problem, but being such, one might predict that the stuttering problem will prove to be a relatively complex problem and thus, perhaps, less amenable to modification. At any rate, the client, by agreeing that his stuttering is his major problem, has indicated that the stuttering is a significant negative factor in the client's life. If the client, following therapy, should no longer consider the stuttering to be his major problem, one might assume that therapy has been beneficial. Scoring of the checklist is achieved by a simple addition of the number of statements to which the client has indicated agreement. It is assumed that the greater the number of agreements, the less desirable are the client's attitudes and feelings. Scoring, however, becomes significant only when the client's scores at various time intervals are compared. While the checklist may provide clues regarding differences between stutterers with respect to attitudes and feelings, it was created to provide the clinician and the client with a means of identifying the individual client's feelings and attitudes. The Stuttering Attitudes Checklist can be used by the clinician both to 1) assess the client's attitudes toward his stuttering before, during and after therapy, and 2) provide the clinician with an entry into a discussion with the client regarding the client's feelings and attitudes.

Situation Avoidance Checklist

Fifty common speech situations are listed on the Situation Avoidance Checklist; the client is instructed to indicate which of the speech situations he "avoids or would prefer to avoid" because of his stuttering. The clinician may read the situations to those clients unable to read the checklist and score the checklist as directed by the client. Scoring the checklist is accomplished simply by counting the number of speech situations the client has indicated that he avoids or would prefer to avoid. The Situation Avoidance Checklist may be used to assist in assessment of the stuttering problem, to determine changes with respect to the client's avoidances of speech situations, and to assist both the clinician and the client in becoming aware of the ramifications of the client's fluency disorder.

Concomitant Stuttering Behavior Checklist

A total of 32 behaviors that have been observed to accompany the act of stuttering in many clients are listed under five categories: posturing behaviors, respiratory behaviors, facial behaviors, syntactic and semantic behaviors (judged to be stuttering avoidance behaviors), and vocal behaviors. Clinicians are instructed to check those behaviors that currently seem to accompany moments of stuttering. The clinician is reminded that these behaviors need not occur during every moment of stuttering but should be in the current repertoire of concomitant behaviors that were observed. The Concomitant Stuttering Behavior Checklist may be used to assess stuttering, to determine change in the client's stuttering-related behaviors, and to assist the clinician and the client in becoming aware of client's stuttering behavior patterns.

Stuttering Frequency and Duration Estimate Record

The Stuttering Frequency and Duration Estimate Record is a single-page form that enables the clinician to record the client's stuttered responses in three conditions: 1) answering questions that typically elicit one- or two-word responses, 2) reciting the alphabet, and 3) reading a 200-syllable prose passage constructed of second-grade level words. The questions, the alphabet, and the reading passage are all included on the single-page form in such a manner as to facilitate the clinician's recording of responses. In the response to questions condition, the clinician counts the number of stuttered syllables and also estimates the average duration of the blocks. In the recitation and the reading conditions, the clinician records 1) the time it took the client to complete the task, 2) the number of stuttered syllables, 3) the percentage of stuttering, and 4) the estimated average duration of the moments of stuttering. The Stuttering Frequency and Duration Estimate Record provides the clinician with one more assessment that should assist him in arriving at some estimate of stuttering severity and might provide one more indication of changes in the frequency and duration of the client's stuttering should he wish to repeat the estimate during and following the therapy process.

Client and Clinician Perceptions of Stuttering Severity Ratings

Apparently simple global judgments of "stuttering severity" continue to be one of the most meaningful assessments of the severity of stuttering. Perhaps because of the marked variability in the frequency of most clients' stuttering both within the same speech situation and between different situations, judgments of stuttering severity generally are more meaningful when they are based on several observations of the client's speech performance in several different speech situations. For this reason, a summarizing or "global" stuttering severity rating by both the client and the clinician would appear to possess a certain degree of face validity in any attempt to assess stuttering severity. The Client and Clinician Perceptions of Stuttering Severity Ratings is a single-page form to be completed by the clinician. In the first portion of the form, the clinician is instructed to read to the client three incomplete sentences dealing with the client's perception of the severity of his stuttering problem. The client is asked to complete each sentence by choosing one of five possible conclusions read by the clinician that indicate how severe the client perceives the problem to be. The clinician records the client's response. The client will have given three indications on a one- to five-point scale of his perception of the severity of the problem. The clinician's portion of the form contains a one- to five-point scale ranging from mild to very severe for each of four aspects of stuttering: frequency, duration, tension, and concomitant behaviors. The clinician is directed to select, on the basis of all the clinician's observations of the client, the scale number that best describes the clinician's estimate of the severity of that aspect of the client's stuttering. In this manner, the clinician makes four estimates on a one- to five-point scale of the severity of the client's problem. The global severity of stuttering ratings obtained through the use of the Client and Clinician Perceptions of Stuttering Severity Scale, in addition to providing more indications of the nature and severity of the client's stuttering problem, frequently provide the clinician with useful comparisons of the client's perceptions of severity with the clinician's perceptions. Clinicians have found a discussion with the client of these comparisons to be a fruitful topic in therapy.

Parent Attitudes Toward Stuttering Checklist

The Parent Attitudes Toward Stuttering Checklist is a 25-item checklist containing statements of attitudes and feelings typically expressed by parents of stutterers. Parents are asked to respond to each statement by indicating if they agree or do not agree with the statement. Responses indicating agreement to the statements are interpreted as being indicative of feelings and attitudes that the clinician might wish either to explore with the parent or to modify. Thus, the greater the number of agreement responses, the greater is the indication that the parent would benefit from instruction and counseling. The Parent Attitudes Toward Stuttering Inventory can be used by the clinician to 1) identify areas of parental concern and parental misperceptions, 2) structure parental therapy sessions by reviewing each item with the parents, and 3) assess changes in parental attitudes as therapy progresses.

Longitudinal Stuttering Assessment Summary Sheet

The Longitudinal Stuttering Assessment Summary Sheet is a single-sheet form that can be attached to the front or back inside cover of the client's file to provide a continuing summary of changes in the client's and the parents' attitudes, feelings, and behaviors as therapy progresses. The summary form provides a space for the data obtained in each of the aforementioned inventories, checklists, and ratings. The form includes spaces for 24 different indicators of client change and four different indicators of parent change. Assuming that the clinician has utilized all of the aforementioned assessment instruments, the clinician will have a "battery" of indicators of client changes with respect both to behavior and to feelings and attitudes.

The above noted checklists and forms are described to indicate those variables that this author contends may assist in evaluating stuttering therapy. As noted previously in this chapter, unidimensional approaches to evaluating pre- and posttherapy differences may be misleading, and they provide little or no information to the clinician as to what aspects of the client's attitudes and behaviors need to be modified in the pursuit of increased fluency.

SUMMARY

Several topics relating to stuttering and about which controversies have arisen were discussed. Early intervention strategies with the young abnormally disfluent child were proposed. Speech-language clinician and parent attitudes toward stuttering and stutterers were observed to be key variables in facilitating fluency in young stutterers. Fluency-initiating gestures and the importance of developing a feeling of fluency control on the part of the child were described, as was the need to attend to the fluency-enhancing feelings and attitudes of the young stutterer. While it was concluded that psychotherapists of all orientations have contributed significantly to the treatment of stuttering, formal psychodynamically oriented, verbal psychotherapy is not perceived as being a necessary ingredient of therapy programs for most stutterers. Long-term nonintensive therapy programs were described as appearing to facilitate the development of an increased fluency that the stutterer is able to maintain following the termination of therapy. The chapter concluded with a description of instruments used to provide a multidimensional assessment of both fluency and attudinal changes during therapy.

Although the author has taken positions on these issues that he perceives to be defensible, he is cognizant of the fact that too much of the defense for the positions is based on clinical observation, clinical intuition, and rational thought processes. Believing that too frequently it may be irrational to be rational in our irrational society, and that by our framework we are sometimes hung, the author seeks compassion from his readers should any of the conclusions reached herein subsequently be found to be indefensible. If the author has developed one piece of wisdom from over 20 years of professional endeavor with the enigma of stuttering, it is that if we just survive long enough, almost all of our conclusions will be supported by somebody's data for at least a brief period of time at one time or another. For fear that a reader might misinterpret the author's intent with the previous statement, allow him to conclude with the observation that he cannot think of a more challenging or exciting problem with which one might be concerned while at the same time experiencing the sense of worth that comes with seeing others benefit from one's labors and attempts to deal with controversies about what one is doing.

chapter THREE

From Psychoanalysis to Discoordination

William H. Perkins, Ph.D.

Two decades ago, I was aligned with the "toilet trainers," the moniker hung on us in those days by "preachers" from the other side of the speech department to which we were attached. Intrigued with the psychoanalytic teachings of Lee Edward Travis and impressed with his clinical results — he and his students had produced the only "cured" adult stutterers I had ever seen — I was determined to treat the neurotic origins of the problem. To do otherwise was thought to be merely symptom management, a lesser business to be avoided if possible.

Thus, I found myself in league with a stalwart band of advocates of psychotherapy whose clinical mission was to relieve neuroses underlying speech disorders. Whether true in fact, we fancied ourselves in loyal opposition to the traditionalists of stuttering theory and therapy: men like Wendell Johnson and Charles Van Riper and their clinical descendants. I doubt that Johnson and Van Riper relished the traditional role, having been young rebels themselves who, ironically, had also been students of Travis in his days at the University of Iowa. That they had turned the mainstream of treatment of stuttering into the channel of learning-to-live-with-it-successfully was a measure of their influence.

Curiously, I still find myself outside this mainstream now navigated by such of my co-authors as Hugo Gregory, Joseph Sheehan, and Dean Williams. Whereas two decades ago I was viewing with alarm their preoccupation with symptoms of stuttering as being too little concerned with the needs of the person who stutters, the shoe is now on the other foot. They view my attention to establishment of normal speech as too mechanical, or as Sheeham would say, as an exercise in false fluency.

This chapter is an effort to set my current thinking as much in contrast with that of my co-authors as possible. In many ways I would have less difficulty pointing out how much I share in common with everyone, but that would be a love-feast and this book is about controversy.

I should note by way of preamble, however, that my turn from psychotherapy to behavior modification over a decade ago was for pragmatic, not theoretic, reasons. Lacking strong evidence one way or the other, I have not abandoned my suspicion that some of the psychoanalytic conceptions of stuttering are probably valid. The hard evidence I do have is that relief of anxiety, whether neurotic, about oneself, or even about speech, provides little assurance that stuttering will improve. The fact that we can obtain predictable results with behavioral tools that can give the most severe or fearful stutterer normal sounding speech provides me with some confidence that a solid treatment for this disorder is within reach.

STUTTERING VERSUS FLUENCY VERSUS NORMALCY

What should the goal of treatment be: fluent stuttering, fluency without stuttering, or normal speech? I opt for the latter but must admit that the closest we can come at present to this ideal is with normal sounding speech, the distinction being one of attitude that we will discuss in the next section. The goal of normal sounding speech differs as much from fluency-without-stuttering, which it resembles superficially, as it does from fluent stuttering, which it also resembles in important ways.

The clinical procedures we use have been evolving since 1964 when I replicated Israel Goldiamond's original experiment with delayed auditory feedback (DAF). I followed the procedures he later reported in 1965 utilizing syllable prolongation and obtained the same results: fluency. Admittedly, the slow, labored drone was a far cry from anything sounding normal, but it was fluent — and for me, it was the first predictable feature of stuttering I had found. Thus began a series of investigations into the nature of fluency and how to shape it into normal sounding speech.

In a preliminary study, we compared these rate-control shaping procedures administered in an operant framework with several popular alternatives, including behavior therapy (Perkins, 1967). This pilot work was not intended to provide a definitive comparison of all these treatments, but it did answer our question. The operant rate control technique worked without exception; its predictable effects contrasted sharply with those of the other techniques, the results of which seemed equally inconsistent.

Anxiety and Stuttering

This preliminary work pointed up a hunch that had been growing stronger during the years I had used psychotherapy as the primary tool to remediate stuttering. I still had no reason to doubt that stuttering is learned, a premise that seemed too fundamental — if not sacrosanct — to even question. But I had begun to doubt that anxiety and apprehension had much to do with the stuttering of most clients I observed. By and large, their disfluencies occurred for no apparent reason. Of course, some saw "Jonah" words and sounds looming ahead which, if not dodged, spelled certain disaster. And for others, speech in general was occasion for apprehension. For the majority, however, they did not foresee most of their bobbles and blocks, so how could they be fearful of stuttering if it was unanticipated?

Margaret Taylor (1966) attacked this troubling question by measuring heart beat intervals and galvanic skin responses before and after moments of stuttering. Her eight subjects varied one from the other in these measures. Similarly, the measures varied from situation to situation. No subject, however, showed significant variation before and after stuttering. Measures during fluent speech were indistinguishable from those during stuttered speech. Moreover, the popular notion that stuttering resembles a startle response was undermined; Taylor found no signs of cardiac acceleration indicative of startle. In brief, she found no evidence from her measures that anxiety triggers stuttering.

About the same time, Burl Gray and Gene England were studying the effects of reducing speech apprehension with reciprocal inhibition procedures. It was their work, reported in 1972, that we replicated as a portion of our pilot study. We obtained essentially the same results as they did: anxiety was consistently reduced, but effects of this reduction in improved speech were seen in only about one-third of the subjects. As Gray and England noted, this is about the same percentage who show considerable improvement with traditional forms of speech therapy. Because these therapies are designed to reduce fear and avoidance and to help stutterers live gracefully with a problem exacerbated by struggles to avoid it, perhaps about one-third of the stuttering population does indeed "hesitate to hesitate."

Fluency

The question of why the majority still stutter was unresolved by our exploratory work. We knew of no theory that accounted for stuttering as we observed it, and so most of our understanding was based on treatment effects. Anxiety and avoidance-reduction therapies were successful with roughly one-third of adults who stutter, so that presumably the underlying theory was appropriate to this group. Although we knew that with syllable prolongation, fluency was almost a certainty (Curlee and Perkins, 1969), we had little more than speculation as to why this procedure was universally effective. That fluency was easy to achieve by a variety of methods merely confounded any explanation of its effects. Reportedly, it could be obtained as readily with various techniques for rhythmical pacing as with rate control (Brady, 1969). Use of masking noise, too, worked well with some, but good results were not obtained as consistently nor did they last as long (Perkins and Curlee, 1969).

Although the reason that fluency was so easy to achieve was far from clear, unpopularity of the results was abundantly evident. Very few of those whom we saw were willing to endure a monotonous drawl as the ongoing price of freedom from stuttering. Early on, it was apparent that two conditions had to be met if we were to offer a palatable alternative to stuttering. The most fundamental one was that the speaker be able to sound normally expressive. Repeatedly we were told by word and deed that these people would rather stutter expressively than drone fluently.

Squarely opposed to the first condition was the second one. It required that the skills for producing the new speech pattern be sufficiently explicit that they could be controlled volitionally at any time. We discovered, to our chagrin, that "lucky-fluency" was easy to achieve and was just as easy to lose. What happened time and again from the beginning, and what still happens routinely despite warnings and admonitions, was that fluency was established at slow rates which permitted direct control of the new skills. Then, as speech approached normal rates, the speakers discovered they could forget their controls and still retain fluency. They thought a miracle had happened. At last they could be fluent like normal speakers without having to think about their speech. If they retained control, they would accelerate from a slow drone to a faster drone. By abandoning their controls, they had not merely increased their speed, they had achieved normally expressive speech. Seduced by their fluency, the honeymoon had begun.

Inevitably, the collapse occurred. The reasons are still as mysterious as how the honeymoon was possible in the first place. One man forestalled his day of reckoning for almost 3 years. For most who abandoned their controls, it arrived within a matter of days or weeks, or occassionally of months.

Stuttering as Learned Behavior

An adequate explanation of fluency and stuttering must account for these inexplicable periods of fluency and their loss as well as for the effectiveness of controls in maintaining normal sounding speech. For this intriguing problem, answers have been sought in every conceivable nook and cranny of the stutterer's soma and psyche. The big-game hunters on these expeditions have more often than not returned with little more to show than field mice. For years, the adaptation effect and consistency effect have been regarded as the most lawful characteristics of stuttering, but there have always been stutterers who did not show these effects. As Dean Williams and his associates (Williams, Silverman, and Kools, 1968, 1969) have been especially instrumental in demonstrating, these effects are also found in normal disfluency.

Having been raised on the premise that stuttering is learned, I found operant theory persuasive at first, and I still see the uses to which stuttering can be put as examples of operant learning. But our experience with manipulation of operant contingencies does not persuade me that the nuclei of stuttered disfluencies are explained adequately as examples of learning. I know that some investigators such as Israel Goldiamond (1965), Eugene Brutten (Brutten and Shoemaker, 1967), George Shames (1970), Bruce Ryan (1974), and Jan Costello (1975) have considerable confidence in operant or learning theory explanations, and so I am withholding judgment until I see how effective their long-term results are with large numbers of stutterers. As you might suspect, however, I no longer think of our treatment program as being "operant," even though we use operant procedures extensively, especially in generalizing new skills to daily life.

DAF Effects and Syllable Prolongation

The possibility that much stuttering may not evolve by learning from normal disfluency began to open with our use of delayed auditory feedback (DAF). Prevailing explanations of DAF effectiveness in establishing fluency suggested that the problem of stuttering might lie in the auditory feedback system, but we could find no way of controlling auditory feedback to instate fluency. Goldiamond's (1965) original suggestion that syllable prolongation is essential to offset the disruptive effect of DAF forecast the direction we took.

In our experience with several hundred stutterers, DAF is effective only as a means of enforcing syllable prolongation. If the rate is too fast for the amount of delay being used, the flow of speech will be disrupted — over and above the stuttering — by DAF effects. In other words, auditory feedback can be manipulated to disrupt fluency, but apparently no one has found a way of manipulating it to improve fluency. Moreover, by modeling the behavior we seek, the same release from stuttering can be obtained with or without DAF, provided the same technique of syllable prolongation is used. Nonetheless, we persist in using DAF at the outset of treatment because its "magic value" gives us assurance that we can obtain immediate fluency virtually without exception. Admittedly, other techniques such as a metronome or masking noise can be used to obtain fluency. In our limited experience with these procedures, however, we have not found that the fluency obtained can be easily shaped into normal sounding speech over which the stutterer has control, and so we continue with syllable prolongation instead.

Stuttering and Articulatory Rate

Doubt about the effect of rate retardation on stuttering was raised in recent studies that showed that slow word rates tend to reduce stuttering, but the effect is relatively weak (Adams, Lewis, and Besozzi, 1973; Ingham, Martin, and Kuhl, 1974). These results puzzled us because they were so discrepant from our clinical experience. We suspected, though, that the reason for such small effects was that these investigators retarded word rate, which offered no assurance that phonetic rate was also retarded. It is prolongation of phones that we thought is essential to reduction of stuttering.

To find out if our suspicion was correct, we devised an experiment in which we used sentences of monosyllabic words that were read normally, at 2-second intervals without prolongation, and at 2-second intervals with prolongation. Two-second intervals were used to simulate the 30-word per minute pace we used clinically to establish fluency. We reasoned that rate could be reduced by articulating rapidly at normal phonetic speeds and then pausing between syllables, or by articulating slowly with syllable prolongation. Clinical experience led us to expect much more reduction of stuttering with the latter technique for retarding rate than with the former. The 19 subjects who met experimental requirements confirmed this expectation. Most showed some decrease in stuttering with syllable rate retarded without prolongation. All showed considerable decrease with phonetic rate retarded; this involved syllable prolongation which practically eliminated stuttering.

Phonatory Discoordination and Stuttering

Why is a slow phonetic rate so powerful a method of obtaining fluency? In an investigation of the adaptation effect as a rehearsal phenomenon (Brenner, Perkins, and Soderberg, 1972), we stumbled onto the lead we have been pursuing. We found the adaptation effect to be reduced by whispering and reduced even more by lipping (voiceless articulation). The explanation for this result, which seemed as parsimonious as any, was that we had simplified phonatory complexity with whispering and had simplified it even more with lipping. By rehearsing these simplified versions of the adaptation trials, improvement in the normally spoken version was less than when the passages were rehearsed with voice.

Confidence that we might be headed in a profitable direction grew as the work of such researchers as Martin Adams (Adams and Reis, 1971, 1974) and M. E. Wingate (1966, 1969) on laryngeal involvement in stuttering began to appear. By then, we had gathered considerable evidence that simplification of phonatory coordinations with respiration and articulation was universally effective in reducing stuttering (Perkins et al., 1976). Our rationale for progressive simplification from voiced to whispered to lipped speech is summarized in Figure 1. As can be seen, the number of physiological adjustments, especially phonatory adjustments, is sharply reduced from the voiced to whispered condition and is minimal under the lipped condition in which articulatory movements need not be

CONDITION	SPEECH ADJUSTMENT	ADJUSTMENT RATE	PHYSIOLOGICAL ADJUSTMENT								
			RESPIRATORY: ALVEOLAR PRESSURE	PHONATORY: TRANSGLOTTAL PRESSURE					VOCAL TRACT MODULATION:	SUPRAGLOTTAL PRESSURE
				Effective Mass	Elasticity	Viscosity	Abduction	Adduction		
VOICED	PITCH	Phrase	▨							
		Syllable								
		Phone		■			■			
	LOUDNESS	Phrase	▨							
		Syllable								
		Phone		■			■			
	VOICED/ VOICELESS	Phrase	▨							
		Syllable								
		Phone		■			■			
	ARTICULATORY	Phrase	▨							
		Syllable								
		Phone		■			■			
WHISPERED	PITCH	Phrase								
		Syllable	▨					▨		
		Phone								
	LOUDNESS	Phrase								
		Syllable	▨					▨		
		Phone								
	VOICED/ VOICELESS	Phrase								
		Syllable						▨		
		Phone								
	ARTICULATORY	Phrase								
		Syllable	▨							
		Phone								■
LIPPED	PITCH	Phrase								
		Syllable								
		Phone								
	LOUDNESS	Phrase								
		Syllable								
		Phone								
	VOICED/ VOICELESS	Phrase								
		Syllable								
		Phone								
	ARTICULATORY	Phrase								
		Syllable								
		Phone								■

Figure 1. Number and rate of physiological adjustments involved in speaking aloud (voiced), whispering, and articulating silently (lipped). The slowest adjustments are from phrase to phrase ▨▨▨▨ , the most rapid are from phone to phone ■■■■■ (about 14 ± 2 per second), and in between are syllable to syllable adjustments ▧▧▧▧ (about 6 ± 2 per second). (From Perkins et al., 1976; reprinted by permission.)

coordinated with either phonatory or respiratory movements. Moreover, the rate at which phonatory coordinations must occur drops from the high speech phone rate to the much slower syllable rate.

The effects of simplifying these coordinations have been so stable that the procedure has become a diagnostic tool for us. Of the 30 subjects in the formal experiment, stuttering was considerably reduced with whispering and invariably was all but eliminated with silent articulation. The only exception to this pattern in over 100 stutterers tested clinically was a woman with a motor speech disorder. When she did not show the expected pattern, we became suspicious that her disfluencies involved something other than typical stuttering. A neurological evaluation revealed that she was suffering from a rare myoclonic seizure disorder.

Admittedly, alternative explanations of these results are possible. We have tested articulatory and grammatical complexity in some unpublished experiments and have found their effects to be slight. We looked at the distraction effect, but it does not explain why lipping is more effective than whispering, unless one is willing to argue that lipping is more distracting than whispering. We considered communicative responsibility, but it requires the assumption that every subject had the same uncontrolled psychological reaction to each experimental condition; this hardly seems credible. Another possibility is that the effects are attributable to reduction in the levels of subglottal pressure required for whispering and lipping. Indeed, this factor does operate and may account in part for the effects, but it does not explain why a retarded phonetic rate using normal voice (with its higher subglottal pressure requirements) is as effective as lipping in consistently reducing syllable disfluency.

We favor a discoordination hypothesis because it encompasses these known strong effects which eliminate stuttering; both retarded phonetic rate and simplification of phonatory complexity facilitate speech coordinations and hence contribute to fluency. This has become a cornerstone in our rationale for treatment. We view stuttering as discoordination of phonation with articulation and respiration. Therefore, we select shaping procedures for their power in facilitating these coordinations.

Facilitating Speech Coordinations

Although a variety of techniques can accomplish this purpose, our original experience was with syllable prolongation, and so we have continued with it as our initial facilitating technique. Basically, we still use the same procedures I described elsewhere (Perkins, 1973a, b). These include management of the breath stream to initiate voice with a soft breathy onset and then to maintain airflow throughout the phrase without any breaks or stoppages in it. Unlike Webster, however, we explicitly avoid having stutterers monitor voice onset syllable by syllable and certainly not sound by sound. Speech sounds spoken at normal rates flow by twice as fast as one can control movement — high speed speech is produced with low speed equipment — and even syllables flow normally at one's upper limits of control. If it is possible to monitor individual sounds and syllables at normal rates without abandoning controls, we have not found the method. Our objective is to teach controls that can be used at normal speech rates so that we can concentrate on dimensions of the phrase that can be monitored, controlled, and still preserve normal rates and expressiveness. In effect, what we seek are controls that, when mastered, will not be apparent when used. In a sense, our most successful graduates become skillful actors whose technique does not show when they sound like normal speakers.

Rhythm and Stuttering

A shift in our emphasis has occurred, however, in the last few years. Increasingly, we have stressed rhythm as the dimension that, more than any other, facilitates speech coordinations. Not that this is a startling direction to take; historically, stuttering is defined as a disorder of rhythm. Nor are we alone in pointing to it afresh; Wingate (1976) has implicated it as the central element of stuttering. The reasons why we have shifted derive from both the research and clinical laboratory. The lead from our own work turned up in the discoordination experiment. One of the alternative explanations for the effect of whispering and lipping was that reduced stuttering was a consequence of increased conscious effort and deliberate articulation. We reasoned that if this were the basis for improvement, then articulatory rate should have been retarded. What we found, instead, was that rate accelerated as fluency improved, suggesting that the rhythm of speech had been facilitated.

This result gave impetus to the clinical impression that rhythm was the key to shaping normal rate and normal expressiveness without loss of control. We concluded that without control of prosody (the patterning of the elements of which make rhythm) we could not systematically produce normal sounding speech. Admittedly, this is the most subtle and difficult of the dimensions of speech to make explicit. Of the elements of prosody — pitch, loudness, and duration — only the latter has proved clinically profitable. Attention to pitch and loudness yields artificial inflections worse than a beginning actor emoting Hamlet's soliloquy. Therefore, we avoid teaching how to stress syllables. Instead, we concentrate on how to shorten unstressed syllables.

We start this instruction early to help offset the typical tendency at slow rates to prolong all syllables equally. Herein lies the origin of the drone, which if left untended is fatal to normal expressiveness. If one learns to prolong all syllables at a slow rate, then that prosodic pattern will prevail as speech is accelerated, and the result will be fast monotony instead of slow monotony. Worse still for permanent results, what usually happens at faster speeds is a relinquishing of controls which frees the speech of monotony and provides an even more rapid rate. This is where the honeymoon with lucky-fluency begins. Thus, what we seek in the beginning is slow speech with natural rhythmic patterns. Just as an orchestral conductor can beat the same rhythm rapidly or slowly, so are we striving for what would sound like a time-expanded recording of speech spoken normally.

Another immense benefit of establishing natural rhythm is that it provides a route to normal sounding speech that does not sound or feel rushed, and it does not require abandoning one's controls at faster speeds. For example, at the beginning, speakers prolong all stressed syllables about 2 seconds each, a duration appropriate to a 30-word per minute rate. They accelerate by shortening the duration of stressed syllables, all the while touching unstressed syllables lightly, even at the slowest rates.

Interestingly, a trade-off seems to exist between rhythm and the other dimensions with which fluency can be maintained. The stronger the rhythmic pattern, the more the speaker can, without disruption, survive hard vocal attacks, rapid rate, breaks in the breath stream, and any other condition conducive to stuttering. Conversely, the poorer the rhythm the more reliance must be placed on slow rate and smooth airflow to maintain fluency.

Normal Sounding Speech Versus Fluent Stuttering

I have gone on at length about the rationale for establishing normal sounding speech because this has been the focus of our clinical and research effort. If we could not shape controlled speech that sounds normally expressive, then this approach would not, in my judgment, be seriously competitive with traditional programs that stress fluent stuttering.

For those who want to sound like normal speakers badly enough to learn the skills of normal sounding speech, and then are willing to use those skills more or less continuously, our alternative to fluent stuttering would appear to have considerable merit. Not that the procedures are that different: in a sense, all we have done is to refine the controls used in preparatory set and pull-out techniques and move them far enough ahead of moments of stuttering that the anticipatory anxieties and "stickinesses" of impending stuttering tend not to arise. For some whose apprehension is great, however, repeated success in their most feared situations is needed before they no longer anticipate difficulty. Instead of using these techniques to cope with blocks after they happen, or are about to happen, we use them primarily to maintain a feeling of fluency and thereby head off stuttering before it starts, a far different matter than suppressing it after it has started. Still, people with mild stuttering particularly sometimes choose to use these techniques only when they become apprehensive or begin to stutter. For them, continuous monitoring of normal speaking skills is not worth the effort, and so they are inclined to rely on lucky-fluency, knowing that if they have trouble they can use their normal speaking skills to recover.

ATTITUDE CHANGE

That attitude is essential to permanent use of normal sounding speech is a conviction we hold with little hard evidence to support it. At least we are in good company: of my co-authors, Cooper, Gregory, and Sheehan have been outspoken about the same conviction. Mainly it is an opinion that rises from clinical experience, buttressed to some extent by research.

Clinical Impressions

A prime impression is that an attitudinal gulf separates fluency, and even normal sounding speech, from normal speech. I have known only one person who was willing to live on a long-term basis with fluent speech that was far too slow and monotonous to sound normal. The vast majority revert to expressive stuttering. Admittedly, they typically perform well when they return to the clinic for follow-up evaluations. But, in daily life, expressiveness seems to take priority over fluency.

Even with normal sounding speech, the temptation to relax the monitoring and controls required to maintain it is great. Many who can pass as normal speakers when using their controls will occasionally lapse into stuttering, and, for some, these occasions occur frequently. These lapses seem to have more to do with the person's sense of identity as a stutterer, and his misgivings about relinquishing that identity, than with inability to maintain the skills of normal sounding speech. One such young man said, "It just doesn't feel like 'me' when I sound like a normal speaker." Thus, the gap between sounding normal and feeling normal is a matter of attitude.

We have probably been as successful as any in helping adults who stutter to sound normal, but few of these people yet think of themselves as normal speakers. Perhaps in time they will, but our guess, which may not be too educated, is that even the most diligent users of normal sounding speech will likely require about 5 years to feel as normal as they sound.

Meanwhile, because we do not know how to achieve this goal with predictable regularity, we have learned to avoid describing what can be accomplished in a few weeks of treatment as being "normal speech." That term connotes sounding normal without having to think about how to achieve it. Success with our treatment requires considerable attention to what one must do; so the best we can offer currently is "normal sounding speech."

We are farther removed in many ways from fluency programs, which superficially most resemble ours, than from the more traditional therapies with their emphasis on change of attitude. We have serious doubts about the long-term effectiveness of any behavioral program that is not systematically concerned with evaluating and effecting improvement in the stutterer's attitude.

Still, we do differ from traditional approaches in that we rely on the old bromide "success breeds success" for much of the attitude change that can be effected. We do not attempt to desensitize a person to the impact of stuttering. At the same time, we do not permit him to avoid stuttering. We try to give our clients mastery of the skills of normal speech sufficient for proving to themselves that with proper use of these skills they can sound normal in any situation, no matter how frightening. Such a demonstration requires stringent resistance to use of the old avoidance tactics.

We have learned, however, that many people will cling to secret doubts no matter how rigorous our attempt to have them demonstrate their new abilities. They will harbor a few Jonah situations that escape detection, and can then tell themselves, "Sure it works most everywhere, but it wouldn't work in a really tough situation." With these people, who permit their doubts to grow rather than trying to expand their conquest of fear, no amount of success in the clinic is likely to lead to permanent use of normal sounding speech.

It is in anticipation of such reactions, which are far from uncommon, that we depart sharply from Webster's emphasis on the mechanics of precision fluency. Granted, the skills must be practiced if they are to be mastered, and so we have everyone engage abundantly in speaking during their 80–90 hours of therapy. Granted, too, that the skills must be practiced accurately if they are to work successfully, and so we monitor their performance carefully.

Practice, however, can take various forms for various purposes. It can involve speaking to an electronic device that provides precise feedback about some aspect of motor speech. Such a technique has merit, in our judgment, as an ancillary method of shaping a skill to be used extensively in the crucible of social communication. As a major focus of treatment, in which a significant portion of clinical speaking time is spent in dialogue with an instrument never again to be encountered in daily life, we cannot resist the impression that this is a computerized version of tongue training, a skill which, mastered in isolation, has little relevance to the pressures of daily speech.

Obviously, such an indictment makes us especially vulnerable in any alternative we offer. Our attempt has been to have the best of both worlds by working in the context of a group. It provides a microcosm of the give and take of social communication. By working in groups of four to seven, everyone has ample opportunity to talk, yet no one is privileged. Quickly, groups become self-monitoring, squelching the talkative and encouraging the reticent. Moveover, they soon pass from mundane topics to gut-level issues bordering on psychotherapeutic encounters. Thus, the clinician is free to concentrate on accuracy of skills used in these 4-hour dialogues three times weekly — this is the other world we seek to perfect.

Division of responsibilities for these two worlds is not formally arranged; it simply tends to happen this way. Group members often monitor each others' speech performances, and they are encouraged to do so. Conversely, the clinician retains responsibility for ensuring that all of the attitudinal topics in need of consideration are explored extensively. We are particularly concerned that the members foresee as many of the pitfalls awaiting them as possible. Some will discover uses of their stuttering that they would just as soon ignore. Most will be tempted by the lure of lucky-fluency. For those who choose not to use controls, stuttering is the alternative if they are unable to retain lucky-fluency. Still, if controls are onerous, we respect the option not to use them, provided the choice is volitional. Sooner or later, most will tire of using their controls, even though they may be elated with the quality of their speech at the end of treatment. If not adquately prepared, the risk is that when they do lapse they will feel guilty, they will feel they have failed, and they will be afraid to return for further help. Especially, they need to become self-reliant, which entails recognizing subtle as well as obvious ways they use to make someone else responsible for management of various aspects of their lives.

Attitudinal Research

What evidence is there that these clinical impressions are anything more than ephemeral hunches and intuitions? Not a great deal, but what does exist is supportive. Probably the most substantial work has been done by Guitar and Bass (1978). They pursued a lead which suggested that, following transfer of fluency to daily life in a treatment program similar to ours, many stutterers' attitudes toward communication changed to those of normal speakers. Attitudes of some, however, did not shift (Andrews and Cutler, 1974). As a consequence, Guitar found, those whose attitudes a year after therapy had not been improved were stuttering significantly more than those who had developed normal attitutes toward communication.

Also, in an earlier study, Guitar (1976) had shown that clients with negative attitudes conducive to avoidance of stuttering, when measured just prior to treatment, were most likely to regress a year later even though they left treatment as fluent as anyone else. He thinks this probably means that these stutterers have become so accustomed to being frightened of stuttering that the limited experience they receive during generalization of fluency is not sufficient to extinguish these old fears. We agree with this possibility, and would add to it another: these people have avoided important occasions to speak for so long they do not know how to cope with them even after they are capable of entering them and speaking normally. In other words, they may not only still be fearful of stuttering, they may also be fearful of not knowing what to say even if they speak effortlessly.

As for our own efforts to evaluate attitudes, the results have been less than spectacular. We sent approximately 150 questionnaires, the results of which are shown in Table 1, to the people we had seen during the 2 years since inception of our 7-week intensive group treatment. To foster honesty, responses were to be anonymous. Therefore, we are unable to say what the quality of speech was for those who did reply.

The exceptions were a few of our disgruntled graduates who wanted us to know their identity; so for them we could correlate their speech performance data with their subjective reports. The comparisons were perplexing. One elderly gentleman replied that his speech before therapy was "poor" and afterward was "terrible." We checked his pre- and posttreatment recordings and found his stuttering at the outset to be severe. After therapy, he could pass

Table 1.   Speech performance questionnaire

	Percentage in each category
Before therapy, my overall level of speech was _____.	
Terrific	0
Good	2.3
Fair	25.6
Poor	39.5
Terrible	32.6
I would rate my current overall level of speech as _____.	
Terrific	0
Good	46.5
Fair	30.2
Poor	18.6
Terrible	4.7
Before therapy, I was _____ with my speech.	
Very satisfied	0
Satisfied	0
Unconcerned	4.7
Dissatisfied	46.5
Very Dissatisfied	48.8
Immediately after therapy, I was _____ with my speech.	
Very satisfied	39.7
Satisfied	41.8
Unconcerned	0
Dissatisfied	16.2
Very dissatisfied	2.3

Presently, I am _____ with my speech.

Very satisfied	4.7
Satisfied	44.2
Unconcerned	2.3
Dissatisfied	32.6
Very dissatisfied	16.2

I now have the necessary skills to control my speech if I want to.

Yes	74.4
No	25.6

I now have the necessary skills to sound normal when I control my speech.

Yes	79.1
No	20.9

I _____ use my speech controls.

Alway	0.0
Almost always	37.3
Sometimes	53.4
Never	9.3

I _____ feel like a normal speaker.

Always	2.3
Almost always	30.2
Sometimes	44.2
Never	23.3

I now stutter _____ than before therapy.

More severely	4.4
Less severely	75.6
The same	20.0

I now stutter _____ than before therapy.

More frequently	4.4
Less frequently	75.6
The same	20.0

I now feel _____ about speaking than before therapy.

Better	68.9
Worse	8.9
The same	22.2

I now feel _____ about myself than before therapy.

Better	64.6
Worse	8.9
The same	26.7

I can speak normally without thinking about controlling my speech.

Always	0
Almost always	27.9
Sometimes	41.9
Never	30.2

for a normal speaker. Clearly, whatever his unfilled expectation was, it had little to do with an objective evaluation of his speech. It is incidents such as these that dampen our enthusiasm for evaluating our success solely in terms of measures of speech performance.

On the other hand, such discrepancies permit us little certainty as to the meaning of the responses that we did obtain. If they are a true sampling of our graduates, then we can find some comfort in knowing that two-thirds to three-fourths of them claim to feel better about themselves than they did before therapy, have the skills to sound normal when they want to, stutter less severely and frequently, feel better about speaking, and, to our surprise, feel like normal speakers occasionally and can speak normally some of the time without thinking about controls.

As for satisfaction with their speech, 95% were dissatisfied at the outset and 80% were satisfied at the conclusion. Unfortunately, this glowing opinion faded for some, so that at the time of reporting only half remained satisfied and the other half became dissatisfied. Whether any connection exists between this slippage and the report by more than half that their use of controls dropped from constant use during therapy to only sometime-use would be conjecture. In any event, the picture would seem clear that many see themselves as having the skills to speak normally, but only occasionally do they choose to use them. This, then, would seem to come down to a matter of personal choice, and the making of that choice would, again, seem to be a matter of attitude.

PSYCHOTHERAPY FOR STUTTERERS

I have little to add about psychotherapy for stuttering that I did not say elsewhere over a decade ago (1965). Those impressions have not changed much, except that I am much less certain now than I was then that stuttering is rooted in neurosis. I must agree with Sheehan that to talk of stutterers needing psychotherapy is to talk of the population at large needing psychotherapy. Flimsy as the evidence is, stutterers do not seem to be any more neurotic than any other group of people. So far as I can discover, no systematic connection exists between personality and stuttering. Still, I cannot discount the connection categorically. The most spectacular improvements in speech I have seen resulted from psychotherapy with no direct attention to speech. The problem is that these are rare exceptions, not the rule. I could not explain my psychotherapeutic successes any more than I could my failures; this was a prime reason for turning to behavioral methods.

Another compelling reason was conservation of effort, time, and money. Whether psychotherapy will effect any change in stuttering is a question that requires many months, if not years, of expensive sessions to answer. If behavioral methods are to be effective, it is apparent within a few sessions. Furthermore, if the results do not last and psychotherapy proves necessary, the investment lost is minimal.

What I will expand a bit is the role of psychotherapy in such a program as we provide. In the first place, we are not equipped to undertake the parental-surrogate responsibilities indigenous to such a relationship when it is the tool with which a personality is to be reshaped. Such relationships, to be effective, require long-term commitments and stability. The recourse, in a transient program such as ours, is to identify people in need of extensive personal help, refer them, and try to follow up on the referral to be sure it is appropriate. Fortunately, we have encountered relatively few who are seriously neurotic.

Like most of us, stutterers, too, could probably use some personal help. We attempt to limit our intervention to the characteristics that threaten the success of the speech endeavor. Two problems arise frequently enough to deserve special mention. One involves operant use of stuttering, the other the dependence of the person who stutters.

If such a thing as a "stuttering personality" does exist, it is probably operantly shaped as a consequence, for most, of having lived practically all of their speaking years with the impediment of stuttering. One way or another, they have had to adapt themselves to the reality of having their speech disrupted in ways which they feel helpless to prevent. Predictably, many find uses that this disorder can serve in helping them cope with daily life. One, for example, is to gain and hold a listener's attention; who but the most callous will turn away from a person stuck in the middle of a block?

Our impression, though, is that stutterers are not likely to be aware of some of the important uses they find for stuttering. An inkling of this is appearing in a study still in progress, some results of which are suggestive of inconsistencies in ways stutterers look at their own stuttering. The vast majority see it as the biggest problem in their lives, and practically none think it is fun to stutter. Yet, they tend to disclaim that their lives are much affected by stuttering, or that they are nervous or anxious. At the same time, they admit more to depending on people because they stutter, and yet they almost unanimously see their speech as being a bigger problem for themselves than for others.

Operant values of stuttering constitute a serious threat to permanent maintenance of normal speaking skills. Where these uses are of more than casual importance, sudden freedom from stuttering can pose serious problems of coping. One man who, through psychotherapy, became fluent literally overnight after a lifetime of severe stuttering, was all but immobilized by the experience. He had avoided facing most of the important issues in his life because, he had explained to himself, he stuttered. Suddenly being unable to stutter brought him face-to-face with the reality of his situation. If these problems are not foreseen and alternative solutions involving normal sounding speech instead of stuttering are not developed, the result is almost certain to be a dilemma for these people. If the new skills are used, they will feel anxious; if not, they will stutter.

As for dependence, people who stutter may show no more of this characteristic generally than anyone else. Still, in relation to their speech, it poses a troublesome problem. Many of the people we have seen have left us with the impression that they feel they have been unfairly afflicted with stuttering, which of course they have. None elected to stutter. It was not by choice that they must suffer the consequences. Only with hard work are they likely to sound as normal as their nonstuttering friends for whom speech is effortless. In this sense, they are indeed afflicted unfairly. They do not state this proposition as a rational argument, nor do they necessarily believe logically that it is true. But their behavior says it in large and small ways. Some, who would hardly blink at a five-figure surgery bill, have begrudged a three-figure bill for their speech. Yet these same people protest that they would do anything to be freed from stuttering. They may demand, sometimes not too subtly, extra time from their clinician beyond that for which they have contracted. They may complain that too much is expected of them, and only carry out assignments when required by the clinician.

These would be minor annoyances at best were it not for their insidious effect on the ultimate outcome of therapy. Our behavioral program, and I presume most others, requires self-directed diligence. If responsibility has remained with the clinician to ensure development of necessary skills during treatment, then with termination of therapy comes termination of enforced usage of those skills.

We have no panacea for these problems, which seem appropriate for psychotherapeutic intervention. We do make certain that each group explores these and similar problems extensively. Whenever the occasion arises, we confront people with the contrast between what they say they want and what their behavior says they want. Further, our most popular maintenance program is devoted exclusively to counseling. Clinician feedback regarding mechanics of speech is prohibited in that group. Beyond this level of encounter, however, we do not feel it appropriate for us to enter into psychotherapeutic involvement.

THERAPY FOR THE CHILD

We have developed two programs for children, one for prevention of stuttering in preschoolers, and one for those of school age whose stuttering has become an established problem. Both of these derive squarely from our conception of the nature of stuttering as having two facets: physiologically, stuttering is a discoordination of speech, and psychologically, it becomes useful and is reinforced as operant behavior. As you might suspect, our recommendations for children seem iconoclastic for those who hold traditional views.

Prevention

Our rationale for prevention of stuttering is twofold. First, we attempt to facilitate the child's coordination of speech. One of our hypotheses is that preschool children showing early signs of stuttering are vulnerable to speech discoordination. When they attempt to speak rhythmically or at rates in excess of those they can manage, disfluency results. Accordingly, our first objective is to reduce pressure on the child for fast or jerky responses.

The other hypothesis related to facilitating coordination is that these young incipient stutterers are entering the social communication contest in a family of fast competitive talkers. If they are to make themselves heard, they must hurry to get a word in edgewise. Obviously, expecting them to slow down and speak smoothly while everyone else is whizzing along is hopeless. Thus, we concentrate on the family and teach them to instruct by example rather than by direction. We try to turn the speaking contest around so that the objective is for everyone in the family to speak slowly and smoothly, and to be a good listener. This program begins on a limited basis at first and is expanded as rapidly as possible to all speech at home. In this way, the incipient stutterer is not singled out for special attention, favorable or unfavorable.

Our second objective is to help prevent these children from discovering payoffs in stuttering, especially the discovery that stuttering grabs attention. Another of our hypotheses is that children who are particularly vulnerable to have disfluencies enlarge into a full-bloom problem of stuttering are the insecure ones who have had little success gaining attention when they speak. Undoubtedly, to attempt to participate in a conversation and have no one listen is as painful for children as it is for adults. Such children are probably candidates for strong reinforcement of disfluencies that their parents respond to with alarm. Even a negative reaction can be preferable to none.

Here is where our approach becomes controversial. Instead of the time-honored dictum to listen attentively to stuttered as well as nonstuttered speech, we instruct the parents in discriminative listening. They learn to attend selectively to their children when they speak smoothly and easily, and to be less attentive when speech becomes choppy and stuttered. Not that they are to punish stuttering or to call attention to it. Quite the contrary: the objective is to call attention to what the child is talking about when speaking effortlessly. It is the content of speech, not the speech itself, that we encourage to be the focus of interest.

We have had only limited experience so far with this prevention program, and so it should be viewed as experimental until far more results have been accumulated. Such experience as we have had has been very encouraging and has given us increased confidence in the hypotheses from which we work. One point has already become abundantly clear, however. Effectiveness of this parent-administered program drops sharply with children who have entered elementary school; parental influence becomes diluted, both in importance and in time spent with the child.

Remediation

We use a version of our adult program for clinical intervention with children who are beyond the reach of our prevention program. Unlike the prevention program, we do work directly with the child rather than exclusively with the family. And unlike the adult program, we work directly with the family as well as with the stutterer.

In other words, we seek adult objectives of establishing normal speaking skills while administering the program within the context of the family.

Our approach with children is to work by example, using members of the treatment group and of the family as models. We are, therefore, just as concerned with having parents master the skills to be learned as with having their children master them. Merely instructing parents is not sufficient; in fact, it can be harmful. We try to avoid the stereotype of the parental injunction, "Do what I say, not what I do." In general, the children who do well have parents who also do well in mastering and modeling the crucial speaking behaviors. This approach avoids the pitfall of placing the child in the dependent role of having something done to him, first by the clinician, then by a parent. Instead, the child is a member of two groups in which he is a fully qualified participant. He monitors the speaking skills of his parents, and occasionally brothers and sisters, as well as being monitored by them. Similarly, he monitors and is monitored by his peers in the treatment group.

TRANSFER AND MAINTENANCE

I doubt that our transfer program differs much from those of my co-authors. This is the operant aspect of our work in which we extend stimulus control of the new skills to daily life. We are as much concerned at this stage with having stutterers demonstrate to themselves that they can sound normal in their most feared situations as we are with ensuring that they can maintain control of their speech in frequently encountered situations. We do not want to leave pockets of doubt that can fester.

Unlike our procedures for shaping and transferring normal speaking skills, with which we are reasonably satisfied, maintenance is another matter. This is the perennial weak link in the therapeutic chain. And judging from the laments of other clinicians, it is as much a problem for them as for us. We tried an abundance of strategies on an exploratory basis: skill-maintenance groups, counseling groups, self-help groups, individual sessions, marathon sessions, refresher courses, family involvement, tape analysis, self-help contracts, prosthetic devices, even hypnotism. Most of these techniques have been helpful to some, but none has approached our shaping and transfer procedures for universal effectiveness. Perhaps other strategies might work better. One that Einer Boberg

(1976) has described to us seems to hold promise. A year after completing a program similar to ours, he has his graduates return for a checkup which includes videotape comparisons of their speech before and after treatment with their current speech. Apparently, this consistently results in marked improvement in previously deteriorating performances.

Criteria of Success

Our judgment at this time is that the problem of maintenance must be viewed in the context of a criterion of success. If that criterion is permanent establishment of normal sounding speech, then without doubt we still have far to go. If, however, the criterion is to demonstrate to each of our graduates that they have the skills required to sound like normal speakers, then we may be within reach of a solution. The issue then would be a matter of personal choice of the people who stutter. With this latter criterion, the clinician's responsibility would be to strengthen and transfer the new skills to those speaking situations most likely to be avoided, and to persevere until the decision whether or not to use normal sounding speech would be a matter of choice, not fear of failure. With this approach, the number of problems becomes delimited to complaints from people such as the ones noted below.

Typical Problems

People Who Have Tried Hard But Failed to Master the Skills The problem in such cases is that although these people may have worked harder than anyone else, they have practiced the skills incorrectly. When carried out accurately, the shaping procedures have proved effective without exception. Good intentions and diligence alone are not enough.

People Who Understand the Procedures Perfectly Yet Cannot Make Them Work This is essentially the preceding problem in a different guise. Being able to describe the skills in no way ensures ability to perform them accurately.

People Who Profess Great Desire to Sound Normal Yet Lose Control of Their Speech in Daily Life This can be either of two problems.

First, if their words reflect their intent, then either their hold on their new skills is too tenuous for adequate transfer, or stimulus control has been lost in the process of generalization. If the former, then shaping is incomplete, as it would be if, as sometimes happens, a person merely listens during treatment and logs only a few hours of actual conversation using normal speaking skills. If the latter, then stimulus changes during transfer have been too large, or practice in difficult situations has been insufficient.

The second possible problem is more difficult. It involves a protestation not matched by performance. The pattern here is of those who may rail loudest against stuttering yet do little that is required to achieve normal speech. These are the people who likely have shown that they have the skills yet avoid doing those things necessary to establish fluency. Typically, these are the people who manage to circumvent all efforts to help them assume responsibility for their own lives. If confronting them with the discrepancy between their words and actions is not sufficient to improve their performance, or to help them accept their true intent, then a referral for psychotherapy is likely in order.

People Who Have Used the New Skills Successfully Yet Prefer to Continue Stuttering   Again, this choice can reflect two possibilities.

One is that so much of their lives has been built around stuttering that, suddenly freed of it, they realize the extensive role it has played for them. When fluent, they feel like unwelcome strangers to themselves. If stuttering has been used as a defense against an unrealistic self-concept, then its removal will arouse anxiety. For these people, psychotherapy is in order. But for some it is more a matter of identity. They wish to feel like themselves, and stuttering is part of that self-image. This choice may be anathema to the clinician who has labored mightily to help establish fluency, but, if it is straightforward, not made out of fear or avoidance, then I see no basis for not honoring it.

The other possibility is that these people tire of using their controls to enable them to sound normal. This is likely to be especially true of severe stutterers, and may account for the greater tendency for them to relapse. They seem to have less margin for relaxation of controls if they are to remain free of stuttering. Lucky-fluency is less likely to be available to them. They are almost certain to stutter if they do not use their controls. In our experience, only the most dedicated will endure this effort without some periods of relapse. What many seem to do is shuttle back and forth — when use of controls becomes too onerous, they abandon them. For many, this means almost immediate return to stuttering. For others, the relapse does not occur for months; but eventually for everyone, it does occur. And when they can no longer endure their return to stuttering, they re-establish their controlled speech. Again, this is a choice that I for one cannot fault.

The above listing is not intended to be a catalogue of all possible explanations for failure to achieve permanent use of fluency. It does not include, for example, husbands whose wives feel they are no longer needed or useful, or wives whose husbands think their stuttering is cute. It is intended, though, to suggest a feasible clinical goal: firm enough establishment of normal sounding speech that it is available as a viable option to stuttering — for those who choose it freely.

MEASUREMENT OF SUCCESS

A definition of success is fundamental to any discussion of how to measure it. By setting stringent or lax criteria of effectiveness, one can turn unimpressive performances into extraordinary achievements, and vice versa. For example, in a 4-year study of clinical effectiveness, when we used the criterion of improved fluency (regardless of how monotonous) to evaluate our results, we had 100% success at the end of treatment (Perkins et al., 1974). Moreover, with this criterion, our results ranged from 92% to 100% improvement on a long-term basis. Using fluency as a standard, we could hardly have hoped to do better; most of our clients should have been jubilant. Unfortunately, many of them were not.

Thus, we decided to use a criterion more revealing of whether our graduates had achieved what they ostensibly came for, namely, reduction of stuttering. With this approach, our criterion was 85% reduction of syllable disfluency. Now, instead of 100% success, by this stringent standard only 70% succeeded.

This standard still did not tell us whether the speech rate was normal or drearily slow, and so we next used a double criterion: normal syllable rate coupled with 85% reduction of syllable disfluency. Now, of those who had achieved no more than fluency, only 44% qualified as being successful. Of those whose speech sounded normal, however, 65% succeeded and retained their improvement better 6 months after treatment.

As far as our research results were concerned, the normal speech group proved superior to the monotonous fluency group no matter which criterion we applied. For this discussion, however, the more important point has to do with the effects of the criteria selected to measure success. With a lax criterion, we were 100% successful on a long-term basis with our normal speech group; with a stringent criterion, applied to the same group and the same performances, we were only successful with 53% of these subjects.

Unfortunately, the criterion of success is rarely considered when therapeutic results are summarized or discussed. Thus, 70% and 80% success rates have been claimed in the press as well as in our journals for some treatment programs. But when we note that the typical criteria used for these reports approximate the lax one by which our clinical results proved to be 100% successful, and when we recall that many of our "successes" were less than awed with their long-term improvement, then we become concerned that such reports are misleading to the public if not to professionals as well.

Difficult as it is to define meaningful criteria for determining clinical success, another troublesome problem remains: how can progress be measured meaningfully? Which scores are valid indicators of improvement? Objective measures of observable behavior can at least be tested for reliability, but are they more valid than subjective opinion, and, for that matter, are they reliable?

Objective Measures

Let us start with the question of what behavior should be measured. The simple answer, of course, is fluency. But even that is not so simple, because if we can have "normal disfluency," then by exclusion we must also have "abnormal disfluency," which presumably is stuttering. If the measure of disfluency is the popular one used traditionally, which ranges from broken words to phrase repetitions, it will likely contain a mixture of normal and abnormal disfluencies. Considerable research has consistently shown that listeners are most likely to judge disfluencies as stuttering if they involve repetition, prolongations, and hesitations in articulating sounds and syllables. Disfluencies that involve larger units such as words and phrases will likely be considered normal. Thus, any measure of disfluency other than in units of syllables and sounds will be contaminated with normal disfluencies and will, therefore, be an invalid measure of stuttering.

Assuming that the measure of stuttering used is the percentage of disfluent syllables, is this sufficient? The answer is yes if one is concerned with frequency of stuttering. If, however, the question of severity is of importance, then the duration of stuttering becomes an issue, and to determine that, a measure of rate is needed. Again, the syllable is the preferred unit for reasons including those presented by Ingham and Andrews (1973). But, as we discussed earlier, it is phonetic rate, not syllable rate, that is vitally connected to fluency and stuttering. To calculate it requires separation of actual speaking time from pause time, and both of these measures must be separated from stuttering time if duration of prolonged blocks is to be reflected in a severity score.

With these as adequate measures of stuttering and rate, the question remains whether or not they are sufficient. Some would argue that they are, and I would agree, if reliability and ease of measurement are prime considerations. The fact remains, though, that these two measures are far from adequate as indicators of normal sounding speech.

For this, expressiveness and rhythm are the crucial observable features. Unfortunately, these are the most complex elements, and they defy a single objective score. At present, the best we can do is make a judgmental evaluation of them. Nevertheless, the fact that they do not permit as precise a score as do fluency and rate in no way lessens their practical significance as indexes of meaningful improvement. Some hold that achievement of fluency at normal rates automatically provides expressiveness; this is true when lucky-fluency is purchased by relinquishing use of speech controls. With retention of controls at normal rates, however, neither expressiveness nor rhythm is ensured. These aspects of normal speech require sophisticated skills to achieve, and they should be evaluated independently.

Now let us assume that we have appropriate scores for all observable aspects of speech. Under what circumstances should they be obtained if they are to be a valid reflection of real-life speech? Reading is easier for most than conversation and is dissimilar enough from it that one has little assurance of the quality of reading being equally good in conversation. Moreover, if conversational situations are used, a host of factors influences the results. Where did the conversations occur? With whom? At what time of day? Stimulus conditions exert such powerful control over behavior that these are anything but trivial questions. Follow-up measures of conversation with the clinician in the treatment room during the hours used previously for therapy may bear little resemblance to those obtained in the home in a family discussion. Perfectly fluent speech in the clinic frequently crumbles with every step taken away from the clinic building.

Obtaining measures of typical speech in daily life is not an insurmountable hurdle, although it can be troublesome. The major dilemma is a legal one: how do you record a spontaneous conversation with a prospective employer, say, and still not violate the law requiring informed consent? An even more difficult problem stems from this same issue. How do you record samples of stutterers' typical performances in daily life? Such evidence as exists consistently indicates that real-life performance is an inferior version of what is seen at checkup times.

One solution to this latter problem, which we are in the process of exploring, is to record the opening remarks of stutterers when strangers call them. Once past the initial amenities in which the interviewers identify their purpose, they ask permission to continue the recording. If it is refused, they erase the tape. This does not give a very large sample of speech that could be considered typical, but when it has been tried, it has given enough to raise serious doubts that what actually goes on in daily life is always revealed by recordings in the clinic.

Then there is the matter of how long after treatment to make recordings that will be indicative of permanent results. We tested our impression that deterioration in performance is stabilized within 6 months. What we found was that such changes as did occur in fluency and rate were between 1 and 3 months following therapy. Changes that occurred during the first month out of treatment and between 3 and 6 months were insignificant. Whether further deterioration occurred after 6 months was not answered by our study (Perkins et al. 1974). Curiously, we also found in this study that measures taken in the clinic before treatment began and 6 months after it ended were reasonably good forecasts of daily life measures (provided the stutterers knew they were being made). In between these times, however, performance within the clinic was a poor indicator of what could be measured outside.

Finally, a comment about participation in follow-up research: the 44 subjects who participated in the study just cited understood they were involved in a clinical experiment. They cooperated well in providing posttreatment measures. Subsequent use of a refined version of the same treatment procedures in group rather than individual settings has yielded more normal sounding speech in a larger percentage of our subjects who were seen with the explicit purpose of clinical service to them. They were charged minimal professional fees. Instead of better cooperation, the result has been just the opposite. For whatever reason, the majority of our graduates has not responded to our efforts to obtain follow-up information from them. Thus, we are particularly impressed, and puzzled, by the relatively high percentage of follow-up returns reported by Webster.

Subjective Measures

By now, it should be apparent that evaluating therapy of stuttering is a prickly problem. Even the most precise and reliable measures seem to be invalid indicators of improvement when seen through the eyes of some of the people who stutter.

We saw this discrepancy in our Table 1 questionnaire responses from some of the stutterers who identified themselves (thereby permitting comparisons of objective and subjective scores); measures of speech indicated normal fluency, but their stated opinions reflected thorough dissatisfaction with the treatment outcome. We also saw it earlier in our clinical effectiveness study (Perkins et al., 1974). In that investigation, we asked undergraduates enrolled in public speaking courses to evaluate fluency, rate, and expressiveness. They showed high agreement among themselves, so they apparently had a clear idea of what they were judging. But when percentage of disfluent syllables and syllables per minute were used for comparisons, they showed almost no relation to judgments of expressiveness or, to our surprise, to judgments of fluency and rate with which they would seem to be obviously correlated.

Why such discrepancies exist can probably be explained, but to my knowledge nothing beyond clinical opinion is available on which to base an explanation. For what it is worth, our impression is that factors such as age, socioeconomic status, job aspiration, and anonymity contribute to measures of objective performance and subjective opinion of that performance. If we could handpick clients with the best chance of permanent success with our method of therapy (as measured by improved performance and their opinion of that improvement), we would choose upwardly mobile young adults striving for a job requiring normal sounding speech. Yet, many who fit this description have not had long-term success, while many who do not fit it have. Interestingly, however, these factors seem to have little effect on shaping and transfer; most of our clients, regardless of background, come out of treatment sounding reasonably normal.

This result is relatively unaffected by any characteristics of stutterers we have observed. Secondary struggle reactions drop out automatically when phonatory coordinations are facilitated, so that we rarely have occasion to work on abnormal articulatory postures or secondary symptoms. Likewise, severity and apprehension do not affect the shaping and transfer results very much, although they do tend to interfere with permanent use of the new skills for reasons already discussed. Because these results are so predictable, this approach would seem to be a logical starting point for anyone who seeks to give up stuttering. In a comparatively short time, effectiveness of the treatment is apparent. With about half of our graduates, this is all the therapy they feel is needed. For them, to have worked long enough on their attitudes to have changed them would have been an unnecessary investment. For those whose attitudes still need attention, the problems that remain lie clearly exposed by the demonstrated ability to speak normally if they choose to do so.

The issue, as I see it, comes down to a choice of purpose for therapy. If improved performance in the ear of the listener is the clinician's major concern, then objective measures of speech can be sufficient. If improved performance in the mind of the speaker is of prime concern, however, then some measure of that speaker's opinion is needed if the outcome of therapy is to be evaluated meaningfully. The first purpose, of sounding normal, is far simpler to achieve, and probably more tempting for most clinicians. The powerful tools of behavioral technology lend themselves to achieving it and to persuading clients that this goal is to be desired. Yet, to say that pursuit of this objective is in the best interest of all people who stutter does not relieve therapists of the ethical implications of their choice of concern. Some clients are likely not to choose fluency. Therapy is a moral endeavor engaged in for the welfare of the people served. I can see no alternative to heeding the wishes of these people, whether expressed overtly or covertly, by word or deed, in determining what is in their best interest. Only they know their deepest needs, and so only they can determine their own meaningful goals.

chapter FOUR

Stuttering Therapy in a Framework of Operant Conditioning and Programmed Learning

Bruce Ryan, Ph.D.

The goal of research and thinking on stuttering should be the development of effective and efficient therapy programs that can be offered by all speech-language pathologists to all people who stutter. We are a long way from that point. Hopefully, by clearing the air on some of these present therapy controversies, discussed and referenced by Gregory in Chapter One, we can move a step closer to that moment in time.

PROBLEMS

We authors in this book face the lack of a common language to discuss what we do, an agreed upon evaluation system, and clear replicable descriptions of what we do in therapy. In addition, there is the conflict, sometimes pretty emotional, between the "operant conditioners" and "the more traditionally oriented clinicians." Someone once compared stuttering theorists to the blind men of India, who, each holding a separate part of an elephant, described what they believed to be an elephant. Each was partly right. We co-authors have an even greater, more important, and less allegorical kind of problem as we face the controversial issues about stuttering therapy. We have not agreed upon an evaluation system. We cannot always, therefore, compare assessments and decide who is right and who is wrong. We are dealing too much in the world of words.

Those of us with a behavioral orientation have attempted to use observations and measurements. We naively believed that the data would make us free and would cause people to change their minds and even their positions. This has not happened to the extent we wished.

Andrews and Ingham (1972a) suggested a therapy evaluation system composed of: 1) measurement of fluency and speaking rate, 2) transfer of fluency, and 3) maintenance of fluency. If more of our colleagues could be induced to collect and share this kind of information along with their speculations, casual observations, incomplete therapy descriptions, and pontifical statements, then there may be a chance to resolve the controversies cited in this book and move on to more substantive activities.

Although the situation is better, there is still a great lack of research data on therapy procedures for people who stutter. There are many books on therapy, but few data are found in them. This means that we are expected to take an authority's word for results with no replicable procedures or data to support or deny the stand. Moveover, it is interesting to observe how many authorities are not bothered by this lack of data. Few authors ever actually discuss their results except in a very general way or through a presentation of selected clients. The authors imply successful results (else why would they have written about their procedures?). We readers are left to assume positive results based upon the author's rhetoric and level of authority.

In the behavioral or operant approach to therapy, procedures are clearly described and replicable, if the replications are done accurately and carefully. Casual perusal of the recent literature reveals a certain consistency across the findings of several different researchers. For example, the work of Martin (1968), Haroldson, Martin, and Starr (1968), Costello (1975), and Ryan (1974) concerning the effects of punishment on the frequency of stuttering behavior all show very similar results.

The data-based operant approach includes measurement systems. This is probably why the operant system has not been well received by the speculators and philosphers who do not see the value of or who do not wish to be bothered by collecting quantitative information to support their speculations and inferences. Then there are the pseudobehaviorists, who use some of the terminology, none of the basic procedures, and all of the old nonbehavioristic therapy activities used before. That is the worst sin. The best evaluation of any theory system is the results of therapy based on it. Unfortunately, all theories and systems claim positive results, but most do not use or report careful measurement or evaluation systems; they simply state, "The stutterers under my tutelage got better."

Another major difficulty is that most written descriptions of therapies for stuttering are so vague that it is virtually impossible to replicate them. Clear descriptions of therapy procedures are critical to the resolution of some of these controversies.

An interesting manifestation of our problem is the clash between the traditional clinical approach and the newer behavioristic or operant procedures. Both groups seem very intent on attacking each other rather than trying to understand each other's viewpoints and analyze the data scientifically, rather than emotionally.

I have been described and categorized by Gregory in the first chapter of this book as being in the behavioristic, operant group of therapists. That is an accurate statement. However, being in this camp does not mean that one loses the right to be human, to think, to analyze, to question, to change, to accept, and to feel real empathy for the people who stutter who need our help.

There have been many attacks on the operant approach (Biggs and Sheehan, 1969; Sheehan, 1970a; Van Riper, 1973). Some of us even changed to using the term "programmed therapy" to avoid the controversy related to operant procedures. However, my basic thoughts and viewpoints about how to solve the problem of stuttering are still unchanged. Operant methodology has much to offer.

The theories and problem-solving strategies offered us within the operant-behavioral-programmed format have not only persisted but have been strengthened by increased activities in so many areas of social services (psychology, education, and even health care). There are continually more reports of behavioral research with stuttering and stuttering therapy.

I have seen the programs I helped to design for stuttering therapy reach, through training other clinicians, hundreds of people who stutter. I have read the data of Haroldson, Martin, and Starr (1968), Martin (1968), Curlee and Perkins (1969), Ingham and Andrews (1971, 1973), Andrews and Ingham (1972b), Van Kirk

(1972), Costello (1975), and Shames and Egolf (1976), to mention a few. I believe these data because the procedures are described clearly and specific measures are reported. In addition, the findings closely parallel those of some of my own work. Finally, these data support the belief, despite what Wingate (1976) has stated, that stuttering may be usefully viewed as learned behavior.

Will the mass of data accumulating in centers using operant learning principles eventually produce the necessary changes in stuttering therapy? Clear goal statements, well planned programs, and the extended efforts of many will be required. Changes will be opposed by the old stalwarts of the field who are still promoting themselves and their interesting, but nonfunctional, theories.

There is a certain rigor required of effective programmed therapy. Compared to the more casual traditional approaches, programmed therapy may provide less creativity, ego-massage, and clinical enjoyment for the clinician. The major reinforcing event in programmed therapy for the clinician is the achievement of fluency by the client. That, indeed, is very reinforcing.

Another kind of problem is the continuing gap between the study of stuttering and the preparation of therapy programs, or, put in another way, the gap between research and "clinicianmanship." It is not enough to continue to study the problem and analyze stuttering behavior through descriptive research. In our own operant efforts, the therapy programs we designed were often also research oriented. For example, the counting of words spoken yielded research information about normal word rate. However, this measure requires a great deal of effort and time to collect. Although it is still a part of the therapy program, its use is questioned. Word rate count has minimal clinical value except in programs involving rate control.

At this time there are three groups vitally interested in stuttering: the researchers who continue to strive for a better understanding of stuttering, the clinician-researchers who study the problem to develop a therapy (the authors in this book are a good example of this group), and the clinicians who must provide therapy for the people who stutter with whom they work each day. The clinician cannot wait until the researcher has completed the research and is ready to provide enough information to develop a therapy. It is the clinician-researcher who must bridge the gap. The clinician-researcher whose goal is an effective therapy has assumed the responsibility and the "glory" to provide not only a theoretical basis for the therapy, but a clearly described, validated, and transmittable procedure. It would be very helpful to the on-line clinician if the clinician-researchers could somehow unify their efforts or at least talk about commonalities so as to present an understandable, cohesive set of information to the clinician.

There undoubtedly is a core of appropriate procedures based on learning theory and aimed toward improving fluency that is part of every successful therapy for stutterers. This is, of course, most true of the various behavioristic approaches. Most therapies give some attention to the speech act. Most therapies do spend some time on speaking fluently, whether it is called controlled stuttering, pull-outs, or whatever. Much of the rest of many therapies is probably unrelated to the attainment of positive results. This core objective of modifying the speech act and improving fluency should make it possible for many different experts in stuttering therapy to share a common ground. It may be extremely naive to think that the various experts in stuttering could agree, but this would be a step toward it. This would not mean, for example, that all the clinician-researchers would be describing similar therapies in different languages. They could be doing different things in therapy, but the common elements could be agreed upon. The noncommon elements should be evaluated to determine their contribution, if any, to the effectiveness of therapy.

For the long-term good for the most people, including both clinicians and people who stutter, the clinician-researchers should take the next step in the sequence after presenting positions on the controversies in this book and work toward cooperative conciliation to present a united effort to solve the problem of stuttering.

PROGRAMMED THERAPY

In an effort to respond to the stated controversies about stuttering therapy, I have developed a basic framework from logic, speculation, observation, experience, and data. My framework is cast in a behavioristic mode. Behaviorism is attractive because it relies heavily on observable events, functional definitions, controlled manipulations of stimuli and responses, and the collection of data from which may be inferred certain information or predictions.

Most of this framework is described in detail in Ryan (1974), but for purposes of offering thoughts on the controversies, that framework is summarized here.

An essential part of the framework is that stuttering is learned behavior. This does not deny that certain physiological or psychological factors play a role in either the development or maintenance of stuttering, but they are viewed as contributing, consequent, or concurrent factors rather than prime causative agents. They are also less well understood and, hence, are less amenable to change.

This leads to the position that the main problem in stuttering is the way the person speaks. Aberrant attitudes and anxiety responses are only concurrent with or results of stuttered speech. Stuttered speech is the problem. The concept of the "stuttered word" is introduced to help define it. Stuttered words are: whole word repetitions, part-word repetitions, prolongations, and struggle. Almost any stuttering behavior may be placed in one or more of these categories. Although more elaborate systems are available, this system has proved functional and adequate in the development and measurement of programmed instructional procedures to help people who stutter to speak fluently.

Measurement of stuttering is reduced to counting these words (counting each stuttered word only once) per time unit of talking or reading behavior. This is "on-line" talk time. Silence is not counted as talking time. From this count and the time of reading or talking a rate of stuttering may be derived, e.g., 10 stuttered words in 5 minutes of talking would equal 2 stuttered words per minute (SW/M) or $10/5 = 2$ SW/M. This measure provides for a simple, easy, relatively accurate, functional count of stuttering behavior. We also count the number of words spoken per time unit, e.g., 725 words spoken in 5 minutes of talking equals 125 words spoken per minute (WS/M) or $725/5 = 125$ WS/M. We may then derive a percentage of stuttering by dividing the number of SW/M by the number of WS/M, or $2/125 = 1.6\%$ stuttering. Normal speech fluency is operationally defined as the absence of stuttered words at a normal rate of speaking. We use 0.5 SW/M (or less) and 130 (plus or minus 20) or 0.4% (or less) stuttering.

Next, it is possible to manipulate (decrease) the stuttering behavior in a number of ways, e.g., slow prolonged speech or speaking only one word at a time. Appropriate fluent, albeit prolonged, speech is rewarded and stuttered words are punished. The latter may be accomplished in a wide variety of ways. If this manipulation is fragmentized, systematized, and organized in a sequence from easy to hard with appropriate consequences, a program is the result. Ryan (1974) identified four such programs; Programmed Traditional, Delayed Auditory Feedback (DAF), Punishment, and Gradual Increase in Length and Complexity of Utterance (GILCU). There are others, or course, but these represent the common programs used in programmed stuttering therapy.

For the therapy sequence we have the establishment, transfer, and maintenance phases of therapy. Establishment refers to development of fluent speech in the presence of the clinician. It is realized that all people who stutter have established fluent speech most of the time. The "average" stutterer is probably fluent at least 90% of the time. The term "establishment" is used simply to describe the initial phase of therapy when the clinician is trying to establish a high rate of fluency and a low rate of stuttering in a therapeutic fluency training program in the clinician's presence.

We use only one of two establishment program for all clients, DAF or GILCU (Ryan and Van Kirk, 1971). There is also a home practice program in each. The DAF program uses delayed auditory feedback equipment, the teaching of a pattern of slow, prolonged fluent speech, and gradual shaping of that response toward normal fluency. There are 26 steps in this program. The program requires approximately 5–10 hours over a 1- to 2-month period, contingent upon the number of hours of training per week. The GILCU program uses a sequence of 54 steps that starts with the reading of one word and gradually progresses to fluent conversation. This program requires 10–13 hours to administer over a 3-month period, contingent upon the number of hours of training per week.

These programs produce comparable fluency. The major differences are that the DAF program requires special equipment, is more difficult to run, runs faster, and is more effective for people who demonstrate severe, long-standing stuttering problems. GILCU provides for better and more spontaneous transfer of fluency sooner than DAF. We have occasionally used both programs in sequence for some clients who demonstrated difficulty on one or the other. Most commonly, we use only one, GILCU for younger clients or those with less severe stuttering, and DAF for older clients or those with more severe problems.

Transfer refers to the generalization of fluency to other settings. This can and does happen spontaneously with some people who stutter; however, all clients are put through the one transfer program. The program consists of 54 steps. Children go through fewer steps. The program requires 10–13 hours to administer over a 3- to 4-month period.

Maintenance refers to the long-term continuance of fluency in a wide variety of settings. The goal should be forever. This program is composed of five steps distributed over 22 months requiring approximately 3 hours of clinician time. All clients are to go through this program.

All of these programs in total require about 20–30 hours of clinician time spread out over a 2-year period. These programs are viewed as being universal in that they are used (the exception is the use of either DAF or GILCU, not both) with all people who stutter regardless of age and severity of problem. These programs have proved to be highly efficient and effective in training of fluent speech (Ryan, 1971, 1974; Ryan and Van Kirk, 1974a, b). They commonly produce speakers who operate at 0.5 SW/M or less or 130 WS/M or 0.4% stuttering. This residual "stuttering" is usually whole word or simple part-word repetition. The speakers appear to have normally fluent speech.

We have been doing research on programmed stuttering therapy for 13 years. At this writing our data base includes 58 people reported in the book by Ryan (1974), five children reported by Ryan (1971), 50 people reported by Ryan and Van Kirk (1974a), and 40 more children reported by Ryan and Van Kirk (1974b). This produces a total of 153 children and adults with written public reports of their performance in fluency programs. There are an estimated 500 or more people on whom we have data that have not been reported.

One of the logic systems we used in the development of programmed instructional procedures (Gray and Ryan, 1973; Ryan, 1974) was that there are three variables: the client or person who stutters, the speech-language clinician or teacher, and the program or procedure. We may characterize the therapy act as the client with a set of problems and skills receiving therapy or training from a clinician or teacher with a set of skills. Together they proceed through a program or procedure. Therapy can only be accurately analyzed within this total context. To talk only about one or two of these variables is not sufficient. We must know something about the client, we must clearly define the procedure, and we must indicate awareness of the skills and attitudes of the clinician. Successful therapy will require a client who is interested in and capable of change; a procedure that has enough appropriate content to provide that change and is relevant to the skill being taught; and a speech-language clinician or teacher who carries out this procedure in the manner described with consistency, reliability, and humanity.

This framework permits clinicians to think positively about help for people who stutter. No longer is the person who stutters doomed to a life of controlled obvious stuttering. How sad! And how unnecessary. It is too bad that our profession was so influenced by authority figures who stuttered and convinced us that there was no hope for the stutterer and tacitly held themselves up as models of what we could and should expect the results of therapy to be. In their effort to point out the "awful truth" about stuttering, they kept us from seeking ways to find the cure.

Another positive result of programmed therapy for people who stutter is the finding that these procedures can be relatively easily shared with and disseminated to others. We have developed and taught intensive programmed 4-day workshops with two follow-up site visits to train clinicians in these programs. At present there are over 300 clinicians in 16 states who are certified and capable of running these programs.

This experience has shown that almost any clinician can, with training and supervision, carry out effective programmed fluency training procedures. People who stutter do not have to go to a distant "Mecca" for their therapy at a great cost of time and money. They can receive training in their own area from local clinicians. This provides for increased ease and effectiveness of transfer and maintenance activities.

The training experience has also provided evidence that programmed fluency training must be carried out in a prescribed manner. The clinician cannot just "wing it," but must follow the program closely to obtain the same positive results as the basic pilot field test studies. Some clinicians found the programs too demanding and too restrictive. Most did not. Most clinicians we have trained achieve very similar positive results.

This then summarizes the basic position and logic of my thinking and experiences. Let us now proceed to respond to the controversial issues in this book. I hope my comments will help shed light on the controversies, provide for better cooperation among the various stuttering authorities, and help us to move toward improvement of the conditions and quality of therapy being offered people who stutter.

TEACHING THE STUTTERER
TO "STUTTER MORE FLUENTLY" VERSUS
TEACHING THE STUTTERER TO "SPEAK FLUENTLY"

First of all, people who stutter should be viewed as just that, not "stutterers." That simple verbal fiat prepares us better mentally to look at the problem. The goal for fluency training (stuttering therapy) should be normal, human speech, operationally defined as a stuttering rate of 0.5 SW/M or less and a word rate of 130 words spoken per minute (± 20) or 0.4% or less stuttering. A speaker who performs at this operationally defined level sounds like the average, normal speaker, or possibly more fluent.

There are three reasons for accepting this objective. The first is that professionally we ought to seek the ideal goal, which is normal fluency. If we do not seek it, we will not find it, except by chance. In my early operant work (Ryan, 1964) the target was to teach the client to stutter more fluently, but the performance of the three initial subjects taught me that normal fluency was a reasonable goal. The literature is replete with references to fluency being easily obtainable, flight into fluency, all people who stutter speak fluently when alone, etc. This concept of fluency later came to be looked upon with disfavor because the fluency obtained was not permanent. The profession then inferred from that observation that normal fluency was not obtainable. The profession should have focused on how to maintain fluency once it was acquired or demonstrated.

The second reason for accepting the stated goal of stuttering therapy is found in the observed ranges of rates and severity of stuttering. Commonly, only severe stutterers are depicted in professional books, shown in videotapes or movies, and written up in sensational newspaper articles. However, the data suggest that there is an "average" rate and that this average is relatively low. Some of these data are presented in Table 1. These data indicate that the "average" person who stuttered was in the mild to moderate catagory (Ryan, 1974). Of interest is the similarity of performance of the two groups though they came from two populations 3000 miles apart and represented two different age groups. As might be expected considering the relationship between age and stuttering rate, sample 1, being older, demonstrated a higher stuttering rate. The major point to be made by these data is that at least half of the stuttering population was in the mild to moderate category. They

Table 1. Average rates of stuttering

Sample	N	Age range	Age mean	SW/M Range	SW/M Mean	WS/M Range	WS/M Mean	Percent Mean
1[a]	50	9–66	27.2	1–30	9.2	59–186	116	8
2[b]	40	7–18	11.1	3–21	7.2	79–149	115	6

[a]Ryan and Van Kirk (1974a).
[b]Ryan and Van Kirk (1974b).

exhibit 92% fluency already. Hence, normal fluency for these people should be a reasonable, attainable goal.

A third reason for our goal comes from the results of therapy. The same clients reported in Table 1 were put through various programmed therapy approaches. For the 45 clients who completed the programs (establishment, transfer, and maintenance) data are presented in Table 2. Again there is remarkable similarity between the two client groups reported, with the major exception being the low pretherapy stuttering rate of group 2 which was composed of younger clients. These offer support for the contention that normal fluency is a reasonable goal for people who stutter. A speaking rate of 128 words per minute is well within the normal range of speaking. A stuttering rate of 0.1 (one stuttered word for every 10 minutes of talking) also is within normal range, as mentioned earlier. These posttherapy stuttered words commonly were whole word repetitions or simple part-word repetitions, both of which are uttered with some frequency by normal speakers (Johnson, 1961a). In addition, these speakers sounded normal to both the trained and untrained ear. The major reasons that clients did not complete programs were scheduling problems, achievement of acceptable fluent speech as judged by the client, moving away, and clinician error in program operation.

Table 2. Results of therapy for clients in Table 1

Sample	N	Pretherapy SW/M mean	Pretherapy WS/M mean	Pretherapy Percent mean	Posttherapy SW/M mean	Posttherapy WS/M mean	Posttherapy Percent mean
1[a]	30	12.5	122	10	0.1	128	0.1
2[b]	15	6.8	122	5	0.2	130	0.2

[a]Ryan and Van Kirk (1974a).
[b]Ryan and Van Kirk (1974b).

Normal fluency is an attainable goal for people who stutter; however, this must be qualified somewhat. The qualifications are couched in the logic of the client-program-clinician variables discussed in the introductory paragraphs of this chapter. For older clients with severe struggle behavior, the client factor concerns the basic physiological and psychological make-up of the client. An older person with a long history of stuttering who stutters very severely, exhibiting extreme, frequent struggle behavior, may achieve fluency at a lower word rate, e.g., 100 WS/M. If he tries to speak at rates above this, he may experience difficulty. A client who is not motivated will not become fluent because he will not follow through on therapy including attending therapy sessions and doing assigned homework. There may be some deep, unclear psychological problems that prevent him from progressing satisfactorily. For some people who stutter there may be a physiological factor related to rate or thought processes. All of these clients can be helped to improve their speech fluency, but they may not attain normal fluency (words spoken rate) for reasons best described as client factors, some of which we do not understand very well. Perkins (1973a) has also commented on this.

A fluency training program suggests a focus on the speech act. A variety of programs (series of steps with appropriate consequences leading toward fluency) have been shown to be effective (Ryan, 1974). A certain number of hours must be spent on monitored practice. Any therapy that does not devote enough time to this will not be successful. To achieve normal fluency, programs must require 10–20 hours or more of monitored normal fluency plus home practice. Programs that are mainly composed of "talk-about-stuttering" activities will probably not produce fluent speech. The activities in the program must include speech practice directly and provide a sequence of activities that enhances the person's fluency and helps him to reach the goal of fluent speech.

At one time I though it might be necessary to develop different programs for different people. Time and experience have shown that there is a universal program that will work for all. We currently use only two different establishment programs, one transfer and one maintenance program for all clients, children and adults, who stutter. There are, in addition, appropriate branching procedures used by the clinicians as needed.

Many nonprogrammed therapy approaches include practice on the speech act. It is speculated that it is this element in these programs that improve fluent speech, not all the other activities that are added to make the therapy more interesting and more totalistic to treat the whole "iceberg" of stuttering (Sheehan, 1970a).

Clinician factors bearing on the achievement of normal fluency cluster mostly around the clinicians' belief and demonstration of that belief in the attainment of normal fluency. The clinician does this through both instruction for fluency and appropriate discrimination and consequation of stuttering and fluency. If the clinician is to carry out a prescribed program, he must have the rigor to do so. He must follow the program. The major reason that validated fluency programs do work is that the clinician follows them very closely.

In summary, I would hope we could all focus on the achievement of normal fluency for people who stutter. It is attainable for most of the people with whom we work. Whether a client is controlling his fluency, or controlling his stuttering, or stuttering fluently is hard to measure and, therefore, hard to know. Normal fluency should be the target. Exactly how the client attains that is decided by the client, the program, and the clinician.

ATTITUDE CHANGE: WHAT IS IT? IS IT NEEDED?

Behavior does affect attitude. Being able to perform an act does affect one's attitude toward oneself concerning that act. People who stutter have certain attitudes toward themselves. Helping them to change their speech does change their attitude (Martin and Haroldson, 1969). Is it enough to change their speech? Most of our data suggest that for many people it is enough. The problem they report is stuttering. If they no longer have that problem, they no longer report a problem. We do not know how long a person who used to stutter has to speak fluently before attitude changes occur. Several people who used to stutter have reported that they almost never think about stuttering anymore.

If we assume that verbal statements about oneself represent attitudes, as do Shames and Egolf (1976), then the following data offer some information about the relation of attitudes and stuttering. In a study of 40 children who stuttered (Ryan and Van Kirk, 1974b), parents, teachers, and children were interviewed pre and post programmed therapy. They were asked several questions. The one of interest concerns the use of the word "stuttering." Parents and teachers were asked, "Does _____ (child's name) ever have trouble talking?" The children were asked, "Do you ever have trouble talking?" The number who used the word "stuttering" or "stutters" was tabulated for pre- and posttherapy periods. The percentage of interviewees who used either word before therapy was: teachers, 23%; parents, 42%; and children, 60%. Posttherapy, 8% of teachers, 30% of parents, and 35% of children used the word "stuttering" or "stutters."

Several tentative conclusions relating to attitude may be drawn from these data. Parents and children used the word "stuttering" more often than teachers in both the pre and post samples. This observation can be explained by the teacher's lack of familiarity with the child's speech. Of most importance to this discussion is the relatively high percentage of parents and children (30% and 35%, respectively) who continued to use the word "stuttering" even after the children were demonstrating very good speech (average less than 1 SW/M) in all samples in the home, school, and therapy room. There are several explanations for this finding. Both the parents and the children may have viewed whatever minor amount of stuttering that was left as significant and reported it. The verbal repertoires of the parents and children concerning the word "stuttering" may have persisted even though the children's speech behavior no longer warranted this. Finally, the children may not have lived down their history of stuttering in either their own eyes or the eyes of their parents. This would fit with the posttherapy observation by the teachers that the children rarely stuttered. The teachers would have had much less history of experience with the child and would be much less likely to operate on past observations and the reputation of the child as a person who stutters.

These data, of course, are not conclusive. Would later interviews after prolonged periods of fluency have produced differences in the interviewees' responses to the questions? This is unknown. These data suggest that, for at least a portion of the children and their parents, some direct work on attitudes, e.g., elimination of the word "stuttering" from their verbal repertoires, might have been of value. The positive aspect of these data is that fully 65% of the children did not use the word "stuttering" after therapy. This represented a change of 25%. This is further confirmation of the observation that improved fluency can lead to positive attitude change.

There are numerous subtle aspects of attitude about which we have only casual observation information. We have a classic post-therapy videotape of a client who continually reports extreme anxiety throughout the 15 minutes of his talking. His talking is extremely fluent (0 SW/M). The only signs of anxiety were a high speaking rate (for him) and a higher than normal pitch (for him). We have seen numerous adults who after therapy continue to report problems with stuttering, but who, when questioned further, report extremely minor incidents. For example, one client stated, "Two weeks ago when I went to the movies, I said, 'Give me two t-tickets'." Another type is the person who stutters who has been to many clinics and has a better verbal repertoire about stuttering than most speech-language clinicians. Often his attitude is one of trying therapy one more time, but commonly his heart is not in it and he does not cooperate. We get the impression he is shopping for a cure that he either really does not want or lacks the personal discipline to acquire. One person who stuttered became extremely angry when he became fluent in only 1 day of progammed DAF therapy. He was angry with all the past therapies that had taken so much time, been so expensive, and produced so little change in his speech. Then there is the situation where a third party is paying for the client's college or other education because he stutters. He would lose financial support if he became fluent. Another client would have been sent to Viet Nam by the army, if he became fluent. Still another type is the client whose parent "buys" the therapy and the client is merely a passive therapy recipient to please his parent. Finally, there is the observation that many people (people who stutter included) become interested in self-improvement and enroll in courses (including stuttering therapy) and never complete them because they are unable to follow through on anything. All of these casual observations have unfortunately not led us to the development of a client attitude measure. Such a tool would be important in both the development of a therapy program and as a measurement of results.

Another related aspect of attitude is the attitude of the clinician. Our logic includes client-program-clinician. Clinician attitudes become extremely important. Effective speech therapy requires more than a "sane" clinician (Walle, 1975). The clinician should have the attitude that the client is a person who stutters. This prevents the clinician from treating the client as if he had problems other than stuttering. This attitude also keeps the clinician from excusing the client from task-oriented activities because of deepseated, albeit unknown, problems. This attitude does not mandate that the clinician treat the client inhumanely. On the contrary, the emphasis is on the word "person." The clinician treats the client as he would treat any person — with empathy, respect, and humanness. Programmed therapy also requires a commitment and followthrough by the clinician. The clinician must have the attitude that the client can and will be helped, and both must stick to the program. The clinician needs a certain amount of consistency and rigor. It is important for the clinician to keep the target in mind and to help the client persist until the target has been reached.

Clinican-client interaction is usually well controlled in the programmed instructional paradigm. In one study (Ryan, 1971) we used seven different clinicians with the same client. There were no observable differences in client performance among the various clinicans. The clinician usually follows the design of the program, which is heavily task oriented. There is not much time for personal interaction except in the moments before and after therapy. Programmed therapy can be run with a heavy, hard hand, but this is not necessary. There are opportunities for the clinician to express interest, warmth, and understanding, especially during the conversational portions where the client may select the topic and discuss with the clinician any of his interests or problems. Casual analysis of tape-recorded sessions of programmed therapy during the conversation modes revealed that the topics were highly varied. They ranged from football to a very personal, deep discussion of how one client felt about accidentally killing his sister with what he thought was an unloaded rifle. Programmed therapy permits the clinician to show his or her normal array of social interaction skills and implied or explicit empathy.

Clinican attitude is a major problem in conducting effective programmed therapy. Specifically, we observed in our study of 40 school-age children who were treated by 20 speech clinicians (Ryan and Van Kirk, 1974b) that the number one problem was consequating stuttered words. The number two problem was consistency in program operation. Both of these problems may be defined as attitude problems. The former, consequating stuttered words, was more of a "won't" rather than a "can't" problem. That is, clinicians could accurately count stuttered words as measured by several different procedures, but under certain conditions in therapy they would not. They often later explained and/or demonstrated that they knew the word was stuttered, but they did not "want" to consequate it.

The second problem, correct program conduct, seemed to be related to the attitude of not wanting to adhere to a prescribed procedure because it was tedious or boring. Programmed instruction can indeed be both tedious and boring, but the clinician with a positive attitude toward helping the client through commitment and consistency will carry it out. The attitude of the clinician is important in any type of therapy for people who stutter. The attitude of the clinician often determines the attitude of the client. In programmed therapy, the attitude of clinician is equally vital.

We do need a good clear definition of attitude. We need further research on the role of attitude of both the client and the clinician in effective training. The future best program in fluency training may involve special client training in attitude of the type which is well described by Shames and Egolf (1976). Of interest in this connection, Guitar (1976) found that attitude measures may be extremely predictive of success in therapy.

PSYCHOTHERAPY FOR STUTTERERS: WHAT IS IT, IS IT NEEDED, AND IF SO, HOW SHOULD IT BE DONE?

It is difficult to define psychotherapy. Definitions range from that of treatment offered by a professional highly trained in psychotherapeutic techniques (a psychiatrist) to support and understanding offered by one human being to another. The simplest delineation of role differences is to say that psychotherapists deal with behavioral and social problems including stuttering in a manner that varies widely among them; speech-language clinicians deal only incidentally with psychological problems (depending on their training) but mostly with the speech act, stuttering (Mowrer, 1977). For people who stutter, psychotherapy per se has never been shown to be particularly successful in helping them to become fluent.

Over the years our casual observation of some 500 people who stutter is that most of them were well within the normal range of personality and social behavior. This observation is supported by research (Sheehan, 1970a). The parents in our study of 40 children who stuttered (Ryan and Van Kirk, 1974b) reported social or personal problems in only 38% of the children. Without normative data for children who did not stutter, it is not known whether or not this is abnormal. However, our own observation of them in the therapy session, classroom, and home did not indicate abnormal behavior or psychosocial problems requiring psychotherapy.

Of those clients over the years who manifested serious psychosocial problems most appeared initially not to have any particular problems. The problems showed up after therapy was underway and usually took the form of poor attendance, lack of cooperation in doing homework and outside assignments, etc. In a few cases we referred the clients for psychotherapy, but only after they demonstrated problems in therapy. Some clients, such as the boy who accidentally shot his sister, had psychological problems but were able to achieve speech fluency in a manner similar to other clients. Psychotherapy may be helpful to a number of people who stutter for reasons other than improvement of their speech. Referral for psychotherapy seems to follow speech therapy when more information is known about the client and his personal needs. It would be very wasteful of professional time to include psychological evaluation as part of every initial evaluation. Our experience has been that a small minority of people who stutter need that type of therapy in addition to fluency training.

Attaining fluent speech for a person who stutters can be a great psychological lift. Fluency is an important social-vocational skill and attainment of normal fluency is "good for the ego." This follows a theory of competence that suggests that building competencies in people improves their self-image and concept. Fluency training may itself be a form of psychotherapy (Van Riper, 1973).

STUTTERING THERAPY FOR CHILDREN

Identification

The major problem in working with children who stutter has been to correctly identify them. At one time in our professional history we were all afraid to work with children for fear of labeling them as "stutterers" and making the problem worse. Fortunately, this situation has changed. To solve the problem of identification, the definition of stuttering (whole word repetitions, part-word repetitions, prolongations, and struggle) was used. The rate of 3 or more SW/M was chosen as the cut-off. Although this rate was chosen somewhat arbitrarily, it did match our casual observation and parent reports. Children brought by parents to the clinic for a "stuttering" problem often had a rate of 3 SW/M or more. Seldom did we see a child with a lower rate whose parent or teacher informed us that the child stuttered. As part of the evaluation we also looked at the topography of the behavior, rating whole word repetitions as the least serious, then part-word repetitions, then prolongations, and then struggle. These are similar to the criteria suggested by Van Riper (1971a). We were prepared to evoke the "topographical" rule: if we saw a child who had a rate lower than 3 SW/M but with prolongation or struggle behavior, we would take this child for therapy. This has not happened. The most difficult situation we experienced was the accurate diagnosis and intervention for the very young (3–5 years) child who demonstrated a rate of 3 SW/M with a topography of entirely whole word or part-word repetitions, the repetitons being short and effortless. We commonly did parent counseling and put this child on a recheck in a 3-month schedule. A rate decrease by the next recheck indicated we were on the right track. If no decrease was evident, we considered direct intervention.

Our attempts to assess the child's awareness of the problem were met with frustration. First of all, how does one define awareness? What must the child do or say to indicate he is aware of his stuttering? Even if the child reports, "I stutter," spontaneously, as many children did in our study of 40 of them, the clinician cannot be sure that the child knows what that means and is not just repeating something he heard someone else say. Children in some of our programs have been notoriously poor at self-identification of stuttering without extensive training, indicating a lack of awareness of specific stuttering. Excessive struggle or tension while producing words is an extremely indirect measure of awareness. Our conclusion was to eliminate assessment of awareness and adhere to the simple, objective counting system described above.

Our next efforts concerned the development of an interview protocol for evoking an appropriate sample of speech. The fourth revision of this Stuttering Interview appears in Ryan (1974). There was a version for preschool and primary children and a version for upper elementary, junior high, senior high, and adult. The major difference between the two versions was greater variety (16 items) in the preschool primary form than the older version (10 items). These tests took approximately 40 minutes of administration time and yielded 20 minutes of talking time. These versions were attempting to sample speech in a wide variety of speaking tasks and situations that ranged from simple counting to conversation to speaking with another adult (usually the parent or spouse). For various reasons, mostly to streamline the process, the older-age Stuttering Interview has been renamed the Fluency Interview and is currently used for all age groups with certain items omitted or modified for extremely young clients. This version (Ryan and Van Kirk, 1971) requires 15 minutes of administration time and yields 10 minutes of talking. It represents an improvement in efficiency without loss of effective sampling of the child's speaking repertoire. The correlation between stuttering rates gathered on the Fluency Interview and from a sample taken of spontaneous speech in both home and school settings was significant (Ryan and Van Kirk, 1974b). This indicates that the present version is adequately sampling the child's speech.

Having both a criterion of 3 SW/M and a reliable protocol for evoking a speech sample (the Fluency Interview) has simplified the task of identifying children with stuttering problems. This seems to be a relatively simple solution for what the literature refers to as a tremendous problem (as exemplified by the large number of pages devoted to this area by Gregory in the first part of this book). Clinicians need a workable procedure for identification. They cannot exist on rhetoric and theory. This procedure seems to have validity. The counts from the Fluency Interview do correlate with parents' statements of stuttering and measures taken in other settings. The procedure is reliable as verified by test-retest experiences. I know of no evidence that indicates we need a more elaborate system to make the determination as to whether or not a given child needs intervention to help with his fluency.

Intervention

The approach to therapy for children with stuttering problems has been to extrapolate the procedures for adults down in age. The two major intervention programs, GILCU and DAF (Ryan, 1971; Ryan and Van Kirk, 1974b), have proved to be useful with children. The DAF Program has been used with children as young as 7 years. The GILCU Program (without the reading mode) has been used with children as young as 4 years. In the study of 40 school-age children (Ryan and Van Kirk, 1974b) we also used the Programmed Traditional and Pause (Time-out) Programs with children as young as 7 years. All four programs have proved to be effective with children with the major difference among the programs being time in therapy (Ryan and Van Kirk, 1974b). GILCU and DAF were much shorter running programs. Data on the outcomes of the programs

Table 3. Data for children who completed establishment, transfer, and maintenance programs

Phase	N	Pretherapy SW/M	Hours of therapy	Posttherapy SW/M
Establishment	35	7.0	9	0.4
Transfer	15	6.8	8.2	0.3
Maintenance	15	6.8	1.4	0.2

with children are presented below and in Table 3. The first set of data, on five children ages 6–9, was first reported in Ryan (1971): the pretherapy SW/M was 11.9; average hours of therapy, 39.3; and posttherapy SW/M, 0.3. These children were in the moderate to severe range of stuttering behavior. Therapy was conducted on three different programs, and the results were quite good, as evidenced by the stuttering decrease to 0.3 SW/M. Some of the children demonstrated spontaneous transfer, and none of them went through formal transfer programs. Three were on maintenance programs. Follow-up at an average of 18 months later revealed that all of these children had remained fluent.

The second set of data includes 40 children ages 7–17 from Ryan and Van Kirk (1974b). These children received one of four establishment programs: Programmed Traditional, DAF, Pause (Time-out), GILCU. The data in Table 3 are shown for establishment, transfer, and maintenance for 35 children who completed establishment and 15 children who completed transfer and maintenance. The children ranged from mild to severe in stuttering behavior. The total three phases of fluency training required about 19 hours (half the time of the previous programs of Ryan, 1971) and were extremely effective. Spontaneous transfer occurred for a number of children. Follow-up indicated the children were maintaining their fluency.

The third set of data concerns children who were 4–8 years of age and participated in the GILCU Program. These data on 14 children come from Arlyne Russo of the Easter Seal Rehabilitation Center of Bridgeport, Connecticut. The pretherapy SW/M was 11.8; average hours of therapy, 16.8; and posttherapy SW/M, 0.2, indicating that the GILCU Program (with transfer and maintenance procedures) was extremely effective for children with moderate to severe stuttering behavior as young as 4 years.

In summary, it can be noted that programmed instruction for children is quite effective and that several programmed procedures have been shown to aid in reducing the frequency of stuttering, if not eliminating it altogether. Much spontaneous transfer of fluency has been observed in working with children. No evidence of any child ever becoming worse after receiving therapy has been uncovered.

The critical event in providing intervention procedures for very young children who stutter (ages 3–5) is to decide whether to provide direct intervention by the speech-language clinician or a parent program. The deciding factor in most cases is the severity of the problem, evaluated in consideration of the child's age. We rarely see 3-year-old children who stutter. Commonly, we are seeing children 4 years and older who stutter. For the youngest children, 3–4 years of age, with mild to moderate symptoms (around 3 SW/M composed mostly of whole word repetitions and part-word repetitions), we usually recommend a therapy program of parental changes in behavior. These changes include being a better listener, reducing complexity of the parents' language, speaking more slowly, not reacting to the child's speech, etc., all of those recommendations suggested by Murphy (1962) and Van Riper (1973). The parents are advised to carry out these procedures and to bring the child in for a recheck in 3 months. If the recheck, based on the Fluency Interview, indicates that the child has improved, the home program with appropriate modification is continued. If the Fluency Interview indicates no change or an increase in stuttering that is substantiated by verbal report of the parent, a direct intervention program by the clinician is initiated. A home practice element in the program is carried out by the parent with supervision from the clinician. GILCU is the preferred program because it requires minimal discussion of the problem of stuttering with the child. It is very important to avoid lengthy discussion of stuttering with children. We run the risk of installing a verbal repertoire that will be hard to extinguish. It seems far better to focus entirely on the speech act and help the child to become normally fluent.

In summary, the Fluency Interview and the two establishment programs, DAF and GILCU, have proved equally if not more effective with children than they have with adults. Direct therapy with children as young as 4 years has been successful. Parent counseling and rechecks have been very successful with even younger children.

Development and Prevention

One of the most exciting and still unresearched areas in the study of stuttering is the development of stuttering. Most studies to date (e.g., Johnson et al., 1959) have utilized indirect and/or post-priori measures for the most part. What is needed are direct observation and measurement of the development of stuttering in young children. There appear to be at least three factors to explore — the speech of parents, parent-child interaction, and language competency — as possible contributors to the development of stuttering.

The speech of parents of children who stutter has not been studied much but may play a major role (Knepflar, 1973). It seems only reasonable to assume that the parents' speech model is an important contributor to the development of the child's speech. The rate of speech, the frequency or topography of disfluencies and stuttered words, and the linguistic complexity of the parents' speech are all possible contributors to the development of stuttering in children. These parameters should be carefully investigated so that appropriate preventative programs involving those areas can be developed.

Parent-child interactions have been speculated to produce fluency problems. Most of the previous information has been extremely indirect and obtained from parent interviews (e.g., Johnson, et al. 1959). Only recently have researchers such as Wahler et al. (1970) and Shames and Egolf (1976) and their colleagues carefully explored the verbal interactions between parents and their children who stutter. Their work has shown that these interactions may play an important role in the development of stuttering. More research is needed to determine if these same factors are in operation for even younger children in the 3- to 5-year-old range. Finally, the language competency of young children who stutter should be examined. Present research (Van Riper, 1971a; Williams and Marks, 1972; Berryman and Kools, 1975) indicates that lack of linguistic ability may be a contributing factor. This would seem especially important in those families where parents use complex linguistic units.

Although many clinicians report success in helping young (3- to 5-year-old) children who stutter through parent counseling, there are few data to verify this and little is known about the actual, causative factors in behavioral terms. Before the development of appropriate therapy programs there is need for such direct, behavioral observation research. In our own experience, direct intervention with young children who stutter has been extremely rewarding and effective. If stuttering is viewed as learned behavior, it is obvious that the problem would be easier to treat in early childhood. The behavior is at low strength, without the years of practice, and has not yet caused the child to experience the serious emotional problems and negative experiences that come with continued stuttering performance.

TRANSFER OF CHANGES TO THE NATURAL ENVIRONMENT AND THE PROBLEM OF RELAPSE

Transfer

The controversy about transfer and relapse essentially concerns the age-old problems of the transfer of the new, better speech to other situations and the prevention of relapse over long time periods. These problems especially apply to fluency training (stuttering therapy), and very little is actually known through research about the parameters of transfer (Mowrer, 1975, 1977; Hanna and Owen, 1977).

One attempt to solve these problems has been to separate transfer from maintenance of fluency (Ryan, 1974). This seemed to follow the observed course of therapy events in that, after fluency was established in the clinic setting, the next phase was transfer of fluency to a wide variety of settings and the last phase was maintenance of fluency over long-term periods. Many clients could demonstrate transfer of fluency, especially with transfer training, but could not maintain their fluency in these settings over long-term periods. The concept and practice of separating these two aspects of stuttering therapy have been helpful.

A major issue in transfer is whether or not to provide such a program. Some authorities, e.g., Goldiamond (1974), believe that establishment of fluency in the client setting is enough. It is then up to the client to decide whether or not to use the new, fluent speech in all settings over a long-term period. A modification of this is to provide within-clinic counseling, advice, or instruction about transfer of fluency, assuming that the client will take this information and act on it. Most therapies provide for some form of transfer, one of the more elaborate being that of Ryan and Van Kirk (1971), with nine subprograms encompassing 54 steps working through a wide variety of speaking situations with the clincian present throughout most of them. These subprograms are: different physical settings, increased audience size, home, classroom, telephone, strangers, work, residual, and 16-hour (all day). The client must "pass" each of these subprograms with fluent speech (0 SW/M) before going on to maintenance.

Given that transfer activities are an important part of fluency training, a number of other issues can be raised. What types of activities are used? Commonly, "speech assignments" are used. The content of these varies greatly contingent upon the philosophy of the clinican (Van Riper, 1973). Our transfer program focuses on the generalizaton of speech fluency because this is a basic thrust of the program in general. A transfer program in any therapy program should have some relationship to the basic therapy being provided.

Another issue is who should be responsible for these transfer procedures: the client, the client's parents, spouse, or friends, or the clinician? The issue is related to self-control vs. external control. We have tried a wide variety of procedures including self-counting of stuttered words, monitoring by parents, friends, spouses, and teachers, the use of home tape recordings, etc. (Ryan, 1970, 1971, 1974). All of these seemed to be helpful to specific clients. However, in our final transfer program (Ryan and Van Kirk, 1971) we basically sort by age, with the younger clients being monitored by the clinician and parent and older clients being self-monitored and monitored by the clinician. We have kept the clinician-monitoring aspect to provide an accurate measurement and consequation system. Our intention has been to be certain that the transfer program is done and to determine its effectiveness. Having this constraint in the program requires more effort by the clinician, but provides for better results. Our observation has been that clients vary greatly in assuming responsibility for their transfer programs, but most of them eventually become involved (become self-controlled) as the program proceeds. They can and do learn to count stuttered words. They learn by doing, as does an "apprentice" clinician.

Where to do the transfer program is another issue. Can role playing or visualization take the place of actual clinician-monitored activities in the field? Probably not, but because of the lack of data this is unknown. Our logic has been to carry out the program in the client's natural environment. What this has meant is that we have a geographical range limit in the clients we can treat. Our experience with transfer programs carried out away from the client's home setting, or by the client exclusively in his home setting, was not positive. The goal, then, is to provide trained clinicians in many geographical settings so that clients can receive their training in their own locale, making local transfer programs possible. This tends to produce better fluency.

Another issue has been how much transfer? We have resolved this by identifying areas of common difficulty, e.g., the telephone. We then set criterion levels for fluent performance and finally test transfer effects by the 16-hour (all day) subprogram, which requires the client to collect 16 hours of consecutive fluency (0 SW/M) or 1 full day of fluent speech in his normal setting. The actual amount of transfer varies with the age of the client and his personal life style or environment. Extremely young children may only go through a few steps of the program. Adult clients may do all the transfer program (54 steps) plus some additional ones related to special speaking requirements, e.g., CB radio communication.

Another issue, or problem, not necessarily controversial, concerns the drop-out during transfer of clients who are doing quite well. This issue was first noted by Ryan and Van Kirk (1974a). A number of clients, giving a wide variety of reasons, dropped out during transfer phases. Reasons varied from "too time consuming" to "I can't take off any more work time." Since these were clients who were doing well on the program, we either could assume they had honest, accurate reasons for their dropping out or we could speculate about why they really dropped out. One such speculation is that since they had become so fluent they no longer saw the necessity for continuing in therapy with its monetary or time cost. Boberg and Sawyer (1977) have reported this. Another is that certain parts of the transfer program were difficult or embarrassing for them to do. This problem did not occur during the transfer phase of the project with the 40 school-age chldren, but it did come up during the maintenance phase. A number of the children no longer wanted therapy and would not show up for maintenance checks. Most of these children were fluent.

One final issue concerns measurement. Commonly, clinicians use a combination of verbal report and actual measurement. Ideally, this should be a covert measure (Andrews and Ingham, 1972a; Guitar, 1976). However, in actual practice this has been hard to achieve, if not unethical. Verbal report of a trained client may be the most simple, efficient method of gathering this information. Unfortunately, not all clients can achieve the level of being an accurate reporter, certainly not most of the children. The measurement system used in our present transfer program consists of direct observation and measurement both within and outside the training setting by the clinician and verbal report of the client. These usually are in agreement. When they are not, verification is done. For example, should all of the direct measurements indicate fluent speech, but the client reports difficulty in a particular speech activity or setting, we do direct observation in that setting or request a tape-recorded sample. This system has proved adequate for the determination of transfer of fluency.

Data to resolve the issues presented above are extremely hard to obtain. Their collection requires portable, wireless microphones and FM radio receivers with tape recorders. The process is extremely time consuming and often frustrating. Tape recordings have to be listened to, data recorded and analyzed, etc. It is not hard to understand why there is such a paucity of this information.

One set of data concerning the value of transfer for 24 clients is shown in Ryan (1974, pp. 108–111). The performance of clients with transfer programs was compared to that of those clients without such programs. The data demonstrated that clients with transfer programs did better. A more recent, larger set of data comes from the study of 40 school-age children (Ryan and Van Kirk, 1974b). These children had been on one of four different establishment programs. Three different measures of stuttering behavior were taken: preestablishment, postestablishment, and posttransfer. The first measure was a criterion test that consisted of 5 minutes each of reading, monologue, and conversation in the presence of the clinician and a tape recorder. The second was a Fluency Interview (Ryan, 1974), which was administered and videotaped by research project assistants with whom the children were somewhat acquainted. The clinician was not present. The third measure, a natural speech sample, was a sample of the child's speech in the home and school setting. These samples were collected by FM microphone and FM radio–cassette tape recorder and by conventional cassette tape recorder. The home settings varied from the teacher and a friend to a normal classroom configuration with the rest of the classmates engaged in a routine discussion or other classroom activity. The data in stuttered words per minute for these three different measures administered three different times in the therapy process for 40 school-age children who stutter are presented in Table 4.

Before these data are interpreted, it should be noted that N varies. The project started with 40 children; 39 children were

Table 4. Transfer data

	Preestab-lishment SW/M mean (N=40)	Postestab-lishment SW/M mean (N=39)	Post-transfer SW/M mean (N=27)
Criterion test	7.2	1.0	0.8
Fluency Interview	7.4	3.7	1.0
Natural speech sample	7.5	3.8	1.6

available for the postestablishment test, and 27 children completed enough of the transfer program to be tested a third time. No effort was made to sort out those children who did not complete and/or pass various programs. This was done so that the analysis had the largest N available, in order to demonstrate the impact of the various programs and their relationship to SW/M rate in the extra-program environments of the Fluency Interview and natural speech samples. The subanalysis of the 15 children who completed and passed both the establishment and transfer programs revealed even lower SW/M rates during the two posttest phases. However, the general trends were the same.

The data in Table 4 reveal a great similarity among the three measures during the preestablishment test period. These were all overt sampling processes, and it is, of course, unknown whether or not a covert process would reveal different rates. During the second measurement period the children performed more fluently during the within-training-setting criterion test with their clinican than they did in the other two settings. The Fluency Interview and the natural speech sample performances produced higher rates of stuttering and were very similar to each other. Also notable is the reduction in stuttering rate of 3.7 SW/M in the extra-program measures (Fluency Interview and natural speech sample), indicating the effect of the establishment programs on the fluency of the child in the extra-program settings. A number of the children demonstrated very low stuttering rates in the first posttherapy extra-program measures. This observation indicates that many children will spontaneously transfer their fluent speech to other settings. A subanalysis of the children revealed that those who had been on programs other than the DAF demonstrated more spontaneous transfer. Many of the children on the DAF Program were using the "pattern" of slow, prolonged speech in the training setting and did not transfer the use of the pattern to other settings. Finally, that the results of the Fluency Interview correlate well with those taken in the natural environment is a great find for the clinician. The collection of natural speech samples is a difficult task, whereas the administration and scoring of a Fluency Interview are relatively easy.

Analysis of the third test period indicates even greater reduction in stuttering behavior in the extra-program measures although they do not equal that of the within-training-setting performance. These data demonstrated the positive impact of the transfer program. For the 15 children who had completed and passed all the programs to that point, performances in all three settings were better and extremely similar among the three tests.

These data demonstrate both the impact of establishment programs on fluency in other settings and the need for formal transfer programs. Some establishment programs such as GILCU provide for better spontaneous transfer. Younger children with milder stuttering problems demonstrated the most spontaneous transfer. Another analysis of these data unfortunately revealed that there was no pretherapy measurement that indicates who would require transfer and who would not. Earlier it was stated that people who stutter vary widely in their ability to spontaneously transfer their newly learned fluency. Two clients demonstrate the present unknown parameters of this phenomenon. The first was an adult, age 35, whom we referred to as the "in-at-9-out-at-5" client. He was receiving an intensive 5-hour daily program. At the end of the first 3 hours on the DAF Program, during which he was speaking extremely fluently at an almost normal rate of speech, he announced, "Is that all there is to it? I can do that." From this point on during the next 2 weeks we never saw him stutter again. He went through the entire transfer program completely fluently. He reported being fluent in all speaking situations, and the report was verified by others in this environment. As might be expected, very few clients have done this. At the other end of the continuum was the young 9-year-old boy who demonstrated excellent fluency 0.5 SW/M throughout the establishment progam in the presence of the clinician, but who demonstrated in all concurrent natural speech samples a continuous, pretherapy rate of 10 SW/M. There was no sign of spontaneous transfer.

The data suggest that transfer programs are necessary to provide for a high degree of effective fluency training that will produce normal, fluent speech in the client's natural envronment. Will better establishment programs someday preclude the need for transfer programs? Azrin and Nunn (1974) think they have such an establishment program. Only further research can answer that question.

Maintenance and Follow-up

Maintenance, or the program to ensure the permanency of fluent speech, is more closely related to the problem of relapse. Most people who stutter have established and transferred very fluent speech in many different therapy programs discussed in this book and elsewhere (Van Riper, 1958; Gregory, 1969; Prins, 1970), but have shown relapse during posttherapy follow-up evaluations. The data from the recent behavioral clinician-researchers are more positive, e.g., Van Kirk (1972), Ryan (1974), Ryan and Van Kirk (1974a), and Boberg and Sawyer (1977).

We have utilized a wide variety of maintenance procedures varying from contacts between clinician and client by way of home tape recordings, post cards, telephones calls, etc. (Ryan, 1974). All of these procedures were helpful to certain clients, but most of them were extremely elaborate and time consuming. Maintenance requires a long-term calendar time commitment to the fluency training process but not a great number of hours. Our present maintenance program (Ryan and Van Kirk, 1971) is designed to operate on a gradually fading schedule for 22 months after the completion of the transfer program. The actual commitment of the clinician is less than 3 hours. During maintenance checks both a sample of speech and a verbal report are obtained. This information determines the course of the maintenance program. The maintenance program has been shown to be of value both in maintaining fluency over long-term periods and in determining the long-term effects of the original training (Ryan, 1974; Ryan and Van Kirk, 1974a, b). Maintenance programs are vital to fluency training and are best carried out in the client's own locale by local clinicians. Occasionally maintenance procedures indicate the need for retraining or recycling, which is also best carried out in the original training site.

A final point regarding maintenance concerns its differentiation from follow-up. Maintenance is viewed as an integral part of the therapy process. The client is considered as still being "in therapy" during the maintenance phase. After this maintenance period is completed and client is formally dismissed from the program, follow-up should take place. Follow-up therefore refers to that measurement or recheck of fluency *after* the formal program, including maintenance, has been completed. These data are extremely hard to obtain. Both clinician-researchers and clients move a great deal. One set of follow-up data will be found in Ryan (1974) and a second set in Ryan and Van Kirk (1974b). These data indicate that most clients have retained their fluency. Follow-up data on behavioral stuttering therapies have been reported by Andrews and Ingham (1972a), Van Kirk (1972), Azrin and Nunn (1974), Mowrer (1975), Guitar (1976), and Boberg and Sawyer (1977). These data also indicate that most of the clients have retained their fluency.

These follow-up data have verified both the positive effects of therapy and the occurrence of some relapse. Most of these studies have shown many clients who have follow-up stuttering rates that are slightly higher than their immediate posttherapy rates, but less than their pretherapy rates.

Behaviorists have not yet solved all of the problems of maintenance and/or prevention of relapse, but they are currently achieving documented positive results and working toward solutions of the problems.

CRITERIA FOR THE SUCCESS OF STUTTERING THERAPY: THE RESULTS OF STUTTERING THERAPY

Prelude

As a prelude to assessing the results of a therapy program, it is important to emphasize again that a clear description of the therapy procedure is a prerequisite to evaluation.

Although the most important measure of a therapy is the results generated, it is still important to have explicit information about the therapy process lest the results be attributable to something other than what was described. Most previous stuttering therapies have been described in very general form, and mostly, therefore, they are not replicable. Some therapies have changed constantly; therefore, tracking of the procedures is impossible. Reports of behavioral therapies of the operant conditioning nature generally include relatively clear, replicable descriptions of the procedures employed. Many therapists have not given, nor do their therapies lend themselves readily to, clear descriptions. One must infer what actually occurred in therapy.

Few therapy reports include precise measurement of results (Ingham and Andrews, 1973). To evaluate accurately programs of therapy, regardless of their nature, it is important to have appropriate evaluation systems. Andrews and Ingham (1972a) suggest three measurement criteria: 1) speech fluency and speech rate, 2) transfer to other environments, and 3) permanence of fluency. I would add four other dimensions: 4) attitude measurement, 5) hours of therapy required to bring about the results, 6) clinician skills and/or equipment necessary, and 7) client evaluation. Other clinicians using other strategies may want to add measures that reflect their individual therapy logic and procedures. For example, those who strive for anxiety reduction should add measures of that. Those who work on dimensions of speech of other than fluency and rate, such as Perkins (1973a, b), should include measures of those variables.

I suggest that the goal for fluency training (stuttering therapy) be a person who used to stutter who not only can speak fluently in all situations but who thinks of himself as a normal speaker and engages in all of the necessary and appropriate speaking activities. With that target in mind let us proceed to discuss the criteria of success.

Speech Fluency and Rate

There are many systems available for counting stuttering behavior (Van Riper, 1973; Mowrer, 1977), from counting each moment ("c-c-car" has two moments) to the simple binary system of counting stuttered words or syllables (Goldiamond, 1965; Andrews and Ingham, 1972a; Ryan, 1974). A given syllable or word either is stuttered or it is not. Counting stuttered words (whole word repetitions, part-word repetitions, prolongations, and struggle) has proved to be a functional, reliable system for us.

Measuring speech rate has involved counting either words (Ryan, 1974) or syllables spoken for a unit of time (Andrews and Ingham, 1972a). We chose counting words rather than syllables because words seem more meaningful and the early influential work by Goldiamond (1965) had used counting words spoken.

Many clinician-researchers like to compute a percentage of stuttering; they believe this helps define the corpus or sample size more accurately than either one or both of the two measures above. The number of stuttered words or syllables is divided by the number of words (often 100 words is used as a set number) and the quotient is multiplied by 100, yielding a percentage. The most recent common solution of the problem is to count percentage of syllables stuttered (% SS) and syllables per minute (SPM), e.g., Andrews and Ingham

Table 5. Hypothetical data for counting stuttering behavior

Client	Number of SW/M	Number of WS/M	Percentage of stuttering $\left(\dfrac{SW/M}{WS/M}\right)$	Subjective severity rating
A	0.5	130	0.3	Normal
B	0.5	100	0.5	Normal
C	5	130	3.9	Mild
D	5	100	5.0	Mild
E	10	130	7.7	Moderate
F	10	100	10.0	Severe
G	15	130	11.5	Severe
H	15	100	15	Severe

(1972a, b), Perkins et al. (1974), and Boberg and Sawyer (1977). These measures provide for an evaluation of speech fluency and rate.

We have commonly used stuttered words per minute and words spoken per minute and occasionally have computed percentages of stuttering by dividing SW/M by WS/M. Hypothetical data presented in Table 5 for 1 minute of speech illustrate those measures and include a subjective severity rating. As can be seen in the examples the number of stuttered words per minute is quite similar to the percentage of stuttering because commonly we are dealing with word rates around 100–150 per minute. In the sequence from mild to severe, which is related to both number of stuttered words per minute and percentage of stuttering, client F, whose rate is equal to that of client E, gains a rating of severe. This is true because the stuttering behavior of client F is probably composed of severe stuttering that causes him to speak more slowly. He is probably engaging in more prolongations and struggle. Percentage of stuttering more accurately represents this exception than does SW/M. Otherwise, SW/M and percentage of stuttering give very similar quantifiable measures of the stuttering behavior of the client, and in 7 out of 8 comparisons SW/M is equal to percentage in estimating severity.

Correlations calculated on clients' performance among the various measures revealed minimal correlation between SW/M and WS/M ($r = 0.18$). Many people who stutter with similar stuttering rates have highly varying speaking rates. There was significant correlation between SW/M and percentage (0.85). The rate of stuttering (SW/M) and the percentage of stuttering were highly correlated with judged severity (0.64) and hours of therapy (0.41) (Ryan and Van Kirk, 1974b). Older children showed rates of SW/M higher than younger children. Another observation was that the rate of stuttering was related to certain types of stuttering. Lower rates usually were composed of whole word repetitions and part-word repetitions whereas higher rates were composed of more prolongation and struggle behaviors. This observation is probably not accurate for adults, who demonstrate a wide range of stuttering rates and word rates.

Contrary to the observation by Ingham and Andrews (1973) that stuttered words per minute may not accurately reflect information on rate and sample size, we have observed that SW/M is an accurate measure of stuttering behavior. In the treatment of over 500 people who stutter we observed only one who demonstrated an extremely low rate of both stuttering and word output. The client's pretherapy rate was 5 SW/M and 25 words spoken per minute (20% stuttering). After a period of therapy his rate changed to 10 SW/M and 75 WS/M (13% stuttering). For the rest of the clients, the measure SW/M did accurately represent the client's stuttering behavior. The problem of sample size is handled by using sampling procedures such as the Fluency Interview, which consistently yields 10 ± 2 minutes, and the criterion tests of 5 minutes each of reading, monologue, and conversation. When other sample sizes are used, we usually report the length of time. When given WS/M over a specific time of sampling, we can easily compute size of total sample; e.g., given 130 WS/M over a 5-minute period we can derive the figure for the total corpus, 650 words (130×5).

A hypothetical illustrative comparison of the stuttered words and words spoken system with the syllables stuttered and percentage of syllables stuttered is shown in Table 6. A conversion multiplication factor of 1.6 was used to convert words to syllables after Johnson, Darley, and Spriestersbach (1963) and Perkins (1973a). The table assumes a 1-minute sample of 102 words spoken.

The comparisons show similarity between the two systems. With the aid of a conversion table or conversion numbers we can translate back and forth between the two systems. For example, Andrews and Ingham (1972a) state their target of fluency is:

> . . . no moments of stuttering, that normal nonfluencies, if present, be controllable, and that the rate of conversational speech be within 200 ± 20 SPM (syllables per minute). (p. 297)

Table 6. Hypothetical comparison of stuttered words/words spoken vs. syllables stuttered/percentage of syllables stuttered

Stuttered words/ minute	Words spoken/ minute	Percentage of stuttered words	Stuttered syllables	Syllables per minute	Percentage of stuttered syllables
0.5	102	0.5	0.5	170	0.3
1	102	1.0	1	170	0.6
3	102	3.0	3	170	1.8
10	102	10.0	10	170	5.9

This translates roughly into 0 SW/M at a speaking rate of 120 ± 12 words spoken per minute. These two targets are quite comparable. Hence, there is reasonable agreement between these two systems at the statistical manipulation level.

Either system is adequate to cover stuttering and speaking rate. Syllable systems are more reliable whereas SW/M are easier to obtain. Andrews and Ingham (1972a, b) commonly present both percentage of stuttered syllables and syllables per minute as a double measure. This is comparable to percentage of stuttering and WS/M. However, we prefer SW/M and WS/M for the reasons described above and are willing to do the translation in order to compare data and results.

All of this discussion is academic when we consider that the goal of therapy is the reduction of stuttering to 0 SW/M or 0% SS. This means that it really does not matter much whether we start at 10 SW/M or 10% stuttering or 6% SS; as clinicians, we still have the goal of reduction of stuttering behavior to zero or the increase of fluency to 100%. The end goal is the most important measurement.

The problem is not one system versus another, but any reasonable system versus none. Only if all clinician-researchers were willing to collect and report data on speech behavior are we ever going to be able to resolve some of the controversies identified in this book.

The unit of measure, SW/M, has proved relatively reliable. We usually achieve 90% or better agreement between independent observers, on SW/M counts, and these measures have been relatively easy to obtain. We have used the measure to monitor program operation. DAF and GILCU should operate at 0.5 SW/M or less per session of therapy. In the sampling process in the environment SW/M provides a simple but reliable process, especially in situations where only small samples are obtainable, e.g., telephone calls. There is relatively little response cost to obtaining SW/M samples with a counter and timing device. This has value for the on-line clinician for whom the clinician program task must be made as simple as possible in order to increase the probability that the clinician will do it accurately.

Word rate data have proved to be a nuisance to collect and often meaningless. Experience has shown that word rates of 100–250 per minute have been perceived by audiences to be within the normal range. The human ear apparently accepts this variance in rate and sorts it all in to a "normal" category. We have continued to collect word rate data simply to verify our results. Word rate as opposed to syllable rate seems to be the less statistically reliable, although we continually achieve 93% or better agreement in word counting between independent counters (Ryan and Van Kirk, 1974a, b). This is less reliable than syllable count (Andrews and Ingham, 1972a), for which reliability of counts is 98–99%. Word count seems to have more communication value and face validity than syllable count. Either syllable or word count does have some value when therapy involves slow, prolonged speech that is designed to gradually shape normal fluency.

In summary, our present measurement system for speech fluency and rate consists of counting SW/M, WS/M, and the time period of the sample. This system has proved adequate and is an integral part of our present fluency programs (Ryan and Van Kirk, 1971).

Transfer to Other Environments

The measurement of fluency in other environments (transfer effects) has been discussed in the previous section under transfer and relapse. An abstract of that discussion is that measurement of transfer to other environments should include at least the client's verbal report, an observed or at least tape-recorded sample of the client's speech in other settings without the clinician, and a verbal report from other members of the client's family or friends. The verbal report from others may be a close approximation of covert measures. These would appear to be reasonable measures of transfer that could be collected relatively easily and give some indication of the transfer of speech fluency. Based on data collected in the study of 40 school-age children who stutter (Ryan and Van Kirk, 1974b), and based on data from Ingham and Andrews (1971, 1973), in-training-setting measures can be interpreted only as estimates of out-of-training-setting fluency. Out-of-training-setting fluency is usually worse. However, some measure such as the Fluency Interview, with a cross-section of speaking events, might provide a reasonable indication of fluency in the out-of-training settings. A measurement of fluency in other environments is provided for or built into formal transfer programs such as those by Ryan and Van Kirk (1971), but these formal programs present a controlled measure and can only be used to estimate fluency in other situations. An extra-transfer program measure is also necessary.

It had been our hope to provide an in-clinic measure of transfer effects that was easy for the clinician to collect, such as the Fluency Interview, but that hope was not fulfilled. Fluency Interview within-training-setting measurements are only estimates of extra-clinic performance of fluency. We may use such measures as an approximation of fluency knowing that stuttering rates will usually be higher in real-life situations.

We need further research to develop measurements such as the Fluency Interview to provide accurate, predictive information on out-of-training-setting performance. These cannot be too elaborate to carry out or unethical to collect. We have the responsibility for solving the problem through research, thus providing the on-line clinician with a simple but accurate procedure for determining transfer of fluency.

Permanence of Fluency

The measure of permanence has been discussed in the section on transfer and relapse. Much of what was said in that section is pertinent here. Also, the information in the section on transfer to other environments applies. In short, a verbal report of the client, an actual measurement of speech fluency, and a verbal report of others in the client's environment should be collected at some time after formal fluency training has been concluded. According to Andrews and Ingham (1972a) and Perkins et al. (1974), there seems to be a stabilization of fluency level at about 6 months posttherapy. This observation matches our own.

The measurement of permanency of fluency (maintenance) seems to be the most valuable criterion of effectiveness of a therapy program for people who stutter. It is, equally, the most difficult to obtain. Two settings where it is relatively easy to collect are in the public school and in the communities with relatively stable populations (of both clients and the clinician). Clinician-researchers who live and/or work in such areas should feel some special responsibility for collecting this kind of information. Boberg and Sawyer (1977) have presented an excellent model of this kind of follow-up activity in their study of 13 people who stuttered. Because of geography and professional diligence they were able to follow up all 13 people. Their results indicated minor relapse in most of the clients, although all of them demonstrated follow-up fluency performance that was much better than pretherapy performance.

Several studies (Azrin and Nunn, 1974; Ryan, 1974; Boberg and Sawyer, 1977) have suggested that talking on the telephone, conversation with strangers, and reading have consistently evoked the most stuttering. Measurement of speech fluency in these three situations posttherapy during follow-up probes may prove an efficient, effective way to collect follow-up data. It is vitally important to collect follow-up data to verify the effects of any fluency training (stuttering therapy).

Attitude

Guitar (1976) and Perkins et al. (1974) have provided data on attitude measurement that indicated the value of such procedures. Guitar found that the attitude measures along with pretherapy stuttering rate were predictive of success in therapy. Perkins et al. advocate the use of therapy procedures to improve attitudes and measures of attitudes as criteria of success.

Our experience with a very simplistic attitude measure used in our study of 40 school-age children who stuttered provided us with some important information (Ryan and Van Kirk, 1974a). From our interviews of parents, teachers, and the children themselves, we found that they liked the therapy, thought it was helpful, and rated the children less fluent posttherapy than we did. This last finding was sobering. We also observed discrepancies among the three groups. The teachers knew the children least well, and rated them most fluent in posttherapy fluency. The major discrepancy between parents and children was that the children reported more avoidance of speaking than did the parents.

Some measure of attitude (including avoidance), such as those developed by Erickson (1969) or Woolf (1967), would be extremely helpful to first, describe the parameters of the problem; second, provide for therapy of attitude change; and third, provide a posttherapy measure of the effects of therapy on attitude. In short, we need to adopt or develop an attitude measure that will be valid and reliable and will have a predictive function for determining the outcome of therapy.

Hours of Therapy

Most reports of stuttering therapy that provide measurement of many aspects of stuttering often neglect to report hours of training or mention them only casually in passing. This criterion is important in the evaluation of a therapy program. Given two programs that produce equal fluency results, the shorter program would be the preferred one. This criterion appears to be a luxury because many altruistic clinician-researchers are more concerned with the fluency effects than with the hours taken to produce them. However, when we remember that we face at least 2 million people who stutter, then our efforts to develop fluency programs that work in reasonable time periods become justified. Also, we observed in our study in the public schools (Ryan and Van Kirk, 1974b) that it was important to complete establishment programs early in the 9-month school year so that the clinician would have time to get to transfer and maintenance before the school year ended. This, of course, is not as critical in other settings. The overall timing of a program is important. Even in a program which runs fast (Ryan and Van Kirk, 1974a), there is still a high degree of dropout during the longer running transfer program.

Our program (including establishment, transfer, and maintenance) currently requires an average of 20–30 hours of clinician time over a 2-year period, the bulk of which comes in the first 6 months. This program produces good effects. In terms of cost-efficency, including computation of either clinician time or clinician response cost, this is an extremely efficient, cost-effective program. Most behavioral programs (Perkins, 1973a, b; Webster, 1975b, c) are conducted in about this time period. Some run even shorter. Azrin and Nunn (1974) described a procedure that requires less than 10 hours of clinician time.

In summary, therapy programs should include hours of therapy as part of their description so that these programs may be evaluated appropriately.

Clinician Skills and/or Equipment

Clinician skills and/or equipment is also a criterion related to the program rather than to its outcome. This criterion is important, if the goal is to provide a large number of trained clinicians thoughout the nation who can and do carry out effective therapy procedures.

Clinician Skills Our observation has been that most clinicians we trained on our fluency programs did not have the basic skills needed to carry out the program, e.g., counting stuttered words, conducting programmed therapy with its high intensity of clinician performance, scoring, or even running a stop watch. The development and consequent evaluation of a therapy program should include consideration of the clinician skills necessary to operate the program. A program requiring high level, abstract performances by clinicians will not be used or, worst of all, will be used incorrectly. This may partly explain why there is such a paucity of widespread effective fluency therapy at this time.

There are some very important issues in this criterion. Clinician-researchers should do task analyses of their program. Can untrained clinicians carry out this program? What skills must the clinicians have? Can the clinician learn these programs by self-instruction? Is the printed description of a therapy program enough to provide for accurate replication? Are there specific clinician attitudes or personality factors that are important to proper program conduct? How much clinician variation will affect the procedure? What are the critical parts of the procedure that must be retained in order to obtain results?

In our study (Ryan and Van Kirk, 1974b) we worked with 20 different public school speech clinicians over a 2-year period. We learned from this experience that answers to all of the above questions were vital to the successful dissemination of the programs. We had to develop training and monitoring procedures to ensure that the programs were operated correctly. Most of the problems that occurred were related to basic discipline, organization skills, and attitudes toward the act of programmed therapy. We had to solve these problems, and some are not yet completely resolved, such as the "can, but won't count stuttered words" performance mentioned earlier.

The laissez-faire, eclectic education of clinicians by training institutions has produced a group of clinicians who are literally unable to carry out effective, highly structured, therapeutic programs because they have so often been left to their own devices and self-instructed. These clinicians also often avoid working with people who stutter because they do not feel adequate because they have not been taught effective procedures. This problem has been produced by our authorities (clinician-researchers) who were so intent on "research" or "writing" or "theory building" that they neglected to clearly describe, teach, and disseminate their procedures. This problem can best be solved by this same group. These clinician-researchers have a responsibility to clearly describe, validate, and teach their effective methods of therapy for people who stutter to as many clinicians as they can, if we are ever to solve this problem.

Equipment   Therapy programs requiring expensive equipment will not be used by many clinicians because of limited budgets. One of the problems in our dissemination of the DAF Program was that the average clinician could not afford the equipment. Equipment-bound programs may be successful, but dissemination will be limited. One criterion for the evaluation of a program should be its cost. There are solutions such as sharing equipment and central placement of equipment, such as at a university that serves a large surrounding area. But, if we are to have procedures carried out by many clinicians in many settings, equipment costs must be minimal. The present costs of our program (Ryan and Van Kirk, 1971) are minimal: a stop watch, a program book, and recording forms; the expensive DAF equipment is optional.

Client Evaluation

The criterion of client evaluation comes last not because I believe it is the least important but because valid measurement for it is hard to obtain. It is included in the interest of stimulating consumer advocacy among people who stutter. The client has a right to effective therapy. Most of them do not know this. The validity of a measure of client satisfaction is questionable. Out experience has been that most clients will give positive evaluations even though they received ineffective therapy. I can still see and hear one of the first stutterers I ever worked with saying goodbye after 2 years of traditional therapy. "Th-th-th-thank yooooooooou for ah, ah, (struggle) h-h-h-helping me," he said.

Many clients are faced with cognitive dissonance at the conclusion of therapy. They have invested much time and, in some cases, money, in the therapy and they often like the clinician. It is very difficult to face up to the fact that this time was wasted, the money ill spent, and these nice people did not help.

Client evaluation must be examined in the total context of therapy. Many teenagers reported not liking certain aspects of the transfer program, especially the classroom activities (Ryan and Van Kirk, 1974b). We ignored this dislike and continued to conduct this program because logic and the data indicate its usefulness. We also observed that many teenagers actually seemed to enjoy the special attention they received by their classmates and teachers during the classroom program, even some who had reported not liking the classroom transfer program.

Client evaluation on the other hand may prove to be very helpful. Certain portions of our program were taken out because both client dissatisfaction and our data indicated that they should be removed. Clients often have good ideas about how to improve a program. With all of its real and perceived shortcomings, client evaluation of therapy should be part of the evaluation system, if for nothing more than to give the client the opportunity to have some say (advocacy) in how treatment is conducted and reasonable expectations of results.

Other Measures

Any clinician-researcher should have the responsibility for providing some kind of objective data regarding the effectiveness of the procedures regardless of the theoretical or philosophical basis of the therapy. If the major part of the therapy is based on anxiety deconditioning or counterconditioning, the data on pre and post levels of such should be shared. It is hard to believe in this day and age of common scientific miracles that any clinician-researcher would engage in, or write about, any therapy program without some kind of objective measurement of effectiveness.

ETHICS AND THE CURE

A final self-generated issue concerns the word "cure" — its meaning, its use, and its potential. The statement from the ASHA code of ethics related to this point (American Speech and Hearing Association, 1975, p. xvii) reads:

> (a) He [the clinician] must not guarantee the results of any speech or hearing consultation or therapeutic procedure. A guarantee of any sort, expressed or implied, oral or written, is contrary to professional ethics. A reasonable statement of prognosis may be made, but successful results are dependent on many uncontrollable factors, hence, any warranty is deceptive and unethical.

This means to me that a professional, ethical clinician does not guarantee his work. It says nothing about cure. To cure means to heal or to remedy (any dictionary). "Cure" is often taken to mean the ultimate remedy, i.e., "the" cure.

We have gotten involved in controversy between professional ethics and the use of the word "cure." We have confused the professional's implicit or explicit guarantee of results with the word "cure." Any use of the word "cure" by any professional is, by association, unprofessional. This is very unfortunate. We should all be seeking the cure for stuttering. We should not feel unethical about engaging in its pursuit. We should continue this pursuit until we find "the" cure for stuttering or, better yet, its prevention.

In the past few years a number of clinician-researchers have come up with very excellent behavioral therapeutic procedures for dealing with the problem of stuttering (e.g., Goldiamond, 1965; Martin, 1968; Curlee and Perkins, 1969; Webster, 1970; Azrin and Nunn, 1974; Ryan, 1974; Costello, 1975; Shames and Egolf, 1976; Mowrer, 1977). Data for pre- and posttreatment, hours of therapy, etc., and clear, replicable descriptions of the procedures have been presented. Although few, if any, of these clinician-researchers have used the word "cure" in describing their findings, the media have. The media thrive on "newsworthy" items. A "good procedure" is not newsworthy. A "cure" is. I have been personally involved in several unpleasant media situations, as I am sure many of my colleagues have. We described our procedures and results in simple, accurate, conservative terms only to find that the media had made the jump to the word "cure." Some of us have received verbal and/or written disapproval from our colleagues for the media's use of the word "cure." This is unfortunate. We were looking for the best therapeutic treatment possible. We were trying to solve the problem of stuttering. We were sharing our positive results with the world and our colleagues. We, ourselves, did not use the word "cure."

What most of us have done is to develop some very accountable, effective procedures for treating the problem of stuttering. These procedures appear to be much better than anything we have had before, although it is difficult to compare them because previous therapies have been so ill described, with little or no objective measurement information presented.

The major ethical issue as I see it is not the use of the word "cure" by either the professional or the media, but the accountability and documentation of present procedures on the market. The ultimate unethical activity is to write or talk vaguely about procedures and results and to imply their effectiveness by our rhetoric or authority. All programs should be produced with specifications similar to those suggested for language by Connell, Spradlin, and McReynolds (1977). We need to develop appropriate evaluation procedures to determine the relative effectiveness of various procedures. We need to work cooperatively to share ideas and data so that we can collectively move toward "the" cure.

Finally, we need to move toward the dissemination of procedures in a manner more effective than convention speeches, 3-hour workshops, and commercial "programs" available from commercial publishers for $59.35 plus postage. There is much more to effective therapy on any level than mere verbal or written statements. It is difficult to become an effective fluency trainer by simply reading a book and/or by buying a canned program. Certain skills are necessary and require "hands-on" training, e.g., counting stuttered words.

We desperately need a collective, coordinated, intelligent, and dispassionate effort to solve the problem. It is unethical to continue in our present way.

Let us spend less time writing critical letters to those of us who accidently had the word "cure" written into a media message concerning our activities and more time in research and communication in concerted efforts to pool our information, solve the present problems of clear descriptions of therapy procedures, and provide adequate evaluation and dissemination of proved procedures to others. We probably could solve the problem of stuttering and find a "cure" if we spent less time promoting ourselves and more time in cooperative problem solving. Incidently, I do not see "one" or "the" program any more than I see one way to teach reading. I see a set of comparable, related procedures, with a core of similarities that are somewhat interchangeable for the client. A good evaluation system would help us determine the basic core.

THE FUTURE

This chapter has been an effort to present thinking, information, and data on the controversies in stuttering therapy identified in Chapter One. The clarification of controversies is only the first step in the achievement of the goal of providing effective, efficient therapy programs for people who stutter. The next step is to resolve these controversies. To do this it will be neccessary to provide clear descriptions of therapy procedures, validate these procedures, share that data, design training programs to disseminate the procedures in both pre-service and in-service settings, and set up research programs to resolve the issues which remain. Clinician-researchers could do this, if they so desired. For the good of people who stutter and the clinicians who serve them let us hope they will.

chapter FIVE

Current Issues on Stuttering and Recovery

Joseph G. Sheehan, Ph.D.

Our knowledge of stuttering is still outnumbered by its mysteries. Despite a vast amount of effort, many fundamental features of stuttering remain puzzling. It is difficult to find easy parallels to stuttering in other disorders — or perhaps we should say that it is difficult to find reasonably true parallels. Against such a background, it is inevitable that controversies should exist.

The behavior called speaking seems so easy to most of the population, once they have learned the speaker role. In a world where so many are glib with nothing to say, what causes an unlucky few to hold back, to falter, hesitate, repeat, struggle, grimace, avoid, and retreat from even the most commonplace situations, such as the

---

Since this chapter was designed and structured primarily to be responsive to the questions posed by the editor, it should not be regarded as either a total or a free standing statement of our own views on the nature of stuttering and its treatment.

Although the chapter has deliberately sought to sharpen the issues and to attack questionable claims or assumptions, nothing in it should be construed as an attack on individuals.

We recognize that perfectly respectable dissent may be offered to the views expressed here. Ours is not the only way of looking at stuttering, even if the conviction implied in our phrasing may have made it appear so. A difference of opinion, Will Rogers once said, is what makes horse racing and missionaries.

The author is indebted to Vivian M. Sheehan for many helpful suggestions concerning the manuscript.

telephone? Why should anyone develop an obvious fear of introducing himself by name, and go through many tortured rehearsals of situations that most people take for granted? The very existence of a problem like stuttering calls into question some of our cherished notions of behavioral principles, such as the law of effect, homeostasis of organismic functioning, the pleasure principle, etc. To the puzzle of persistence of stuttering must be added the puzzle of its apparent nonpersistence in four out of five cases in which the problem begins and develops sufficiently for label identification. Some of the recoveries may appear more puzzling than the onsets. However, most recoveries in the absence of formal therapy, for which we have been driven to the term "spontaneous recovery," do mesh well with our own principles of therapy when the common or underlying behavior patterns are examined.

So, many issues remain in the dim light of our present knowledge on stuttering. In addition to the reinforcement or persistence of the law-of-effect problem alluded to in the foregoing, there are issues such as these: Is stuttering a unitary disorder, or do several possible subtypes exist? Should all stutterers get a similar approach in therapy? Are there some stutterers who are better off without therapy, as currently practiced? Why is there a pattern of familial incidence — 12% or 13% when first-order relatives only are counted, and twice that when all known relatives are considered (Sheehan and Costley, 1977)? What accounts for the startling sex ratio in stuttering — about five times as many males (Schuell, 1946; Sheehan, 1975)? Why is there a lack of identifiable underlying predisposing differences between stutterers and nonstutterers? In the light of evident effects of self-esteem on stuttering, and other social psychological variables shown to govern its immediate frequency, why are there not more identifiable personality traits? Do some stutterers stutter more with punishment, and others with reward? In the absence of definable or systematic personality difference, for what does a stutterer require psychotherapy? How are we to account for the novel-stimulus effect, or disruptive stimulus effect, sometimes called the distraction principle? Are there quick cures that can be authenticated? Recovery implies permanence: but how permanent can be said to be the psychological well-being of any human being? Is recovery a term borrowed heavily and inappropriately from the medical model? Is the latter model appropriate, or is stuttering primarily a matter of disordered behavior? Etc., etc., etc.

The six questions posed by the editor have relationship with many of these issues. He has posed them well, capturing in the process many of the current concerns of beginning and not-so-beginning therapists. Some of the questions we see as subsidiary to others, so that the space requirements are unequal. For the organization of this chapter, question number six on success criteria and results has been moved upward to second position, while the questions on attitude change, psychotherapy, transfer, relapse, and child therapy are covered in the context of the larger question of success criteria and results: what are the goals of therapy, and what kind of product are we attempting to produce?

ALONG THE GREAT DIVIDE: AVOIDANCE VERSUS ACCEPTANCE

The question on "stuttering fluently" vs. "speaking fluently" is faithfully reflective of current literature in three respects: 1) the issue is misleadingly stated; 2) it focuses unduly on fluency per se, as though that were the only variable that therapy for stuttering need be concerned with; and 3) even when stripped of false verbiage, it is most clearly seen as a part-question of a much larger issue, the "Great Divide" in therapy for stuttering.

On one side of the Great Divide are clinicians who ask stutterers to accept for purposes of therapy the role of stutterer long enough to study, recognize, monitor, modify, and eventually eliminate the false-role behaviors that comprise the vast bulk of the stutterer's handicap.

We should stress that it is the *role* the stutterer is being asked to accept, not the original behavior. Most of the original behaviors are destined to go. Otherwise, there would be no point to the therapy.

Confusion on this point is pervasive in the literature. A recent reflection of it is in Culatta's "Fluency: The Other Side of the Coin." He charges that contemporary therapeutic philosophy is "illogical and failure oriented . . . because it holds as a final goal a still deviant behavior . . . Milder stuttering can be viewed as pathological behavior approved by speech clinicians" (Culatta, 1976, p. 795).

Let us emphasize, it is the *role* that the stutterer is being asked to accept, not the original stuttering pattern. No clinician we know of has ever proposed that as a serious goal of "therapy," for then therapy would be an exercise in helplessness. But the acceptance of the stutterer role in itself reduces many of the false behaviors and the struggle and tension that lead to and accompany each moment of stuttering.

In avoidance-reduction therapy, two kinds of acceptance are asked of the stutterer. First, he must develop sufficient acceptance of himself as a stutterer to stop concealing the problem from himself and others — long enough at least to undertake a systematic weakening of the handicapping behaviors via principles of learning. Second, he must accept the goal of less than perfect fluency, for no one has that. In some cases, those with a history of lifelong stuttering are going to continue to show more than the usual amount of disfluency. To plan otherwise is to deny experience and to court disaster.

We have elsewhere (Sheehan and Voas, 1957) made a distinction between the therapeutic handling of primary stuttering behaviors of repetition and prolongation, as compared to the behaviors Van Riper has designated as secondary — avoidance, postponement, starting, antiexpectancy, and release. It is the latter that are slated for elimination in therapy. Repetition and prolongation involve approach behaviors with respect to speaking, at least in a manner that is different from secondary behaviors. Sheehan and Voas found that practice of primary behaviors facilitated improvement, while practice of secondary behaviors retarded it (see Figure 1).

Avoidance-reduction is a keynote of this approach, a common theme that runs through the therapies of Van Riper, Johnson, Dean Williams, Bloodstein, Ainsworth, Emerick, Luper, Gregory, Bryngelson, Sheehan, J. D. Williams, and various others of Iowa persuasion or influence. It should be noted that there are significant individual differences among those just listed, in theory, in conceptualization of therapy process, and in methods emphasized. Whether there is currently enough shared commonality to call it the Iowa school is open to question, as Bloodstein, who has used this term, has also indicated.

In our own view, stuttering is false-role behavior arising out of a multilevel approach-avoidance conflict, of the double kind.

Consistent with this view, we set the primary task of therapy as reduction of avoidance or holding-back tendencies with respect to communication, and sufficient self-acceptance to eliminate the need for shallow pretense and false-role behaviors. The stutterer is asked to stop hiding the problem from himself and others, for so much of the immediate fear, shame, guilt, and manifest tension comes from

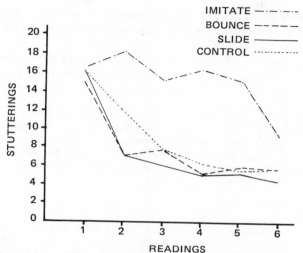

Figure 1. Comparison of the reduction in stuttering produced by three therapy methods. (From Sheehan and Voas, 1957, p. 717.)

efforts to conceal the stutterer role. It is assumed that no miracle or program can forever eliminate the possibility of the experiencing of a moment of fear in the future. What is the person to do when fear descends? He cannot run back to the laboratory to reenter a program claiming to "establish" fluency. Attempting to deny the anticipatory cues does not work; if it did, there would be no such thing as an adult stutterer. Unless he has learned to stutter more easily, openly, and simply in response to the old fear cues, he will revert all the way back to ground zero. He will fall flat on his facial contortion.

Unless the stutterer has learned a different and more effective style of stuttering, when the inevitable moment comes he will stutter his old way. The result is as though he had learned nothing at all — worse, for the shame and guilt can be devastating.

The stutterer comes into therapy feeling that his stuttering is something entirely horrible. When the clinician merely strives to keep him from ever doing it again, teaching him voice-from-the-tomb breathy onsets or offering to sell him gadgets to prevent moments of stuttering, the clinician thereby endorses the horribleness of it all.

Consider the contrast to an experience with a clinician who shows interest in the components of the behavior itself, an acceptance of the social reality that one who comes in with a lifelong stuttering problem will not have it immediately stop, and a genuine and abiding interest in the person not just in his degree of fluency. Van Riper, who epitomizes these clinician characteristics, employed an apt quote from Travis and included it in the very first edition of his textbook. To a field that sometimes seems to have lost sight of the clinical relationship, Travis' thoughtful words were:

> The primary concern of speech correction is the person.... It is not enough to know what sort of a speech defect a person has. In addition, one should know what kind of a person has a speech defect. The speech defect has no particular meaning apart from the person who presents the defect. We are not interested in speech defects but in speech defectives. (Travis, 1936, p. 1)

Van Riper added:

> Speech correction is but one small area in the field of clinical psychology, and the speech correctionist who thinks that he deals with lisping rather than lispers, and with stuttering rather than stutterers, will find discouragement at every turn. (Van Riper, 1939, p. 62)

One of the features of avoidance-reduction therapy is that most of those who utilize this approach tend to take the person and his life style into account. The handicap that a stutterer experiences depends upon more factors than the stuttering behavior itself. There are some seriously disturbed individuals whose stuttering is the least of their problems. In the economics of mental health, they are often referred to speech clinicians. If the latter are not merely to pass the buck via a referral to mostly nonexistent general psychotherapy facilities, they need sufficient capability as counselors or psychotherapists to offer some help for the larger problems in living — not just the disfluency count.

The other school, and a much older one, is the avoidance-cultivation, or distraction, method. It aims to prevent stuttering through active interventions to induce immediate fluency, to "establish" or nurture fluency in a sheltered "laboratory" environment, then to transfer programmed fluency and to maintain it.

In the days of Demosthenes (2,000+ years ago), or of Avicenna (1,000+ years ago), or of Bogue (50 years ago), the methods of fluency induction were fairly unsophisticated: for Demosthenes, the legendary pebbles; for 10th-century Arabian philosopher Avicenna, a deep breath before speaking; and for Bogue, a drawling chant while rhythmically swinging dumbbells. The "octave twist" was also employed.

The twin introduction of modern technology and the operant conditioning movement bestowed a more sophisticated image upon the distraction or avoidance-cultivation school, though its underlying premises remained unchanged.

Since we only recently described the salient characteristics of the distraction, or avoidance-cultivation, or suppression-of-stuttering school, we trust that we may be allowed an excerpt:

> The older school has typically employed distraction or disruption devices in an effort to first produce and then extend a fluency acquired through some special means. Fluency can be produced temporarily by hypnosis, confidence-achieving suggestions, and various mechanical devices. So prevalent have been machines for curing stuttering throughout history that an enterprising lawyer who is also a member of the Council of Adult Stutterers in Washington, D.C., catalogued a whole array of patents obtained to cure stuttering (Katz, 1977). Some older examples are variants of Itard's fork, which distorted the tongue position sufficiently to produce distraction-based fluency for a time. More recent patents have included portable masking and modified hearing aids, now so expensive that the effects are not likely to outlast the schedule of payments . . . Direct fluency methods characterize the older therapies. Often it is assumed that the stutterer needs to learn to talk all over again, or that he needs to use some special kind of control system. Or, an attempt is made to suppress the stuttering behavior through punishment for stuttering ("contingent" punishment). (Sheehan, 1975, p. 147)

We also offered a critique, one part of which follows:

> With therapies that aim at the prevention of moments of stuttering, and the stretching of fluency through the cultivation of avoidance of difficult situations, there is never an assurance of a method for meeting future fear and failure. By their very nature, such therapies increase the penalty on stuttering, the avoidance component, and the conflict. That they work for awhile at all is probably due to the novel-stimulus effect, or distraction principle. This means that their half-life is far less than the stutterer's full life.
>
> The cultivation of fluency and suppression of stuttering behavior appeals to the worst in the stutterer: his tendency to deny the problem, to cover up, to conceal. And unless the cover-up is complete — in itself a fantastic and unlikely achievement — the stutterer will be worse off. His avoidance tendencies will have been strengthened. If "programs" of such elaborate nature aim at pushing stuttering down under the surface, then the behavior must be shameful indeed. (Sheehan, 1975, p. 148)

The contrast between the opposite poles of distraction therapy and avoidance-reduction therapy may be illuminated by the set of

Table 1.   Contracts between distraction and avoidance-reduction therapies

Distraction	Avoidance reduction
1. How quickly can I make him fluent?	1. How can I prevent false fluency and flight into health from obscuring the problem and delaying real therapy?
2. How can I prevent instances of lapse into stuttering behavior?	2. How can I reduce general tendencies toward avoidance and attempted concealment of the stuttering behavior, so that he can begin to exercise his normal capacity for speaking more normally?
3. How can I get him to speak perfectly — total elimination of all stuttering behavior?	3. How can I get him to speak acceptably — within the normal range of normal speaker disfluency?
4. How can I get fluency "evoked" (or nurtured?) in the laboratory to transfer over to real-life situations?	4. How can I reinforce working on real-life situations all along throughout therapy?
5. How can I suppress fear?	5a. How can I help change the feelings and attitudes underlying fear?
	5b. How can I teach a more adequate response to fear that will inevitably arise?

contrasting questions listed in Table 1. Avoidance and holding back from speaking are core perpetuating factors in stuttering. The socially damaging and stigmatizing struggles, pretenses, tricks, crutches, and habituated mannerisms or shallow disguise are to be reduced along with the avoidance tendencies that produce them. Eventually, they are to be eliminated, and will be if the stutterer can give up his pretenses. Focusing on fluency does not really work, unless, as both Van Riper and Dean Williams suggest, the experience of speaking fluently can be given some stimulus value. But even then, the person cannot count on a magic reach to it.

Provisions for future fear and future failure possibilities are sound psychotherapeutic features of therapy for stutterers; if they are not there, the therapist is merely being repressive. A basic feature of all psychotherapy is that the therapist dissociates himself from societal demands that have caused the client to fail in the past.

The therapist needs to be on the side of the id, to accept the fears and failings of the client, not just to demand more perfection in performance. The stutterer has already had plenty of that. If it worked, he would not be there for therapy. Aiming for perfect fluency and encouraging denial of the stutterer role is merely a way of ensuring that the behaviors will continue. When a clinician sets goals and suggests methods that a stutterer has failed on all his life, he is being foolish and unrealistic. If the stutterer could talk better, he would. But he has gotten himself into a vicious circle. The clinician's role should be to help him out of it, not to strengthen the perpetuating forces.

It is not true that a stutterer "can speak if he wants to." The effect of motivation increase for a naive stutterer is to increase the avoidance tendencies, i.e., to make him hold back more from the act of speaking. Conflict theory and avoidance-reduction therapy can turn it around: motivation increases can strengthen approach drives for speaking without asking the client to tread lightly lest he stutter.

WHAT SHOULD BE THE END PRODUCT OF THERAPY? — SUCCESS CRITERIA, OUTCOME EVALUATION, AND FOLLOW-UP

The "Experimenters" Are Always Successful; But Are the Stutterers?

The sixth of the principal questions put to contributors to this book is of such breadth and importance that we have decided to move it to the number 2 position. Accordingly, this section takes up with the matter of outcome: the assessment of success or failure in therapy, and the definition of the end product that therapy must aim to produce.

Outcome evaluation and follow-up are excellent vantage points for other issues, for a number of reasons: 1) we must thereby define therapeutic goals; 2) these goals in turn reflect the context in which the stuttering and its treatment are embedded; 3) outcome evaluation and follow-up are difficult problems methodologically and clinically; 4) the current rash of competing claims for high success rates may be placed in perspective; 5) studies of recovery in the absence of therapy throw new light upon old claims and old methods, including those reappearing in new guises; 6) the fact that adequate follow-up is nonexistent can be brought into clear focus; 7) groundwork can be laid among students, stutterers, and their parents to develop a consumer awareness of rampant and escalating fraud; and 8) this book can become more than a showcase for aggressive competition among the contributors for ever higher and higher percentages of claimed rapid cures.

If we compare the newest generation of speech pathologists with that of Iowa in the 1930s, or Michigan in the 1940s, it is clear that there is a shift toward more strenuous exploitation of claims. It is difficult not to view this development as a huge retrogression. Controversies regarding ideas, concepts, and theories are probably healthy; they illuminate alternative ways of looking at the problem of stuttering. Even the nitpicking on pseudomethodological issues is probably some sign of a move toward professional maturation. But competition on claims for recovery, "establishment" of fluency, or cure, or fluency maintenance percentages, reflects a backward trend in ethical sensitivity as well as scientific caution. Beware of the numbers game! By the time you can do a follow-up, the pea is under a different shell. A new program will have replaced the old one, with a new and bigger claim to match it.

Follow-up on the kaleidoscope of constantly improving claims reveals that though the "experimenters" have a never-ending stream of successes, the stutterers have a never-ending stream of failures. Thus the operant conditioners boast of having "evoked fluency" more than "previous pessimism would have imagined." But we do not hear this operant fluency evoked at ASHA meetings or at other public gatherings. Instead, privately arranged "surprise" phone calls are offered as an ultimate criterion of stutterer success. And every time a really independent follow-up study is undertaken, by a disinterested third party, the program changes faster than that at your neighborhood rerun theater.

Only the Claims Are New, Not the Methods

One of the most dismaying features of currently evolving tales of quick and permanent cure is that only the claims are new, not the methods. We hear of stutterers cured in half an hour through "discovery" of an airflow technique or operant program that turns out to be an elaboration or variation on discredited breathing exercises. After all, the stutterer has been breathing a long time without programmed instruction.

When we keep hearing of startling new results based on tired old methods, we have a right to be skeptical. Where are all these phenomenal successes? We would like to see, hear, and authenticate. We are tired of hearing *about* all these cures. We want to hear *from* them. Let them speak for themselves — if they are able to do it. Recently, at the 1977 American Speech and Hearing Association meetings in Chicago, we were to have had an opportunity. But fluency-shaping's star pupil failed to show for the panel of "recovered" stutterers. Another panelist, who was laboring visibly to use "airflow technique," had an uncomfortably tense and difficult time. Since this man had the courage to go ahead and speak in the presence of obviously strong fear, he should eventually improve — not so much from airflow as from strengthening approach tendencies toward speaking. However, we believe he would have been more comfortable and freer from tension — and so would his audience — had he accepted the likelihood of stuttering in the situation and accepted that reality enough to stutter openly and easily (cf. May, 1968). Instead, his struggling, partially successful efforts to cover up or suppress every looming moment of stuttering made everyone more tense.

If we re-examine Wendell Johnson's classic series, *Studies in the Psychology of Stuttering,* we note that many of the techniques whose effects he studied with admirable scientific caution, such as masking, choral speaking, rhythm, etc., are reappearing today. But the difference is that Johnson had the scientific sense and ethical integrity to recognize that experimentally induced reductions in stuttering frequency are not cures. As a stutterer himself, he knew that today's fluency interval is followed by tomorrow's relapse. Fluency attained under conditions of laboratory isolation typically has no effect on the stutterer's responses to the fear-arousing situations of everyday life. In order to recondition, the clinician must do so under similar stimulus conditions; otherwise, he merely has an exercise in discrimination learning.

Stutterers tend to get better in the clinic, perhaps through situational adaptation, or because the initial authority threat posed by the clinic diminishes with time and familiarization. There is also, in learning terms, the matter of simple habituation. As a situation becomes more familiar, the elements of stimulus complexity and overload diminish. The artificial improvement that stutterers are subject to in the clinic we refer to as "clinic voice." In one sense, it derives later from a selective use of therapeutically effective methods within the clinic that the stutterer does not bother to make himself use outside. Even with a punishing handicap, it is easier to fall back into old habit patterns than it is to monitor one's speaking processes. Having to "work on one's speech" is always a nuisance, and the stutterer may be pardoned for occasionally lapsing into a quite normal preoccupation with the content of one's communication. However, the principle of reinforcement is not equally forgiving.

The stutterer must go through a learning period, as any of us must when undertaking a change of entrenched attitudes and strongly reinforced habit patterns. Deep-seated feelings of shame, guilt, and unworthiness in the speaker role comprise part of the attitudinal constellation. Instrumental acts of word avoidance and situational avoidance, as well as the grimaces, tricks, crutches, and accessory mannerisms, tend to make up the idiosyncratic features of each stutterer's pattern. The former is a matter of Pavlovian or classical conditioning. The latter is a matter of instrumental or Thorndikian (trial and error, maze learning, etc.) conditioning. There are always two sides to the stutterer's handicap, and two sides necessary to his therapy. Therapy may require instrumental changes along with changes in feelings.

The "Laetrile Effect" in the Treatment of Stuttering

It was easier to be a stutterer in the days when we grew up with the handicap. It was also easier, much easier, to be a student of speech pathology. The quacks were more obviously identifiable as such. Those running the commercial "stammering institutes" that guaranteed a cure usually did not have academic degrees, even though their literature proclaimed that they had the problem of stuttering solved. For a stutterer, "cure" is a forgivable fantasy, even though it must be relinquished before sensible therapy can begin. For a speech pathologist with years of training to hold Laetrile-like fantasies on the problem of stuttering is much less forgivable. We have researched the problem long enough to know better.

Stuttering is a complex problem whose nature forever tempts people to offer simplistic cures. Neighbors and casual acquaintances usually do not offer advice on treating cancer or diabetes. But stuttering has a persistence along with a now-you-see-it-now-you-don't quality, so it fosters irresponsible and/or fraudulent claims for easy solution. Simplistic "cures" abound, and the history of medicine is littered with them. Even intelligent people who should know better are taken in, or ensnare themselves. So we have copper bracelets for arthritis[1] and Laetrile for cancer. A generation ago it was Krebiozen.

By "Laetrile effect" we mean the persisting and unreasonable belief that a problem with known complexities must have a quick and easy solution. If someone could come up with a simple answer to the complex problem, and if the answer really "solved" the problem, we would certainly have no objections. But that is not going to happen. Too much is known of the complexities of the disorder — and for that matter, of human nature — to entertain that hope intelligently. If only it were so, we could cheerfully turn our attention to problems other than those of the stutterer. But self-presentation via speech is always going to be difficult for some, depending upon how they feel toward themselves and toward significant others. That kind of problem will and can never be "solved" by a simplistic gimmick — or even a complex gimmick.

Among the human complexities that render simplistic solutions impossible are the array of problems that can confront a stutterer as a result of his therapeutic improvement. Have people forgotten preparation for recovery? Loss of the defensive function? The need for stuttering? Problems that surface only after speech improvement? The notion that the stutterer's problems are located in the vocal tract is hopelessly naive. So is the notion that stuttering may ever be "solved" by a vocal tract gimmick, or by laryngeal surgery, a horrible throwback that has recently become a tangible danger to the stutterer.

On the Trail of Rapturous Testimonial

Nothing is more pessimism inducing than to have your hopes dashed. But that has happened to stutterers for centuries. Throughout the sorry history of the treatment of stuttering, many have prematurely uttered a loud "Eureka," as Van Riper has pointed out (1973). No doubt each would-be discoverer of "the cure" benefitted immediately from his claims. The sociology of quackery could be studied quite effectively via "cures" for stuttering. Katz (1977) has recorded with illustrations a whole chronicle of patents issued through the history of the United States Patent Office.

---

[1]As an exercise in therapist self-disclosure, Yalom (1975) confessed to one of his therapy groups that the copper bracelet the member had spotted on Yalom's wrist was for arthritis. This from a medical man! The group was taken aback — how far back was not disclosed.

Against this background, we offer advice to the young student and to the speech clinician:

First, beware of all claims for sudden and sensational cures. Individual variations in motivation are such that no one can ethically guarantee a cure. Recognition of this fact has led to the incorporation of a prohibition against guaranteed cures into the American Speech and Hearing Association code of ethics.

Second, reports in "scientific" journals that claim high percentages of persisting recovery must be examined in the light of 1) knowledge of spontaneous recovery figures, and 2) independent follow-up by third parties not having a stake in the outcome of the claimed recovery rate.

What Therapy Is Commonly Used?

"Traditional" is always the other fellow's therapy. "Innovative" is always our own — no matter how hoary, ancient, and bearded. The literature is constantly being cluttered up with self-serving proclamations of a "new" therapy, while anything already published becomes "traditional." The dizzying confusion that results for the new student of speech pathology has been eloquently stated by Bloodstein, in his foreword to Reiber's recently edited book, *The Problem of Stuttering:*

> To begin with, there are the monumental contradictions that preclude any simple outlook on the problem and make it so intractable. To speak fluently is such an easy accomplishment for most stutterers that they almost always seem just a short step away from becoming normal speakers. Yet once they have begun to speak normally they seem to be almost continually under the threat of imminent relapse. As a result, stuttering can give the bewildering impression of being at once remarkably easy and very difficult to treat. In our groping toward an effective approach to therapy, we seem to value nothing as much as a new method, unless it one that is very old. That is, we properly distrust every measure that seems to us to be "traditional" and until it becomes all but extinct, and then we revive the suffering old bag of bones with an enthusiastic whack and march it off the replace the point of view that has most lately become traditional. In this way the new often becomes old and the old new with a whimsy that can be startling to all but those who have just arrived on the scene. (Bloodstein, 1977, unpaged)

Of late it is the operant conditioners who have been busily trying to dismiss anyone else as "traditional." Ingham and Andrews (1973) exemplify the fad. In much more lurid commercial form, so does Schwartz (1976), although the operant conditioners are not to be saddled with his simplistic claim of having "solved" stuttering through "discovery" of the airway dilation reflex.

What can properly be called traditional? What therapy has been most widely used? The most substantial data on these points come from an earlier comprehensive survey by Jackson (1949), who found that most centers used what we have been describing as distraction or avoidance-cultivation therapy. In addition, results of the Sheehan-Martyn studies (Sheehan and Martyn, 1966, 1970; Martyn and Sheehan, 1968) throw light on the distribution of therapy approaches more recently used in the population of those who stuttered as they grew up. For example, therapy methods associated with Van Riper, Sheehan, and others who have advocated some degree of self-acceptance in the stutterer role were not represented anywhere in our three samples. Reports by Cooper (1972), Dickson (1971), Shearer and Williams (1965), and Wingate (1964b, 1976) present the same general picture.

There must be some reasons why a therapy that had proved so successful for me and for so many others has not become more widely employed. The mythology of the last few years, catalyzed by the operant conditioners, is that it has. Ingham and Andrews (1973), for example, have so written. They have called therapies that have involved avoidance-reduction, acceptance of the stutterer role, and teaching new patterns of stuttering by a name that coincides with the promotion of their own therapy far more than it coincides with reality. They have called it *traditional*, a term that suggests it has been widely used and is now old hat. But the term is far more appropriate to the newly packaged old therapy that operant conditioners are dispensing.

Avoidance-reduction therapy has never been tried on any kind of large scale, or for that matter, tried widely at all. The 147 stutterers and former stutterers we carefully interviewed in our series of three samples of entering University of California students gave no indication they had ever received any but the most superficial kind of distraction-based, avoidance-cultivation therapy.

There is no question that the textbooks of Johnson and Van Riper have sold widely and have had pervasive influence on issues such as disfluency, stages of stuttering, and other matters of theoretical interest. But somehow the message on therapy has never come across. The therapists on the firing line have simply not used the therapy. Ask any stutterer who has had years of public school therapy, and you will hear a lot about breathing, "gentle onset," slowing down, relaxing, and reading poetry, but not much else. Ask any stutterer who has had his fluency "established" or stretched through operant conditioning, and you will hear pretty much the same thing. More objective evidence that clinicians have not used avoidance-reduction, or acceptance-and-modification of the stuttering pattern type therapy, comes from the finding we alluded to earlier: it was unrepresented in the sample we took from 5138 entering students at UCLA and at the University of California, Berkeley. How is it that a therapy so widely preached has never been practiced? The tenets of Van Riper therapy have been observed about as faithfully as the Ten Commandments.

So much for the tradition of labeling the other fellow "traditional."

In the Footsteps of Assaultive Therapies

Much behavior therapy as applied to stuttering tends to fall within the tradition of the assaultive therapies — electric shock, metrazol shock, tranquilizer dosage, lobotomy. They are mechanical assaults administered routinely to the person, regardless of his individual life style, interests, needs, and personality dynamics, and regardless of the significance of stuttering in his life. Motivation for recovery consists in showing up and undergoing the assault. It is the "experimenter" who counts, not the person. The client is a nonperson — an experimental subject, an S. His only individuality is a small percentage contribution to commercially inflated outcome claims. It is the program that counts!

The Cult of Operant Behaviorism

As Staats (1977) has pointed out, for some operant conditioners not only is the person and his life style ignored, but even the vast literature on emotion is ignored. Even Pavlovian or classical conditioning is "treated as a species of operant conditioning of a noncontingent type (where the consequence occurs whether or not an instrumental response is made)... In Skinner's operant behaviorism, emotions and classical conditioning are in effect eliminated as important, by excluding emotions as a causal circumstance for instrumental behavior. On a more general level this can be seen by an almost total ignoring of classical conditioning in animal and human research" (Staats, 1977, p. 231). Staats further points out that formal operant analysis leaves out consideration of how emotional responses affect instrumental responses, in animals as well as humans. He goes on to suggest that "operant theory, which attempts to isolate instrumental conditioning and raise this principle to unique importance, produces inconsistencies with the empirical world" (1977, p. 231).

Recent syntheses of the relevant literature have been undertaken by Hessell (1971) and by Van Riper (1973). Many other writers, such as Ainsworth (1975), Bloodstein (1975a, b), Johnson (1959, 1961b), and Wischner (1969), have written of the relationship between stuttering and anxiety.

The central role of fear or anxiety in producing conflict in stuttering is too evident to overlook, yet some operant conditioners have tried to blindfold themselves to consideration of such concepts, as applied by operant workers to stuttering. This has led to the unspoken premise that recordable fluency equals improvement no matter how bizarre the conditions under which it is obtained. Denying oneself the use of constructs such as anxiety or self-esteem leads inevitably to the fallacy that the stutterer's problem may be meaningfully measured by the proximate fluency count. But the problem of stuttering cannot be meaningfully defined in this manner, nor can meaningful improvement be validly inferred from such local measures as fluency count. Artifacts of all kinds may be reflected in the fluency count — novel stimulus effects, attentional shifts, reduced propositionality, reduced stimulus complexity, and the like.

Socially disruptive stimuli can produce immediate fluency while at the same time rendering it meaningless.

Concerning Transfer

"Transfer" is a fallacy. It really does not happen. To the extent that there is a transfer problem, the therapy has been deficient. In action-oriented avoidance-reduction therapy the changes are going on via assignments and role enactments in outside situations all throughout the therapy. We do not regard improvement within the clinic as much more than an artifact — contrary to the operant conditioners, who have the unscientific habit of claiming thereby to have "established" fluency. It is merely habituation to that restricted and essentially meaningless set of stimuli.

In avoidance-reduction therapy, a transfer problem is only a symptom of ineffectuality of the therapist to bring about assignment fulfillment within the outside world during the course of the therapy. Transfer is a manifestation of something lacking in the therapy. But with many operant conditioners, it is a planned after-thought.

The clinic is like a capsule, a microcosm revealing what happens when you are completely open. Stutterers sometimes need to be reminded of this test-tube function of the clinic — of what ease and fluency result when you become open enough to reduce situation and word avoidances.

Attitude Change

So much has been written of the malattitudes stutterers are supposed to have toward their problem that we frequently lose sight of the fact that the vast majority have already achieved a partial acceptance. A person who grows up with a visible, though variable, flaw in the social presentation of the self inevitably comes to terms with it to some extent. We first became aware of this principle in observing the reactions of normal speakers in an introductory communication disorders class, in which two assignments were given which asked that the normal speakers portray themselves as stutterers in various public situations. Most became quite involved and quite upset. The assignment appeared to tap their general insecurities concerning their own self-presentation. In contrast, a majority of the stutterers, given a comparable assignment, had a comparatively easy time.

The stutterer feels guilty and then begins to cover up a vague something he perceives to be wrong with him. Guilt over the concealment (secondary guilt) is then added on to guilt over the vague something (primary guilt). The vicious circle of self-reinforcing stuttering is created by self-revealing efforts at concealment.

A human being's defensive effort, his effort at concealing what he feels guilty about, is the most revealing facet of his personality. Consider the list of developments based on this principle: the lie detector, the word association test, the Rorschach test, etc. Through his behavioral defenses, aimed at preventing or covering up instances of blocking, the stutterer gives his feelings away. As the stutterer is robbed of the basic human dignity of respectful self-presentation, guilt becomes translated into shame.

Psychotherapy and Speech Therapy

The relationship of psychotherapy to speech therapy, and the degree of compatibility or coexistence of both behavioral and psychotherapeutic approaches, has long been one of our chief interests. Through conflict theory, the two are potentially and logically compatible in conception, if not always as practiced.

In Chapter One, Gregory has pointed out that speech pathologists share techniques in common with counselors and psychotherapists. While, as he points out, there are differences in background and emphases among these three disciplines, it is important to recognize that all therapy with a stutterer involves the role of psychotherapy to some degree.

"Attitude work" and supportive therapeutic functions are basic to the treatment of most stutterers. Since the speech clinician is likely to be the most available hope of a stutterer, it is vital that he not pass the buck too readily to those in allied fields. A clinician who hits the panic button and makes referrals outward at the drop of a cross word cannot be counted on to help many stutterers.

For the future, certain speech clinicians may become specialists in treating stutterers with added psychological training relevant to that role (Ainsworth, 1975; Van Riper, 1975). Specialists or not, speech pathologists need to recognize that they are exercising an essentially psychotherapeutic function, as that would be broadly defined. But that does not have to be frightening to the speech clinician.

Offered a chance to break out of the vicious circle via avoidance-reduction therapy, the stutterer for whom the behavior is serving a neurotic or defensive function will reveal these deeper levels of his conflict. Many stutterers need help in adjusting to the emergence of fluency and the loss of "giant in chains" protective functions (Sheehan, 1954b). In the light of approach-avoidance conflict theory, such psychotherapy shares common goals with therapy for stuttering, since reduction of the avoidance gradient is the dominant feature of each. Since we have developed this theme fairly extensively in many previous publications (Sheehan, 1951, 1953, 1954b, 1958b, 1970a), we see no need to duplicate it here.

Who Should Be the Therapist?

Every stutterer grows up with the naive advice of neighbors and casual strangers ringing uselessly in his ears: "Relax, think what you have to say, slow down, take a deep breath, did you ever try to talk with pebbles in your mouth, etc., etc. . . . ." Surely this is one of the sources of fundamental discouragement to be observed clinically in so many stutterers and in the prevalence of stutterers who "turn off" early and give up the quest for a satisfactory therapy. There seems to be something about the intermittency of stuttering, especially its amenability to endless new distractions, that seduces the listener into a ready conviction that he can deliver an offhand suggestion that will unlock the key to what is an obviously habituated behavior.

Perhaps, then, it is not surprising to find professional therapists with massive ignorance of the stuttering problem stepping eagerly into the role of expert on the treatment of a disorder they never bothered to study. While M.D.'s have been especially prone, so have quite a large number of inadequately trained speech clinicians. But the growing army of behavior therapists have set new milestones in overreaching their capacities. Experimental psychologists who have obviously never bothered to inform themselves of the vast existing literature on stuttering turn up reporting fast cures in behavioral journals. We have already seen several, reportedly cured by operantly cosmetized breathing exercises, again stuttering convulsively but still clutching their reprints from *Behaviour Research and Therapy* — and sometimes even *JSHR*.

What Is a Satisfactory Therapy for Stuttering?

In these days when we hear reckless talk of "stuttering solved" and quackish claims for half-hour cures, we may well examine what must be minimum criteria for a satisfactory therapy. Here are some we have distilled from years of therapeutic contact with stutterers:

1. Individual differences in motivation must be recognized.
2. Individual differences in the nature of stuttering behavior itself must be recognized.
3. Consideration should be given to the type or subtype, for stuttering is by no means a unitary disorder, and different kinds of stutterers may require different emphases in therapy.
4. Quick cures, or total cures, or promises of perfection in fluency should not be held out as ethically realistic possibilities.
5. Not everyone should be treated solely by a single program.
6. The ultimate focus of therapy should be the person and his possibilities for self-growth, not just his disfluency rate.
7. The probability of other problems resulting from improvement in speaking must be anticipated, and the person should be offered help with these problems, within reasonable limits.
8. The clinician should be prepared to cope with the possibility of neurotic resistance, flight into health, and self-sabotage.

9. Relapses should be prepared for, and means for coping with relapses should be a part of joint planning before therapy is terminated. In some cases, small relapses should be clinically induced, so that the dread of future relapse may be mitigated.
10. A sustained period of follow-up should be provided.
11. Therapy should teach the person sufficient clinical competence regarding his own problems so that he may in the future be better able to cope with them, to become his own clinical resource. At least, his knowledge of stuttering should be developed sufficiently for him to become his own clinical resource on that problem.
12. Like a good parental relationship, a therapeutic relationship may result in an independence and self-sufficiency that is only relative. In therapy, as at home, the door should always be open as a transitory base for self-renewal.

PATTERNS OF RECOVERY FROM STUTTERING[1]

Since this is a book on controversies regarding therapy for stutterers, we should take note of methodological issues regarding data on improvement and recovery, especially with respect to the series of studies that have now been carried out yielding data on spontaneous recovery. We have included a clarification of the procedural record, along with a comparison of longitudinal with cross-sectional and retrospective methodologies.

Some Historical Background on Recovery

We have long been fascinated by processes associated with recovery from stuttering, beginning with our own. In a doctoral dissertation submitted at the University of Michigan in August, 1949, we noted, "...it has always been easier to account for stuttering than for its disappearance" (Sheehan, 1951, p. 61). In 1950, we initiated at UCLA a Student Health Service survey that found that the number of recovered stutterers outnumbered the number of stutterers in that population still actively stuttering. In 1957 we organized and chaired a "Symposium of Recovered Stutterers" at the American Speech and Hearing Association meetings in Cincinnati, in the hope that light might be thrown on recovery processes, through a series of personal accounts by those sufficiently improved to give them.

---

[1]Margaret M. Martyn, Ph.D., aided significantly in the preparation of this section, and in the collection of data upon which it is based.

Our desires to follow up on these intriguing leads had to wait until the spring of 1964. At that time, we received from the director of the Student Health Service at the University of California, Berkeley campus, a most welcome request. Dr. Henry Bruyn contacted us prior to establishing a speech pathology service at Cowell Hospital on the Berkeley campus.

As a first step, we proposed a systematic survey of all students entering Berkeley for the first time in September, 1964. Following this, a second survey was scheduled at Berkeley for February, 1965. Since the earlier survey at UCLA in 1950 had shown the presence of a substantial number of recovered stutterers, we planned in connection with each survey to gather systematic additional data on both recovered stutterers and active stutterers. Because of the time pressure on Student Health Service examinations, our general speech screening procedure had to be brief.

Four speech pathologists from the San Francisco Bay area participated with the investigators in both surveys. All were qualified as speech diagnosticians. As we have reported the procedure in detail in three previous publications (Sheehan and Martyn, 1966, 1970; Martyn and Sheehan, 1968), only the barest outline is covered here. The initial determination of present or past speech handicap was made by the subjects themselves, who were asked to rate themselves as conversational speakers, and whether they now had or had ever had a speech problem or had ever taken any special speech training for such a problem.

In the screening interview, a speech pathologist conducted a brief speech examination and asked whether the student had ever had a speech problem or had one currently. As we have described, each was asked to read a speech screening passage, *My Grandfather.* Those who reported a present or past speech problem or who gave evidence of either during the interview were then referred for two separate interviews with each of the co-investigators, Sheehan and Martyn. Each interviewed the subject long enough to make a determination as to whether the subject was either an active stutterer or a recovered stutterer, had some other speech problem, or displayed speech within the normal range. In the case of either an active or a recovered stutterer, one of the investigators, Sheehan or Martyn, conducted a 20-question structured interview, writing down the subject's responses on a form for this purpose. Except in a few instances, when time pressure prevented, complete duplicate interviews were conducted as a reliability check.

It should be noted particularly that each subject included in the study had to have been seen for diagnosis and evaluation by at least three speech pathologists separately. Initially, the subject was seen during the speech screening and was diagnosed as a stutterer, present or past, active or recovered. Next the subject was seen separately by either Sheehan or Martyn, then (except as noted above) separately by the other.

Inadequate comprehension of our criteria for inclusion as either a stutterer or a recovered stutterer is evident in recent literature suggesting that our findings might be accounted for by the laymen's use of the term stuttering, or by "family legends." We did not, of course, take just anybody's word for it. A potential subject had to show that he knew "the inside of stuttering," to describe characteristic symptoms such as preformations, syllable repetitions, grimaces, and fear of stuttering on certain words or in certain situations, such as reciting in classes or answering the telephone. Moreover, most recovered stutterers were able to demonstrate their old stuttering pattern; in this respect they differed markedly from the active stutterers who showed great resistance to such a demonstration. Further, any subject included had to have been labeled a stutterer by others, as well as by himself.

Of course, nearly any normal speaker, when asked if he had ever stuttered on a word, will answer affirmatively. But that ancient fact has zero relevance to our findings.

Results of the First Berkeley Study

The principal finding from our first Berkeley sample (Sheehan and Martyn, 1966), that 80% of those determined to have been stutterers had recovered on their own, or "spontaneously," both astonished and intrigued us. We had not expected the proportion of those who had recovered to be so high. Moreover, they had done it on their own, without professional intervention. Not one achieved a recovery during a period of enrollment in public school therapy. Not one would recommend public school therapy for another stutterer. Instead, they attributed their improvement to speaking more, to not avoiding, to going ahead anyway, to resisting time pressure by speaking at their own pace, and similar phrases. One advised, "Fight it as you would an enemy."

It was striking to us that these stutterers had successfully utilized, without professional guidance, the avoidance-reduction methods that, along with others, we had been advocating for years.

The stutterers who remained active intrigued us, too. Mostly, they were not seeking treatment. They had reached the conclusion that no one they were likely to contact understood the problem well enough to offer competent help. They had decided to live with it, though with a continual struggle to keep it hidden as much as possible.

Further Studies of Spontaneous Recovery

So intriguing were the results of the first Berkeley sample that we decided to check the findings via two further samples (Martyn and Sheehan, 1968; Sheehan and Martyn, 1970). Most important, other investigators independently gathered data. Obtaining data through interviews with parents of school children rather than stutterers themselves, Dickson (1971) obtained results in close agreement with ours on important variables such as recovery rates (allowing for age differences), age of onset, severity, sex ratio, and many other factors related to recovery.

Using our methodology, Cooper (1972) conducted a series of studies whose results square well with our own, allowing for age level and for mean differences to be expected of successive samples from the same general population. Even assuming possible regional differences, there is substantial agreement among Dickson in New York, Cooper in Alabama, and Sheehan and Martyn in California.

For example, in one study Cooper (1972) reported a 36% spontaneous recovery ratio for junior and senior high school students in Alabama public schools. While at a superficial glance the figures appear discrepant with our 80% for entering undergraduate and graduate students at the University of California at Berkeley and at the University of California at Los Angeles, the studies actually corroborate one another. Data from the three Sheehan and Martyn studies synchronize with data from Cooper and his group when differences in the demography of our respective samples are taken into account. For example, the Cooper, Parris, and Wells (1974) sample consisted entirely of University of Alabama entering freshmen. In the University of California, Berkeley, and in the University of California, Los Angeles, the number of entering juniors tends to be greater than the number of entering freshmen. This circumstance is due to upper class transfer from California junior colleges or from California state colleges. Moreover, our samples had a heavy percentage of entering graduate students who were necessarily older. For

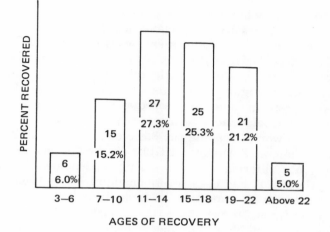

Figure 2.   Ages of recovery, at 3-year intervals, of the 99 stutterers who recovered and were able to recall the age of recovery with sufficient precision to be included in the data on this point. Of the 147 stutterers turned up in the interviews, 31 remained active and the other 17 had recovered but could not with certainty recall the age.

our combined samples as published in "Stuttering and Its Disappearance" (Sheehan and Martyn, 1970), the mean age of the recovered stutterers was 23.7, while for the active stutterers it was 22.6. This is 4–5 years older than the likely mean age of Cooper's 1972 sample, which consisted of entering freshmen at the University of Alabama. When these demographic differences are taken into account, and the percentages in Figure 2 are examined, it may be seen that Cooper's results correspond quite well to those of Sheehan and Martyn.

In Figure 2 we have constructed a histogram showing ages at which our subjects reported recovery. As Figure 2 (combined data from all of our surveys) shows, by age 14 the cumulative proportion who had recovered up to that time is about one-half.

Data reported by Gillespie and Cooper (1973) show that the junior high school grades reflect a dropping off of the proportion of stutterers that is quite consistent with the Sheehan and Martyn data reported in Figure 2. Again, if we look at the senior high level, the spurt in recovery rate at ages 16–18 in Figure 2 corresponds reasonably well with Gillespie and Cooper's findings, which show a substantial drop in the percentage of stutterers by the time the twelfth grade is reached.

The data do not show, as is commonly believed, that spontaneous recovery occurs "especially in childhood." Rather, as Figure 2 reveals, it is the adolescent years that provide the peak times of recovery. Before gathering actual data, we shared the common impression that many recoveries occur soon after the child first begins to stutter. Figure 2 indicates that for those who developed enough of a problem to be categorized as stutterers, relatively few recoveries occur before adolescence.

It may be worth recalling the basic data on which Figure 2 is based (Sheehan and Martyn, 1970). We had interviewed 5138 University of California students during student health examinations. Of these, 147 had been severe enough to have been categorized as stutterers at some time in their lives. Thirty-one had remained as active stutterers at the time the survey data were taken, providing an overall 80% spontaneous recovery rate. Of those who recovered, 17 were unable to give a time period for their recovery with sufficient precision so that they could be included in the data on this factor. The percentages in Figure 2 are therefore based upon 99 recovered stutterers who had recovered and were able to remember the age. The Figure 2 percentages are probably a lower bound on recovery, because they include only those who recover and remember the age. It is likely that more of those who could not specify an age had recovered at younger ages that were more difficult to recall.

Similarly, the figures on ages 19–22 and 22–27 are likely to be a lower bound and an underestimate. Since some of those studied had not passed through the age intervals in Figure 2, it is possible that some of the 31 active stutterers not included in this histogram might become recovered stutterers at later ages. Therefore, it is quite likely that the ultimate spontaneous recovery rate for stuttering is higher than 80%, rather than lower.

The columns for age intervals in Figure 2 are probably all too low, especially at the low end and at the higher end. As stutterers advance in age, they have less time to recover and begin to fall into age intervals at which their recovery chances are reduced. There are also conditional probabilities, such as that the subject is able to recall the age, and these tend to be lower than the overall probability of recovery. The reason is that they do not include the people who recovered but could not recall the age with sufficient specificity.

In Figure 2 the last column, "above 22," is almost meaningless, because it is an artifact of the ages at which the data were taken. However, it was included to make the data presentation as complete as possible. If we were able to interview subjects at the ages of 30, 40, or 50, it is likely we would have found additional spontaneous recoveries from among those 31 who were still active stutterers at first enrollment in the University of California.

We also found that severity as a variable was unrelated to age of recovery. However, severity was negatively related to probability of recovery and positively related to enrollment in public school speech therapy. These twin relationships help to account for the otherwise dismal finding on the effects of public school therapy. Another factor in the latter was that the public school clinicians covered in the study did not seem to be giving therapy a fair chance, for the methods they were reported as using bore little relation to established therapy procedures (Sheehan and Martyn, 1971).

The age level data in Figure 2 are to be interpreted with the precaution that there are probably less precision and more room for error at the lowest age level, since the subject was recalling earlier experiences over a longer period of time. The data from late childhood and adolescent years appear to be relatively more secure. Presumably, this precaution would not apply to the Andrews and Harris (1964) data, for their study was longitudinal and observational rather than retrospective.

Longitudinal versus Cross-Sectional Study

In this section, we examine the assets and liabilities of partially retrospective studies, such as those of Sheehan and Martyn, Cooper and his group, Shearer and Williams, Dickson, Patricia Johnson (1951) and Wingate, in comparison to partially longitudinal studies as exemplified by the Andrews and Harris report (1964).

Much misunderstanding exists concerning the relative merits of longitudinal studies as contrasted with cross-sectional and retrospective studies. On a priori grounds, the longitudinal approach appears preferable, as we noted in an earlier discussion of methodology:

> The most substantive methodological limitation in the Sheehan and Martyn study, equally present in the Wingate study and in the Shearer and Williams study, has not been mentioned but should be. All of these are *ex post facto* studies and are based upon recall data. Yet we

have to make a beginning, to break ground somewhere. What we need most for the future, however, are long-term followup and longitudinal studies. (Sheehan and Martyn, 1967, p. 400)

Though longitudinal studies may *eventually* provide more permanent answers than are possible through a retrospective approach, experience shows that they are rare and difficult to accomplish. Moreover, the time span of longitudinal studies introduces special methodological problems. It is difficult to maintain the same criterion of who is considered a stutterer over a long time span, for the field itself may shift somewhat. Practical necessity may dictate that different judges are used in the later sample than in the earlier phase of the study, so that interjudge reliability looms as a larger problem. Intrajudge or test-retest reliability may also be reduced by the passage of time. Inevitably, even longitudinal studies involve some degree of retrospective search. What has happened in the intervening time? Should the investigators ignore these possible events? If they do not, they find themselves engaging in retrospective activity.

In response to a comment by Bandura (1969), we have pointed out that portions of the Sheehan and Martyn data are not based on the subjective recall for precise events (Sheehan and Martyn, 1970). We did observe the subjects directly in the face-to-face structured interview situation, and the determination of recovery status, degree of improvement, and probable degree of severity at worst were made on that basis. Bandura's (1969) coverage of our studies showed that he did accord the research considerable credibility.

Since longitudinal studies are actuarially rare, we may learn from more immediately feasible retrospective studies. Among the disadvantages of the latter are that second-guessing becomes so easy that the literature is soon cluttered with it. No originality is required for pontificating that there is danger in going backward.

The most substantive longitudinal research published to date on recovery rates is that of Andrews and Harris (1964). They conducted an observational study of roughly 1000 children in Britain, from birth to 16 years. Ingham (1976) has pointed out that "1000 children" is not a precise figure, and that the Andrews and Harris study suffered an approximately one-third attrition of the children for whom data were gathered in the initial phases. With longitudinal studies, attrition is an inevitable problem — illustrating the principle that longitudinal studies have severe problems of biasing sample shrinkage.

The sampling characteristics of the three Sheehan and Martyn studies (Sheehan and Martyn, 1966, 1970; Martyn and Sheehan, 1968) are far superior to those of any longitudinal study anywhere. That is not as bold a claim as it seems. Over time, people die, move away, become uncooperative, or are otherwise inaccessible. For longitudinal studies, this is par for the course. From Ingham's criticism, it would be easy to infer that the Andrews and Harris data were particularly deficient and invalid. But that would be unfair. Theirs is a good study; they merely lost subjects at the going rate for longitudinal studies.

The three Sheehan and Martyn samples (Sheehan and Martyn, 1966, 1970; Martyn and Sheehan, 1968) were uniquely free from sampling bias, for those examined were not treatment-seekers, nor were they those who had selected themselves into a clinic for a problem. Fairness would dictate that while second-guessing the partially retrospective aspects of our studies, critics should at least acknowledge the freedom of our data from clinic bias or sample shrinkage.

As it happens, the Andrews and Harris recovery ratio squares well with the Sheehan and Martyn recovery ratio, even though the data-getting process was totally different. Their reported recovery rate is 80%. Correcting for age differences, and comparing these figures with our Figure 2, it is clear that the principal longitudinal study that does exist reports a recovery rate close to but somewhat higher than our own.

Spontaneous Recovery Studies and Their Implications

Since our data on ages of spontaneous recovery show clearly that many of a group or sample of stutterers are on the verge of recovery from changes in their life situations (Sheehan and Martyn, 1970; Sheehan, 1975), it is almost inevitable that cures are attributed to ongoing therapies that actually have no permanent efficacy. Wischner (1969) posed the issue that the 80% spontaneous recovery figure reported in our research suggested a possible standard against which recoveries during therapy might be evaluated. Methodological problems related to outcome research on stuttering have been thoroughly discussed by Gregory (1969, 1972) in connection with a systematic comparison of modern therapies.

Here are a few of the more salient findings from the growing literature on recovery from stuttering.

1. No authenticated quick cures that hold on follow-up.
2. Recovery has been uniformly shown to be a gradual process.
3. Huge differences exist between those who recover and those who do not, depending upon what they have done about the problem — depending upon the course of action they had taken. How have they tried to cope with their stuttering — by approaching speaking situations or by avoiding them? When we interviewed recovered stutterers, who substantially outnumber active stutterers in a college population, we learned that they had taken some action. They decided that they would "go ahead and take part in life anyway." They somehow reduced what is easily recognizable as "avoidance behavior."

SUMMARY AND CONCLUSIONS

1. Stuttering is a complex problem whose nature forever tempts people to offer simple solutions.
2. Our knowledge of stuttering is still outnumbered by its mysteries. But we do know enough to reject simplistic gimmicks, quick-cure claims, and "success" percentages based on laboratory fluency counts.
3. The problem of stuttering cannot be adequately defined in terms of disfluency counts or speech interruptions.
4. Stuttering is always the problem of a person. Unless we understand the person, we will not understand the problem.
5. In many cases the frequency of stuttering is a trivial fact with reference to the totality of problems the person has.
6. To understand the person, the stuttering behavior is not the only behavior in which we should be interested.
7. Ultimately the person must speak for himself. No one else can do it for him. How effectively he can express himself depends upon the kinds of growth experiences he has had through therapy and through successful role enactments beyond it. He will speak fluently or haltingly, depending upon how he feels toward himself and how he feels toward his listeners.
8. Stuttering commonly begins in a young child communicating upward toward adult authority. Everyone else has more authority than he has.
9. Therapy for a stuttering child must inevitably involve the family, since members of the family are members of the problem. Instead of merely focusing on the child's speech behavior,

the clinician should center on the triadic relationship of mother, father, and child, as well as on related concepts in family therapy.

10. Both in its origins and as an ongoing process, stuttering is best understood as double approach-avoidance conflict, stemming from the role uncertainties of the child, against a predisposing background connected genetically with maleness in a significant number of cases.

11. Social penalties and punishment for stuttering behavior exacerbate and perpetuate the problem for most stutterers.

12. The immediate frequency of stuttering is highly susceptible to change through the introduction of novel or disruptive stimuli. The false, artificial, and temporary fluency that frequently appears has had the effect of hopelessly confounding contingent "punishment" experiments with a built-in artifact.

13. The "Great Divide" in therapy for stuttering is between distraction or avoidance-cultivation techniques, as contrasted with avoidance-reduction or role-acceptance methods. Distraction therapies frequently aim for quick and perfect fluency via "experimental" suppression of stuttering or its anticipation. They have the adverse effect of increasing the stutterer's belief that the moment of stuttering is a horrible event that he must go to great lengths to avoid, while offering essentially no means of coping with future fear and relapse.

14. Distraction or avoidance-cultivation therapies tend to cultivate intolerance for the chance bobbles of normal speech, the disfluencies. Avoidance-reduction therapies aim to promote acceptance of normal disfluencies along with easy, effortless, and nonhandicapping stutterings en route to the banishment of secondary or struggle behaviors.

15. Under avoidance-reduction therapy, a stutterer's eventual success is bounded only by his courage. But distraction therapies waste the stutterer's potential for courage while promoting cowardice and cover-up, for cover-up characterizes the problem and makes it worse.

16. Since only the claims are new, not the methods, the current rash of sensational claims for fluency maintenance, "cure," or "success" reflect not a scientific breakthrough but a deterioration of ethical standards in publication. By the time an independent follow-up can be done, the program has changed and the pea is under a different shell.

17. Avoidance-reduction therapy cannot accurately be called "traditional," for it has never been tried, really tried, on anything like a wide scale. Behavior therapists have called others traditional in an effort to make themselves appear innovative. Yet their methods turn out to be variations of long discarded breath-control techniques that were traditional when Aristotle was a boy. If anything is traditional in stuttering, it is the attempt to suppress.

18. Much of current behavior therapy applied to stuttering follows in the path of assaultive therapies, such as electric shock or tranquilizer dosage, in that they are mechanical methods routinely administered to the person without regard to his life style or individual motivations.

19. "Transfer" is a fallacy, for solid improvement must occur all along during therapy in "outside" situations if it is to occur significantly. To the extent that there is a transfer problem, the therapy has been deficient.

20. Many adult stutterers have already achieved a partial acceptance of their stuttering, a fact that can be built upon as a basis for therapy.

21. Since therapy with stuttering necessarily involves psychotherapy to some degree, it is not too much to ask of the clinician who would work with stutterers that he become reasonably knowledgeable on both subjects. A therapist with such twin knowledge is the best hope of the stutterer.

22. A satisfactory therapy must recognize that stuttering is not a unitary disorder, that stutterers are not interchangeable "subjects" drawn from a homogeneous population, that quick cures or perfection in fluency may not be ethically proffered, that individual motivations and needs differ, and that the ultimate focus of therapy should be the person and his possibilities for self-growth, not just his disfluency rate.

23. The process of recovery from stuttering has now been studied by a sufficient number of investigators so that important conclusions may be drawn. Among these are that recovery is typically a gradual process and that cross-sectional and retrospective studies of recovery may sometimes be methodologically superior to longitudinal studies, because of less sampling bias and the elimination of heavy attrition commonly found in the latter. Moreover, studies of recovery accord well with one another, despite inaccurate reviewer comment to the

contrary. Approximately four-fifths of those who have at some time been diagnosed and considered stutterers recover by the time they reach University of California admission criteria. The vast bulk of these recoveries take place during the adolescent years. Data from Cooper's (1972) Alabama samples on younger subjects are supportive of our ages-of-recovery data. Severe stutterers and those with a family history of stuttering have a lower recovery probability. A most important finding was that huge differences appear between those who remained as stutterers and those who recovered, depending upon the pattern of action taken with respect to the problem. Those who recovered decided to go ahead and speak anyway, even if they stuttered in the process. They refused to let stuttering keep them from taking part in life, and they largely rejected false pretenses that they did not have the problem. Since these behaviors involve reducing avoidance and increasing approach tendencies toward speaking, this most important result, from studies of those who have recovered on their own, provides empirical support for both conflict theory and for avoidance-reduction therapy. Those who have recovered in the absence of therapeutic intervention have provided us a naturally occurring experimental group.

chapter SIX

Empirical Considerations Regarding Stuttering Therapy

Ronald L. Webster, Ph.D.

A HISTORICAL NOTE

This publication was stimulated by a special anniversary symposium presented at the 50th Annual Meeting of the American Speech and Hearing Association. Passage of the first 50 years marks a special time in the development of a discipline. Perhaps we now have sufficient continuity of effort to initiate an assessment of developmental processes that have been and are at work in shaping our form and function. In particular, I wish to examine briefly the relevance of scientific development in the analysis and treatment of stuttering. This preliminary discussion will aid in establishing the point of view from which I am responding to the issues under examination in this book.

Dating from the middle 1600s with formal recognition of the intellectual endeavors designated as science, methods of objective, scientific investigation have been extended from physics and chemistry to the life sciences, and more recently, to behavior. Human behavior has come within the purview of science for about the last 100 years (Boring, 1950). The application of scientific methods to the study of stuttering is a relatively recent endeavor, having a history of around 50 years. This means that we might expect to witness certain characteristics of work on stuttering that are typical of early stages observed previously when methods of science were first applied to new problem areas.

Beginning stages of scientific work may approximate the form of science prior to the emergence of methods that provide substantive empirical and theoretical information. At first, basic constructs in an area are likely to be defined rather loosely. Progress typically occurs when constructs become tied more firmly to empirical observations or are replaced by those which are suitably tied to observables. Improved power in definition leads to improved tests of constructs, and this, in turn, leads eventually to a better quality of scientific knowledge (Stevens, 1939). The essential idea is that reliable, empirical events lie at the heart of scientific methods and scientific constructs. This lesson is one of the most important in the history of science (Butterfield, 1957).

Work on stuttering seems to be representative of early stages in scientific development (Webster, 1974). Our predecessors have done their work well in creating the *form* of science and the beginnings of its substance. They have defined issues, have started the exploration of stuttering, and have begun the structuring of therapeutic methods (Webster, 1977). Contemporary work begins from a favorable vantage point because of the efforts of our forebearers in stuttering research.

While we acknowledge the importance of prior work, we must also accept the fact that our responsibilities lie in continuing to strive for improved knowledge. This means that we ought to examine closely our cherished assumptions and methods and perhaps develop increased sensitivity to their scientific merit. Such a course of action cannot be taken without some threat to what our teachers have so painstakingly learned and taught us. Methods and concepts which we previously accepted may require revision and/or replacement. Knowledge of the history of science should prepare us for this possibility.

I believe it is fair to state that work on stuttering is frequently characterized by a substantial amount of speculation and subjectivity (Webster, 1974). I also believe a reasonable first step in seeking improved knowledge of stuttering is to search for more comprehensive and complete ties between constructs and the observable aspects of stuttering. We are likely to benefit a great deal by improving the rigor, objectivity, and reliability of both our constructs and methods. It appears as if the time has come for a strong, careful, empirical approach to the study of stuttering and to the development of empirically validated therapies for the disorder. The point has been reached where theory for theory's sake cannot be legitimately sustained as a true form of scientific endeavor. There must be a concentrated search for empirical laws that will ultimately create the scientific base from which solid growth can occur.

POINT OF VIEW

Controversy is fueled by two or more sets of divergent ideas which bear upon a common issue. Differences between and among such ideas are typically reducible to differences in methods used for their development or support. Thus, we can suggest that the resolution of controversy is ultimately to be found 1) in the examination of methods from which concepts are derived, and 2) in tests of the scientific adequacy of these methods. My purpose here is not to stimulate controversy, per se, but to excite interest in the issue of methods used in the development of stuttering therapies. I have taken this approach because in my own work I have found that fidelity to the methods of empirical science has been fruitful in elucidating instances of lawfulness within the domain of stuttering.

Sir Francis Bacon once remarked that, "Nature to be commanded must be obeyed." Bacon's observation has considerable contemporary relevance for work on stuttering. One implication is that our methods of therapy should be grounded in the empirical search for lawfulness rather than in theories, the teaching of experts, or subjective clinical experience. My personal bias has been to conduct careful, controlled manipulations of speech response details in an effort to isolate those elements that generate the reliable acquisition and maintenance of fluent speech in individuals designated as stutterers. By searching for and identifying those elements of response which generate fluency, I suggest we are in agreement with Sir Francis' dictum that nature must first be obeyed. When we arrange the results of these studies into a stuttering therapy that reliably leads to the acquisition and subsequent retention of fluent speech, we are beginning to approach the command of nature. I would agree with Sir Francis that the adequacy of our commanding is largely a function of the adequacy with which we have listened to the messages concealed in nature's processes.

My responses to the issues under discussion in this book are based upon my experiences in the development of a detailed objectively based speech reconstruction therapy for stutterers. This therapy has been designated as the Precision Fluency Shaping Program (Webster, 1975b, c). The therapy program is based on a series of operationally defined target behaviors that appear to be antecedents to the production of fluent speech in stutterers. Targets are defined very specifically at the level of articulatory gestures, respiratory responses, and voice onset characteristics. They are taught as elements of response in the context of isolated sounds and syllables and are then instated within the speech flow. Distinctive physical operations define each of the targets and the permissible variances in the targets. Correct sequences of target acquisition and specialized instructional procedures have been arrived at on the basis of substantial empirical testing. Targets link together efficiently and reliably. Therapy procedures are arranged so that clients overlearn target behaviors. At each stage in treatment, the client is aware of those explicit details of response which produce fluent speech. Targets are transferred systematically to a wide range of extra-clinic settings as a normal part of the therapy process. It should be noted that the therapy program is a standardized therapy and is used routinely in the same format for all stutterers. Individual variations in properties of stutterers are accommodated by varying the amount of time clients spend at each therapy segment. Transfer of target behaviors to extra-clinic settings also involves standard procedures that are routinely accomplished by clients in treatment. The therapy program is normally administered over 19 consecutive days. In this time, clients practice their new skills for a total of approximately 100 hours.

A comprehensive report on the Precision Fluency Shaping Program is currently in preparation. A figure has been borrowed from the report for purposes of illustrating results obtained in therapy with this program. Figure 1 represents data summarizing results obtained in a comprehensive study of some 200 randomly selected stutterers. The clients were evaluated with objective assessment procedures 1 year prior to the admission to treatment ($N=100$), at the entry of therapy ($N=200$), at the end of the 3-week therapy program ($N=200$), in a follow-up study conducted an average of 10

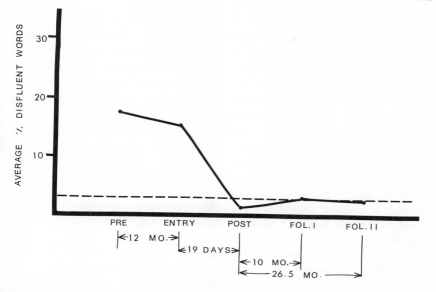

Figure 1.   Mean disfluency scores for participants in the Hollins College Precision Fluency Shaping Program.

months following the completion of therapy ($N=200$), and again 26.5 months following the completion of therapy ($N=100$). The response measure shown in Figure 1 is a count of spoken words on which at least one disfluent event was observed. Results are expressed in terms of the average percentage of words scored disfluent on standard oral reading and conversational tasks. All follow-up samples were derived through surprise telephone calls to clients. While a single figure does not completely describe the results of the program, sufficient information is presented to indicate the base from which I will be responding to the issues under discussion in this book.

A WORKING DEFINITION OF THE STUTTERING COMPLEX

It is axiomatic in science that the unity of nature is probed by isolating, manipulating, and observing those elements within the whole that are of interest and are accessible to the scientist. It is simply not possible to deal successfully with the entirety of nature. This lesson has not been entirely heeded by those who have chosen to study the phenomena of stuttering. There has been a reluctance to adopt even beginning working definitions that fail to deal with "the whole problem" (Beech and Fransella, 1968; Van Riper, 1971a, Webster, 1974). Clearly, it becomes necessary when approaching stuttering from an objective, empirical point of view to establish tentative working definitions that can successfully guide current research efforts and that can be expected in time to yield definitions of greater precision, resolution, and comprehensiveness. Thus, not only must we begin to examine specific components of stuttering, but we must start to make assessments regarding the relative importance of their contributions to the definition of the problem. All aspects of a set of phenomena may not be of equal importance. Again, scientists necessarily must make judgments about the relative significance of events in structuring a problem. With these concepts in mind, I shall summarize the events we regard as relevant to the definition of stuttering, to research on the problem, and to its effective clinical treatment.

A schematic representation of the phenomena that we see organized around the concept of stuttering is presented in Figure 2. This definition of the stuttering complex includes: 1) speech events that are originated by the musculature of the larynx and upper vocal tract and are perceived by external observers as phonatory blockage, prolongations of sounds, and repetitions of sounds, syllables, or words; 2) accessory speech responses that involve struggle with the speech musculature, substitutions, silent stops, starters, and respiratory distortions; 3) accessory nonspeech bodily responses that involve changes in overall muscle tension, postural changes associated with attempts to produce speech, facial posturing, and autonomic nervous system arousal; and 4) the personal reactions of the stutterer to himself and to other individuals. This "hierarchical features" representation of the stuttering complex is consistent with observations made during the development and continued use of our therapy program.

The essential characteristic of this definition is that central features of stuttering are found directly and only in motor events which occur at the level of the larynx and vocal tract. Work on the development of our therapy program has led us to believe that the primary events of stuttered speech involve distorted activities in the muscles involving the onset of voicing and the control of articulatory gestures. The three central features in the complex include phonatory blockage, repetitions, and prolongations. These three types of distorted responses seem to share a common feature in which target positions, response speeds, and forces overshoot

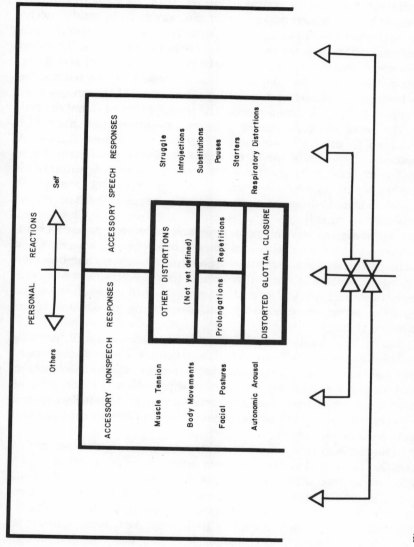

Figure 2.   Organization of the stuttering complex.

normally attained values. Much remains to be learned about the frequency with which these distortions occur and about their specific manifestations. It does appear, however, that work such as that of Freeman (1975), which makes direct measurement of muscle activity, is relevant to improving definitions of distorted events. In addition, work on the development of our therapy program has indicated that target behaviors directly counter the forms of distortion noted. Information about the characteristics of these distorted responses has been generated by manipulating tiny details of speech gestures and identifying their impact upon the propagation of fluent speech.

The presence of the distorted speech events noted cannot yet be accounted for clearly by variables identified at the present time. A reasonable hypothesis would be that organismic properties figure heavily in the determination of stuttered speech. Even though learning is very much involved in the process of therapy via speech reconstruction, it does not seem prudent to assume that the distortions are "learned."

The accessory speech responses and accessory nonspeech responses may very well represent learned behaviors that become tied to the distorted speech gestures. Some information that bears on this interpretation is derived from our therapy program. We commonly observe that accessory behaviors of both types drop out as correct articulatory, phonatory, and respiratory responses are acquired in therapy.

Learning is likely to be involved in the acquisition of personal reactions of the stutterer to himself and others. The great variety of reactions manifested by individual stutterers to their speech distortions would seem to support this interpretation. In addition, as noted later, a tight focus on the reconstruction of distorted speech gestures normally produces positive changes in self-perceptions and relationships with others.

The working definition of the stuttering complex suggested here also implies that the manipulation of peripheral features may in some way feed back to increase or decrease characteristics of the central speech distortions. As an example of this point, we might expect that increases in muscle tension throughout the body might be responsible for increases in the frequency with which distorted speech events occur, and concomitantly, decreases in muscle tension might lead to some reduction in the frequency of stuttered events. In addition, instruction in how to reduce struggle behavior or how to alter respiratory patterns may in turn produce some slight changes in properties of speech production. It seems reasonable to suggest the importance of exploring interactions among various levels of this model. At present, the properties of the hierarchical features representative of the stuttering complex support the merit of working closely and carefully with the distorted events designated as central features. For us, stuttering consists of distorted speech gestures. The stuttering complex refers to central features and the associated features that appear to be organized around them.

STUTTER FLUENTLY VERSUS SPEAK FLUENTLY THERAPIES

My personal preference is for the concept of "speak fluently" therapy. However, I do not see all such therapies as being equally powerful or equally desirable. For example, I am not in favor of trying to reinforce fluency as a class of behavior with praise, M & M's, or pats on the head. Because of my early experiences with such therapies, I no longer favor those which rely on fluency-forcing stimuli, such as delayed auditory feedback, masking, or rhythm. It has been my experience that these therapies have difficulty achieving reliable transfer and retention of normal fluency (Perkins, 1973a, b; Ryan, 1974; Ryan and Van Kirk, 1974a; Webster, 1974; Shames and Egolf, 1976). The probable reason for this difficulty is that the stutterer does not learn enough about those specific aspects of his behavior that actually generate fluent speech. These therapies tend to work with long, complex response chains. Thus, it is difficult for the client to discover what he actually must do to generate fluent responses. I do not mean to rule out the potential of these therapies; however, I think there are problems of focus remaining to be solved. The main drawback, I perceive, is that the definition of response units for successful speech reconstruction has not been adequately carried out. During the development of our therapy program, we attempted to use a delayed auditory feedback based procedure. Eventually, dissatisfaction with "fluent speech" as the operant to be used in therapy stimulated our work on the identification of more basic and potentially more useful response elements. We were successful in this search. Rather small response units now assume the form of targets in our present therapy program.

I prefer the form of therapy that provides the client with a well developed knowledge of fluency targets; correct, structured practice in the acquisition and linking together of targets; and transfer activities that are closely integrated with clinic training. Some of the attributes of such a speech reconstruction procedure seem to be as follows: 1) the client learns a set of responses that yield immediate improvement in fluency; 2) he also discovers that he has control over details of responses that generate fluency and that he can reliably command fluency; 3) the client finds that fluency targets generalize effectively to nonclinic settings and to difficult speech circumstances; 4) usually the client becomes more motivated to work on his speech because he is clearly aware of the progress he is making in therapy; 5) the client and clinician can expect therapy to last for a standard amount of time in most cases; and 6) if the clinician is working on the reconstruction of physical properties in speech, then modern technological developments such as computers can be used to improve the efficiency, accuracy, and reliability of clinic training. Our program now relies on a specialized computer, referred to as the Voice Monitor, to facilitate acquisition of target behaviors by our clients. We have found that the cost effectiveness and reliability of therapy have been substantially enhanced by objective response specification and computer assessment of behaviors being acquired in therapy.

There are several important points of contrast between our current therapy procedures and the methods advocated by those who use "stutter fluently" therapies. Although space restrictions preclude a thorough analysis of these points, a series of brief statements will suffice to establish the essential nature of the contrasts.

It has been common practice in "stutter fluently" therapies to emphasize the client's study of his disfluent speech as a condition of therapy. In our treatment program, all efforts are directed toward the stable use of fluency-generating target behaviors that involve details of respiration, voicing, and articulation. The goal in therapy is to bring speech gestures to target values and thereby propagate fluent speech. We have found that time allocated to the examination of disfluent speech is time removed from our therapeutic process. Although knowledge of targets may be facilitated by familiarizing clients with properties of their disfluent speech, we have not witnessed evidence that supports this notion.

There is another contrast to be found between treatment procedures of "stutter fluently" therapies that emphasize the assumed identification of what each individual "needs" and the development of a well standardized treatment program. It has been our experience that when the behavioral analysis that defines the essential responses to be at the focus of therapy is incomplete, then there is necessarily an emphasis on identifying "needs" of each individual. This apparent requirement for meeting individual needs can be attributed to deficiencies in what is in fact taught during therapy. The clinician, aware of deficiencies in client performance, searches for more useful information. The high frequency of client self-reference to attitudes and feelings encourages exploration of such dimensions. The symptoms of client personal discomfort are likely to be varied and possibly interesting. The clinician is almost automatically drawn into the attempted analysis of the client's individual needs. If indeed there are core features to stuttering, and if these core features share certain common characteristics across stutterers, then we might expect to find that a standardized treatment procedure would be effective with a larger number of stutterers than other forms of therapy. In the development of our program we have found that individual variations within the therapy process are largely tied to the amount of behavior a given client must learn, his diligence in practicing and monitoring those behaviors being learned, and his ability to observe details of his own muscle gestures. Individual differences are readily accommodated within a standardized therapy by adjusting the amount of time each individual spends at given stages in the therapeutic process.

There is another contrast related to the previous point. A rather dominant belief exists among the proponents of "stutter fluently" therapy that rapid acquisition of fluency leads to rapid failure of fluency (Van Riper, 1973). I think this belief represents a rather impressive overgeneralization and does not take into account the practical power of new methods involved in the establishment of fluency. We have found that 19 carefully structured, consecutive days of treatment provide a standard interval that is effective with a large majority of cases. While not all individuals can be expected to complete the program in a standard interval, it is reasonable to expect more than 90% of the cases to complete therapy in this standard interval.

There is still another contrast that involves a recurrent theme in the "stutter fluently" therapies. In all fairness, the theme is not restricted only to "stutter fluently" therapies but is also found in the work of some of the behaviorally oriented clinicians (Brutten and Shoemaker, 1967). It is reasonable to suggest that a component of therapy might involve desensitization as part of the overall process. I cannot agree with those individuals who repeatedly stress the potential role of anxiety as an enhancing factor in stuttering. In fact, from the current experimental base of our therapy program, it seems as if the issue of additional therapy involving desensitization procedures as a corollary to fluency training represents a superfluous issue. We are discovering that when the client has achieved control over fluency-generating targets, he can normally speak fluently in spite of fears, anxieties, and life stresses. I believe the move to supplemental desensitization methods as part of fluency training is unnecessary. Inadequate knowledge of how to generate viable fluency patterns with techniques in use could motivate a search for other therapy variables. I would encourage the search to be directed toward enhanced knowledge of responses involved in speech production. It has taken my colleagues and me a long time to recognize the primacy of the central features of the stuttering complex previously remarked upon in this chapter. It has also taken a substantial amount of time, effort, and relearning to develop sensitivity to nuances of response that are normally not attended to in traditional approaches. I cannot stress too heavily the potential merit of studying observable behaviors.

An additional contrast between the "speak fluently" and "stutter fluently" approaches involves the possibility that there is an overemphasis on fluency in the former approaches. Certainly, this represents a logical possibility and requires examination. I believe that an emphasis on fluency would indeed be strongly misplaced if the clinician asked the client to speak fluently and, in fact, did not provide tools of sufficient power to help him attain that goal. I must report that during my early work with stuttering, I had a very strong emphasis on "fluent speech" as the response to be modified and enhanced in therapy. The practical deficiencies in this level of response specification soon led to efforts to find more satisfactory response units for use in therapy. As a result of developing the target concept, and as a result of empirically tested instructional methods, we have evidence that we are providing clients with tools that are effective in producing fluency. The tools are the target behaviors that propagate fluent speech. The focus in therapy is upon targets, not upon fluency. Targets represent very specific response elements that can be discriminated readily, learned well, and generalized on a practical basis into everyday life.

There is an additional comment I would like to make with respect to the issue of "stutter fluently" versus "speak fluently" therapies. This comment does not involve a contrast, but instead represents a report on our experiences with our current therapy program. Even in the instance when little progress is shown by a client in therapy, we usually observe that the quality as well as the quantity of disfluencies has changed substantially. Usually, we find that disfluencies are reduced in number and those that occur are less pronounced and involve much less physical effort than they did prior to treatment. Thus, my point is that even when this form of "speak fluently" therapy does not live up to our expectations, it may achieve the level of performance which is sought in the "stutter fluently" therapies.

I believe it is useful to once more comment upon the importance of method in analyzing various therapeutic approaches. There is one essential procedure that will rapidly lead to the definition of effective therapeutic practices: the systematic development of standard forms of speech performance and self-report data from stutterers prior to treatment, following treatment, and again in follow-up studies. Without an increasingly developed sense of professional responsibility in providing our peers with objective data regarding the outcome of therapy, we are doomed to live forever within the jungle of opinion. No science can long endure under such conditions.

ATTITUDE CHANGE: WHAT IS IT AND IS IT NEEDED?

The methodological issues involving attitude manipulation in therapy require careful examination. There are formidable technical problems in measuring attitudes and in determining their relationships to overt actions (Anastasi, 1976). It is incumbent upon those who stress the importance of attitude change procedures to demonstrate the relationship of such procedures to the efficacy of therapeutic practice. It is not clear to me that this has been accomplished in the existing literature (Van Riper, 1973; Bloodstein, 1975b). Advances in the understanding of issues, such as the role of attitude change in therapy, are eventually dependent upon the demonstrated results of such manipulations. Assumptions about the importance of attitude change in therapy may have substantial face validity; nonetheless, documentation of the role of attitudes is a requisite condition if scientific advances are to occur.

If stuttering therapy is sharp in its focus on speech details, properly comprehensive in its choice of physical responses to be changed, and suitably administered, then the issue of attitude change as an active component in therapy may be largely tangential to the main course of treatment. Attitudes, emotional responses, and self-perceptions of stutterers could be determined by the fact that these individuals display certain characteristic forms of speech disruption. If this is the case, it follows that if we can establish reliable patterns of normal speech fluency, we should expect to see positive changes along attitudinal dimensions, even if there are no direct attempts made to shift attitudes. The definition of the stuttering complex provided earlier in this chapter shows this as a possible outcome. My observations on fairly large numbers of stutterers treated with our program lend credence to this hypothesis. Our therapy program deals directly with the details of speech production and does not involve systematic attempts to manipulate attitudinal characteristics.

Some data bear on this point. We administered the Adjective Check List (Gough and Heilbrun, 1965) to 100 stutterers immediately before and again at the end of therapy. At the end of therapy, results obtained in fluency measures were comparable to those shown in Figure 1. Attitudinal factors shifted markedly as a function of therapy. Significant (0.01 level) changes occurred on 15 of the 24 scales. Two additional scales showed changes significant at the 0.05 level. It is important to note that the direction of these changes was positive in all cases. For example, the number of favorable adjectives increased, the number of unfavorable adjectives decreased, and scores improved on self-confidence, self-control, personal adjustment, achievement, endurance, nurturance, affiliation, and autonomy.

We have also collected self-report data with the Perceptions of Stuttering Inventory (PSI), a 60-item checklist developed by Professor Gerald Woolf (1967). The PSI gives information on struggle, avoidance, and expectancy behaviors. The reliability of PSI scores is quite good. An analysis of 100 PSI scores randomly drawn from pretreatment testing of stutterers showed split-half reliability of 0.93 for the total test. Stability of PSI scores over time was also quite good. Another sample of 100 pretreatment cases was analyzed with a mean interval of 9.5 months between first and second administrations of the PSI. The correlation between total test scores was 0.72, a respectable value for the long intertest interval involved.

We administered the PSI to 200 stutterers before treatment, immediately at the end of treatment, and in a follow-up study conducted an average of 10 months after the completion of therapy. Before treatment, only three stutterers showed PSI total scores in the normal range (10 or below). This constituted 1.5% of the population studied. At the end of the treatment program, 89% of the cases had PSI scores of 10 or below, and in the follow-up studies, 72% of the cases maintained PSI scores of 10 or below. Adjective Check List and Perceptions of Stuttering Inventory data suggest that clients experienced rather profound attitudinal and emotional changes as a function of acquiring improved speech fluency.

At the time the follow-up study was conducted on these 200 cases, a questionnaire was also answered. Ninety-three percent of the cases reported more confidence in their speech than they had prior to treatment, and 80% of them indicated that they had more self-confidence. Clinical observations indicated that there was an increase in the sociability of clients, a greater tendency to express ideas, and a much greater willingness to undertake activities that were previously closed off because of stuttering (i.e., returning to school, changing jobs, participating in public speaking courses).

We normally see substantial changes in attitudes that appear to be propagated by processes of the speech reconstruction program. I think it is fair to suggest that there is tentative evidence for the hypothesis that attitudes, emotions, and self-perception are symptoms of stuttering. Therapies which direct their attention toward properties of attitudes as primary components in treatment may very well be providing a "symptomatic" form of treatment.

PSYCHOTHERAPY FOR STUTTERERS: WHAT IS IT, IS IT NEEDED, AND IF SO, HOW IS IT DONE?

I find it very difficult to respond in an affirmative way to the issue of psychotherapy. There is a serious lack of reliable and valid outcome data that might serve to implicate the relevance of psychotherapy for the treatment of stuttering. There are a great many psychotherapies. I see no clear evidence, based on my work with stutterers or derived from my reading of the literature, that would suggest the need for *any* form of psychotherapy as a standard component in the treatment of stuttering. I have a feeling that psychotherapy, as part of stuttering therapy, is likely to serve a greater number of needs for the clinician than for the client.

I also have serious concerns about the legitimacy of attempted psychotherapy by clinicians who normally have little or no formal supervised training in the conduct of such procedures. The use of possibly irrelevant procedures by poorly trained clinicians cannot bode well for either the client or the profession. There is also a substantial possibility that clients may have their motivation to seek therapy reduced by negative results of psychotherapeutic efforts.

It would be cavalier to discount completely the possible role of psychotherapy because it might be relevant to some individuals who stutter. Certainly, investigators should be free to search in all areas for new knowledge. However, I would suggest that there is a very great need to recognize that we may not have explored sufficiently those avenues of treatment that have a direct impact upon the production of speech. Until it is clear that deficiencies in speech reconstruction procedures are largely responsible for deficiencies in therapy outcome, I believe it is unwise to adopt an alternative procedure based on psychotherapy. One rarely progresses in the analysis of nature's problems by employing levels of observation that lead to reduced objectivity and decreased resolution of observation.

STUTTERING THERAPY FOR CHILDREN

I have relatively little to say about stuttering therapy for the young child. My colleagues and I have not studied the developmental aspects of stuttering. We have had experience in working with children between the ages of 5 and 12 years. These children, about 30 in number, have shown disfluent word scores ranging from 3% to 67% and PSI scores ranging up to 39 out of a possible 60. Children seem to acquire fluency skills quite readily when the tasks are made simple enough for them. We use procedures of the Precision Fluency Shaping Program with simplified instructions and therapy materials keyed to the verbal skill levels of the children. Our results are comparable to those achieved with adults. For a random sample of 23 children, the mean pretherapy disfluent word frequency was 17.5% and the mean posttreatment disfluent word score was 1.2%. All PSI scores after therapy were 10 or under, and 15 of the 18 were at 5 or below.

I believe careful, tight focus speech reconstruction therapy is particularly appropriate for young stutterers. However, work with children must be done using a light touch and with a great deal of attention to providing positive feedback to the child as he is working with fluency skills. We normally require that one of the child's parents attend a sampling of therapy sessions and learn how to provide support for the child who is acquiring fluency skills. We have also found that children respond well to the use of the Voice Monitor in therapy. Computer assessment of speech characteristics and feedback of information serve to sustain children's motivational levels in treatment and enhance their independent use of target behaviors.

TRANSFER OF FLUENT SPEECH TO THE NATURAL ENVIRONMENT AND POSTTREATMENT RETENTION OF FLUENT SPEECH

Transfer of behavior changes to extra-clinical environments and the maintenance of such behavior changes following a treatment program represent topics of substantial significance. In this area in particular, methodological adequacy is requisite. The relative merit of different therapy procedures for producing transfer and maintenance of behavior change must be established with procedures that are both reliable and valid. In addition, we must be particularly sensitive to the nature of interpretations that are made regarding observed results and their possible relationship to therapy procedures. The importance of quantification in attaining these goals is not to be underestimated.

The topic of discrimination has been studied as a dynamic behavioral process by researchers in the area of learning. Highly specific procedures have been created for probing and explicating different facets of discriminative processes. A related behavioral process, generalization, has been treated historically as a passive event which more or less just happens. Attention has recently been given to the possibility that generalization is also an active process that can be differentially influenced by specific experimental manipulations. Stokes and Baer (1977) call attention to developing techniques for facilitating transfer of behaviors from one environment to another. In their initial description of generalization technologies, Stokes and Baer list nine general headings. These technologies range from the simplistic approach of "train and hope" to more sophisticated procedures which involve specialized training in how to generalize. The body of literature reviewed by Stokes and Baer supports a suggestion that the problem of transfer in stuttering might very well be examined in terms of the adequacy of the underlying technologies embodied in the therapy program. The concept of "preparedness" as discussed by Seligman (1970) may also be relevant in the search for basic response units to use in therapy and for the development of specific transfer technologies.

Our experience in the development of the Precision Fluency Shaping Program has indicated that rather specific technological considerations are significant for attaining effective transfer and long-term maintenance of fluent speech. Our work to date suggests that success in transferring fluency to everyday speaking situations and the ability to sustain fluent speech after the completion of therapy are a direct function of the client's explicit knowledge of *what he does* to generate fluent utterances. Some years ago, when we were working with delayed auditory feedback-prolongation therapy, we had substantial difficulty in identifying activities that would increase transfer of fluency from clinic to outside settings. Each client appeared to respond to different efforts to implement transfer. We began to speculate that a "menu" of transfer techniques might be required as part of therapy (Webster, 1974). This did not work out well.

We later developed a new perspective on the matter of transfer. After observing clients in transfer and listening to their reports, we grew to suspect that the existing transfer technology was not well matched to the overall requirements of therapy. We also began to recognize the possibility that the fundamental events in our therapy were not matched to the learning capabilities of our clients. Client reports repeatedly indicated that instability in transfer performances was attributable to deficiencies in knowledge of what to do in order to speak fluently. It seemed as if clients in transfer were trying to recreate the physical sensations they experienced during therapy, but were unable to identify and sustain the relevant responses. As we explored this problem a breakthrough of sorts occurred in the structure of therapy that had important implications for transfer. When our behavioral analyses of the skills to be learned in therapy began to isolate small, identifiable response components at the level of speech gestures, the target concept emerged. As we learned about target definitions and the sequences involved in the assembly of targets into fluent speech, we simultaneously developed a technology for transfer that became part of the existing therapy program. We refer to this technology as the "parallel transfer process." Fluency targets are taught one by one at the level of sounds and syllables and are stabilized in the clinic. A series of very simple transfer steps is included in the client's training with each of the targets. Thus, the client learns a small number of readily discriminable response elements that are generalized one at a time to nonclinic settings. As therapy progresses the elements are blended together systematically in the speech flow and more complex transfer activities are introduced. The integration of target and transfer training means that the client is never asked to move suddenly to the use of a new and complex speech pattern in situations that are likely to interfere with his ability to attend to the act of speaking. By the time targets are used in the speech flow at normal rates, the client has already become proficient in transferring them to various settings. We have found that it is not necessary to have a menu of transfer routines that are attempted on a trial-and-error basis in an effort to find a match with what a given client might require. The standard transfer procedures are used with all clients and are the most reliable methods with which we have had experience.

I believe I can say with some reliability now, whenever there are problems in achieving fluency from our clinic to outside settings, it is most often because we have misinstructed the client. The failure is quite likely to be in the application of method rather than in basic properties of the method itself. The accuracy of target-training procedures must be maintained throughout therapy. More information on this topic appears later in this section. I reiterate the point that if the primary characteristics of stuttering are to be found in speech gestures, transfer from therapy to extra-therapy settings is more likely to be achieved by a specific transfer technology that takes into account the nature of response details being learned in treatment.

Much of what we see in current efforts to achieve transfer in stuttering therapy seems to reduce to variations on the "train and hope" method. A great deal remains to be achieved in the development of technologies for attaining transfer. I do have one comment about a developing trend in some stuttering therapies. There seems to be a tendency to segment the treatment of stuttering into a therapy component and a long-term transfer component. It is misleading to then talk about the results of therapy in an affirmative manner and to discuss transfer as a separate and muted problem. If the therapeutic processes are sufficiently powerful, therapy should ultimately prove to be a one-time event for most stutterers and transfer should be a normal component of the process.

While it is easy to overgeneralize, I think it is fair to suggest that any type of therapy that is going to improve speech fluency

Table 1. Percentage of clients retaining normal disfluency scores in reading and conversation measures 10 months posttherapy and percentage of clients receiving supplemental treatment for four different clinicians

	Percentage of clients (normal range)	Percentage of clients returned for refresher training
Clinician A	43	44
Clinician B	65	39
Clinician C	69	23
Clinician D	81	11

must either directly or indirectly serve to mo.⁄e the physical properties of the stutterer's utterances toward the target values appropriate for fluent speech. My bias is to suggest that the direct, careful manipulation of speech details represents what is potentially a reliable and efficient approach to attaining positive long-term therapeutic results.

Given the fact that the primary focus of our therapy program is upon responses to be learned by stutterers, it is reasonable to expect that there will be some relapse based on forgetting of skills, interference among responses learned, or inferior learning in therapy. If the behavioral analysis that precedes development of a therapy program correctly identifies the critical response elements to be learned in treatment, then the problem of developing technologies for generalization and maintenance of fluent speech can be identified and dealt with more effectively than if these conditions are not met. A report of some of our experiences may be relevant here.

The problem of relapse in our clients seems to be related to at least several specifiable variables. The first factor has to do with how well we trained the person in the use of fluency targets during treatment. In the case of this variable, the technical competence of the clinician in knowing target values and permissible tolerances for targets, as well as the adequacy of instruction sets, is highly important. Table 1 presents a summary of observations made with respect to the variable of clinician competence and the issue of relapse following our therapy. Four different clinicians are represented in this summary. Each of the clinicians treated a total of at least 32 clients in the same working environment. At the time these data were collected, clients had been out of therapy for an average of approximately 10 months. The disfluency measures were average scores obtained from oral reading and conversational speech samples collected through surprise telephone calls to the clients.

Details of data-collecting procedures appear elsewhere in this chapter. Note the substantial differences in results obtained by the clinicians. If you were a stutterer who had chosen to participate in this specific therapy program and you had freedom of choice with respect to the clinician who would work with you, whom would you choose? The data suggest it would be wise to choose clinician D. I should note that the differentiating variables with respect to the efficacy of the clinicians in using the program were in the area of technical competence. Based on assessments by the author, the clinicians were rank ordered rather neatly in terms of their knowledge of targets, target tolerances, and instructional clarity.

As a result of 4 years of work on training clinicians, we have been able to develop a structured training program that keys on those specific elements in our therapy that require specialized professional skills. The development and empirical validation of clinicians' training programs are of substantial significance if we are to obtain widespread dissemination of any effective stuttering therapy.

I feel very strongly that the definition of clinician technical competence has been given insufficient attention in the development and dissemination of stuttering therapies. Textbooks, lectures, and clinical observation may, in fact, not do enough to facilitate the high level technical competence that is probably required for reliably effective stuttering therapy. We should be prepared for the likely possibilities that: 1) the objective definition of technical competence for a given therapy will require substantial research, and 2) specific technologies will be required for the efficient development of relevant technical skills. The test of these points will be in the adequacy of performances manifested in stutterers treated by clinicians whose training embodies the concepts just noted.

The points just made regarding clinician technical competency do not represent idle speculation about how things might be. We have now trained approximately 125 speech clinicians with different versions of the training course. We have repeatedly tested and revised training materials and methods in an effort to improve clinician technical competencies. Revisions have been guided by the results of tests during training and also by measures of speech performance and client self-report data collected from cases treated by clinician trainees. At the present time there are two forms of the clinicians' training program. The first is a 3-week course conducted at Hollins College in parallel with the stuttering therapy program.

The second is an intensive 5-day course. Approximately 100–120 training hours are involved in the former course and approximately 40 hours are required for the latter course. Both courses are effective in bringing clinicians to the minimum skill levels necessary for beginning use of our therapy. The longer training program provides the trainee with an opportunity actually to observe cases in treatment and to participate in the administration of the program. The definition of relevant, objectively specifiable clinician skills and the development of effective training technologies are demanding of substantial time and effort, both on the part of researchers who conduct the basic work and on the part of those who participate in the training. This is not a minor point. Clinicians who have not been instructed in use of our program have not been able to use it effectively.

Let us return to the issue of relapse. It is also clear to us that client regression toward pretreatment disfluency levels is not entirely attributable to a lack of clinician technical competence. Another factor that enters into relapse has to do with the client losing discrimination of target details. Targets involve subtle aspects of gestures in respiration, voicing, and articulation. If the client loses the discrimination of given targets, regression toward disfluency will occur. Several targets are likely to be poorly discriminated before serious retrogression occurs. We have found that in most cases fairly short periods of additional training can usually overcome the effects of lost discriminations. Refresher training for stutterers who have minor problems normally can be completed in from 1 to 3 days.

Relapse also occurs in some individuals who decide after they finish therapy that additional practice is simply not necessary. In these cases, it is possible that the amount of effort required to sustain fluency with our current technology is too great. Finally, there are a few stutterers who apparently derive social benefits from stuttering and who decide not to use fluent speech. The number of such cases, in my experience, is very small, but, nonetheless, this factor is relevant when the issue of relapse is discussed.

CRITERIA FOR SUCCESS IN
STUTTERING THERAPY: THE RESULTS OF THERAPY

Science advances as a function of the improvement in observational power and the increased application of quantitative methods. The history of work on the evaluation of stuttering therapy is weak in both reports of high resolution observation and the effective use and quantification (Van Riper, 1971a, 1973; Ingham and Andrews, 1973). Progress in research on stuttering and the evaluation of therapy outcomes may be expected to occur as more adequate procedures are developed for obtaining answers to the classic questions of science: How many? Of what magnitude? Of what kind? Under what conditions?

The usual assessment of stuttering is made through the direct perceptual processing of an observer. Different processing levels are available that range from overall subjective estimates of severity based on properties of speech, nonspeech responses, and client reports (Van Riper, 1958) to detailed counts of speech and speech-related events by class (Brutten and Shoemaker, 1967). Subjective verbal descriptions yield information that is primarily applicable to a nominal scale of measurement. Even though attempts are often made to use subjective estimates of severity, the lack of meaningful, objective anchor points and the unknown properties of observer reliability render the procedure of little use for either research or serious clinical purposes. Highly differentiated descriptive methods that attempt to measure all potential relevant aspects of stuttering pose different problems. There are practical difficulties encountered in observing so many details of behavior with relatively large numbers of stutterers (as may be required in evaluating the effects of therapies), observer reliability for many categories of responses must be determined, and much of the data collected may be only incidentally related to the evaluation of central features of stuttering.

A practical, meaningful, and reliable measure of central features in stuttered speech can be obtained through frequency counts of disfluent events which occur in association with standard speech units. Response frequency is a common and useful dependent variable measure in behavioral research (McGuigan, 1968; Hersen and Barlow, 1976). Frequency is also one of the most widely reported indexes of stuttering severity (Van Riper, 1971a).

The primary response measure used in our work has been the number of words on which at least one disfluent event was observed. Disfluent events include struggle with speech onset, silent stops followed by audible struggle, forced breathing, and repetitions of sounds, syllables, or words. Words omitted from reading passages, substitutions within reading passages, and words in repetitions of phrases or whole sentences are also scored disfluent. A reliable measurement procedure can be established by scoring *all* instances of disfluency and avoiding the selection of assumed "stuttering disfluencies" and the rejection of assumed "normal disfluencies." This measure is reliable, can be obtained easily with large behavior samples, and co-varies well with clinical estimates of stuttering severity. Our clinic staff members routinely yield agreement scores on total frequencies of 95% and over. Words common to the scoring of two independent, trained observers is normally over 90%. Clinicians in training quickly reach these levels of scorer reliability. Disfluency scores are derived from standard 500-word reading passages and from the first 300–500 words spoken during standard interviews. Speech rates are also determined.

The choice of behaviors and procedures to be used in the assessment of stuttering therapy presents a difficult problem. For example, a clinician is generally not in a position to use a procedure that might be desirable, such as collecting continuous records of client speech on a long-term daily basis. The real-time, continuous tracking of human behavior requires technologies that are not commonly available. The next best step involves some form of client behavior sampling that relies on standardized methods. Behavior sampling requires an inference that the client is showing "typical" behaviors at the time of sampling. The reliability of this inference can be estimated by repeated sampling of the same cases under the same circumstances or by sampling a large number of different cases under the same conditions. If measures made under the same conditions cluster together and if the frequency distributions of the measures have similar forms, then there is reason to believe that under those specific conditions the behavior samples are reliable. Thus, to provide effective assessment of stuttering, clinicians must determine both scorer reliability of disfluent events and behavior reliability.

In our own work we have chosen to make repeated measures on large numbers of stutterers under a variety of conditions. An example of these points is represented in Figure 3. Frequency distributions of average disfluency scores for reading and conversation for 100 stutterers are shown 12 months before treatment and again at entry to therapy. The preentry mean score was 17.3% and the entry mean score was 15.6%. Medians were 14.3% and 11.2%, respectively. It should be noted that the frequency distributions were similar even though the measures were made many months apart and under different circumstances. Preentry measures were derived from tape-recorded speech samples made by clients in their home environments. Entry measures were made in our clinic on the day

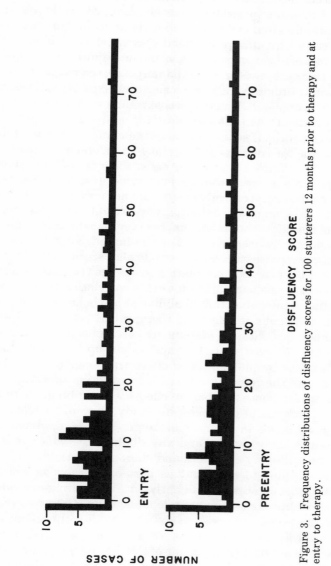

Figure 3.   Frequency distributions of disfluency scores for 100 stutterers 12 months prior to therapy and at entry to therapy.

therapy was to begin. The Pearson r for these scores was $+0.68$. All stutterers in the original sample remained stutterers a year later. While there were slight variations in level of stuttering, the essential properties of the group remained very much the same.

An additional example is shown in Figure 4. Frequency distributions are shown for 200 randomly selected cases at the end of our therapy program and again an average of 10 months after therapy was completed. The respective means were 1.3% and 3.2% disfluent words. The medians were 0.5% and 1.3%, respectively. Posttreatment measures were made in the clinic on the day following the last day of treatment. All follow-up behavior samples were made through surprise telephone calls. Clients had no time to prepare for the reading and interview tasks presented. Almost all calls were made by staff members who had not treated the clients involved. In this manner, potentially powerful stimulus control variables of the clinic that might have served to enhance the production of fluent speech were reduced or eliminated. There was a close agreement between posttherapy and follow-up scores. The Pearson r was $+0.43$. This is a good correlation given the truncated distributions involved in the computation of this correlation coefficient. It is reasonable to infer that the reliability of the behavior sampled is quite good and that the effects of therapy had been well retained. More detailed, quantitative statements can be made by comparing characteristics of posttreatment and follow-up measures for individual cases or by plotting cumulative frequency curves (Figure 5). Inspection of the cumulative frequency curve permits determination of the approximate numbers of clients who retain given fluency levels. For example, in the follow-up study, 78% of the clients retained fluency levels in the normal range. That is, disfluent word counts were at or below 3% and any disfluencies which occurred tended to be relatively effortless and short in duration.

It is important to note that as part of therapy we normally observe our clients speaking fluently in a wide range of outside situations including classrooms, telephone calls (100 or more calls as part of the transfer process), in speeches before other clients, and in stores or other local businesses. As noted earlier, intensive outside transfer is a routine component of the therapy program. Clients progress from very simple activities to more complex activities as they move through the transfer sequences. Success with simple transfer tasks is requisite for advancement to difficult tasks. While we have not attempted to use covert recording procedures, our ob-

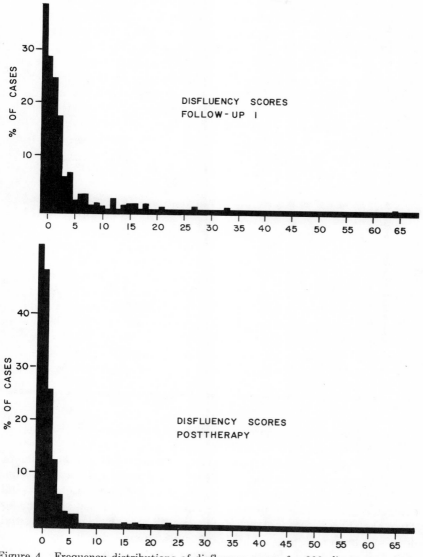

Figure 4. Frequency distributions of disfluency scores for 200 clients at end of therapy and 10 months posttherapy.

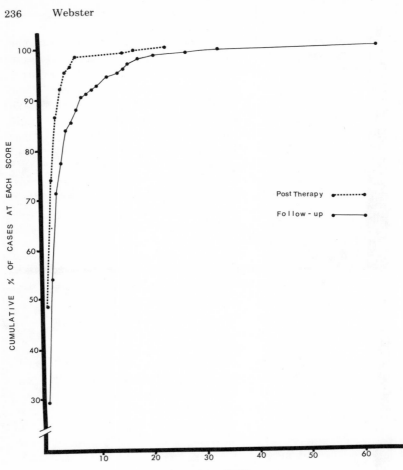

Figure 5. Cumulative distribution curves for disfluency scores for 200 clients at the end of therapy and 10 months posttherapy.

servations and the reports of others indicate that the transfer of fluent speech is successfully made even to stressful speaking situations outside the clinic. We do not mean to imply here that all clients are 100% fluent in transfer, but in the majority of the cases they are able to demonstrate fluent speech that is clearly at normal levels in both ordinary and difficult speaking circumstances.

The overall reliability of therapy effects can be enhanced or diminished by systematically derived client self-report data. If there is agreement among speech performance measures, self-report data derived from standard instruments, and third-person observations, then the reliability (and concomitantly, the validity) of the therapeutic process is enhanced. For example, PSI scores were obtained on the 200 clients already mentioned in this chapter (Figures 1, 3, 4, 5). The pretreatment mean PSI score was 30.4, the posttreatment PSI mean score was 5.7, and the follow-up PSI mean score was 9.2. The substantial drop in expectancy, avoidance, and struggle scales supports the findings shown by speech performance measures. In addition, third-person reports from wives, husbands, and employers generally confirm high level performance when PSI scores, self-report information derived from questionnaires, and speech performance measures cluster in the normal range. When either speech performance measures or PSI scales are outside the normal range, third-person reports generally confirm instability in the use of target behaviors which generate fluent speech.

When multiple response measures and repeated response measures yield the same general findings, an inductive schema is established. The concatenation of specific, diverse instances of lawfulness in dependent variable measures adds to the probability that the overall therapy effects are in fact what they seem to be (McGuigan, 1968). The permissible inference from the data discussed in this chapter is that most treated clients have demonstrated shifts from a position on the disfluent side of the fluency-disfluency continuum to a position on the fluent side of the continuum and have remained at approximately the same location on this continuum with the passage of a substantial interval of time. All indications are that for approximately 75–80% of the cases the magnitude of the stuttering handicap has been reduced to a low level.

There is a great deal more information that is generally relevant in assessing the overall efficacy of a stuttering therapy program. The characteristics of a given therapy can be further described by noting the number of clients who drop out of the therapy program during the interval studied. In our program, during the interval covered by the study of 200 cases, three individuals failed to complete the program. One might reasonably ask for the number of clients who seek additional therapy with the same program and the number contacted in follow-up studies who have sought other forms of therapy. In our study of 200 clients we found that 16.5% of them sought refresher training with us and 0.5% sought another form of therapy. The proportion of clients available for follow-up study is also of interest. During the interval covered in the study noted here,

323 stutterers were treated by our professional staff members. Complete data were obtained on 200 clients at the time the study was terminated, and incomplete data had been obtained on approximately half of the remaining cases. Characteristics of incomplete data were not noticeably different from those of the completed cases.

Therapy is also properly evaluated in economic terms. The comparison of both the real dollar costs of therapy and the results obtained permit rough determinations of the cost effectiveness of a given therapy. This becomes a most important topic in terms of today's economy. The replicability of therapy results is also important. If therapy results are clinician specific, the general applicability of a program might be extremely limited. If, on the other hand, the details of method are generalizable across other trained clinicians, then evidence is provided for the efficacy of the method. We are finding that clinicians are replicating our results.

I believe it is extremely important to note that, at best, the current level of stuttering therapy evaluation is exceedingly primitive. It will probably remain at this level until such time as we have available instrument-based procedures for assessing the nature of specific distortions found in the speech of stutterers. The development of a "speech microscope" and associated data analysis procedures should be a matter of high priority in research on stuttering and in the development of more effective diagnostic and treatment procedures. It is quite likely that relatively minor advances will be made without the development and rather widespread use of objectively based response-measuring apparatus. It would be premature to settle for current methods used for the assessment of stuttering therapy, even when the very best available methods are used.

FINAL COMMENT

I want to end my discussion of the issues by calling attention to a brief description of technological development in medical treatment presented by Dr. Lewis Thomas, president of the Sloan Kettering Cancer Center in New York, in his book *The Lives of a Cell* (1974). The first level of development is what Thomas refers to as "nontechnology." At this level, efforts of practitioners are directed toward comforting, reassuring, and in other ways providing support for patients. Treatment approaches are usually quite varied and not particularly effective. The practitioner must be a strong individual, for there are many more defeats than victories in treatment with therapies at this level.

The second level of technology represents what Thomas calls a "halfway technology." Here fairly reliable compensatory efforts are made with various maladies. For example, he mentions heart surgery, organ replacement, and irradiation treatment for cancer as such halfway technologies. Great skill and substantial resources are frequently required to achieve correction or compensation for the basic disorder. There is enhanced reliability in treatment at this level, but costs are relatively high and well trained specialists are necessary for employment of the technology.

The third level of technology represents for Thomas a "decisive technology." At this level, methods are characterized by comprehensive knowledge of causal factors behind disease entities. Here he includes methods of immunization against diphtheria and polio and the decisive technologies for treating bacterial infections such as syphilis and tuberculosis. He points out that at this level of technology, effectiveness of treatment is quite good, costs of treatment fall, and time for treatment is much reduced. He also adds that there are relatively few treatment procedures that have attained this level.

It would seem to me in making a candid assessment of development of work in stuttering that our first 50 years have been spent largely at the level of nontechnology. This is not to be interpreted as a pejorative comment; it simply describes an epoch in the history of work on stuttering. I think there is clear evidence that we are moving toward halfway technology. Halfway technology, while less than perfect, represents a step in the right direction. Often the work with halfway technology provides groundwork necessary for the eventual attainment of a comprehensive understanding of a problem.

chapter SEVEN

A Perspective on Approaches to Stuttering Therapy

Dean E. Williams, Ph.D.

The purpose of this chapter is to discuss my views about the nature of stuttering and of stuttering therapy in relation to the questions posed by Gregory in Chapter One. It is obvious that the questions are interrelated and that a person's general orientation toward the problem of stuttering will determine the thrust of the discussion for all of them. Therefore, before discussing the questions posed, I will state some important assumptions about the nature of stuttering that affect my approach to therapy.

ASSUMPTIONS

Assumption 1

The stuttering problem we are concerned with here begins in early childhood (Williams, 1978d). It develops as a negative reaction by the child to disfluencies while speaking (Williams, 1971, 1978a). The form of the negative reaction is one of "trying not to" talk wrong and/or of "trying to keep from" talking wrong. From this coping approach there develops a general orientation toward talking of "What can I do to *not stutter*?" instead of "What can I *do to talk*?"

Assumption 2

The behavior of stuttering is purposeful. It is done by stutterers because they believe it "helps to get the word out." Or, said in another way, they believe they have to do it in order to say the word. The struggling behavior is not involuntary in the same sense that it is "out of control" and hence must run its course regardless of what the person does. This can be tested in two ways. First, stutterers can be given the following instructions: "When you begin to stutter, stop doing what you are doing. Don't finish the word." I have never met a stutterer who cannot do it. Second, stutterers can be instructed as follows: "When you begin to stutter, continue to stutter but do not finish the word until I signal you to do so." When they begin to stutter, tensing and struggling cease and they have to "fake" stuttering to continue doing it.

The tensing, struggling behavior of stuttering is intricately tied to a purposeful effort to "get out the word." It most certainly is not a spasm in the medical meaning of the term.

Assumption 3

Nothing causes the fluency breaks other than what the stutterer is *doing* or *has done* to interfere with talking. When the listener, and indeed, the stutterer himself, considers the "stutter" to be a *beginning*, the person actually *has already* interfered sufficiently with the talking process so that he can no longer continue without obvious breaks in fluency. In summary, when we consider a person to "begin" to stutter, we are, in fact, hearing and seeing the consequence, the end result, of what the stutterer already has done to interfere with talking.

Assumption 4

The motivation for the behavioral pattern described in assumption 3 is to be found under the general umbrella of anticipation. Stutterers attend to internal cues, i.e., "feeling of stuttering" or "feeling of fluency," for signals as to whether they will stutter or will be fluent. If their feelings signal "stuttering," they begin modifying their speaking behavior in an attempt to keep from stuttering. This is the pattern described in assumption 3, which results in stuttering behavior. If their feelings signal "fluency," they continue talking. An interesting clinical observation supports this assumption.

Historically clinicians have observed that if stutterers honestly try to stutter they cannot do it. A certain amount of negative reaction associated with the anticipation of stuttering must be present to create the stuttering response. The behavior we label as stuttering represents, for the adult, the behavioral correlates of a fear-motivated reaction pattern.

Assumption 5

Stutterers come to believe that an instance of stuttering just "happens" in spite of everything they do to prevent it — or to get the word out without it. This belief develops because of the stutterers' reliance on their internal feelings to tell them whether they will stutter. A person's emotions are for the most part controlled by the autonomic nervous system and therefore are not readily and quickly controllable. Inasmuch as stutterers consider the emotional response to be an integral part of the overt struggling response (both representing a "stutter"), they feel helpless to control the emotional part of the stutter. Their only recourse is to keep the impending overt part as inconspicuous as possible. In short, they use the muscles, airflow, etc., they need to use to talk in an effort to fight the "erupting stutter." When stutterers swing their arms or jerk their heads, they are attempting to change the "feeling of being stuck" to one of "feeling" that now the word will come out.

Assumption 6

The fears of stuttering, although not quantifiable, are important determinants in motivating the "trying not to" or "keep from" response that is basic to stuttering. Too often, the fears of stuttering are considered in a singular, global way as a general, unspecific "fear of stuttering." Or, they are subsumed under the vague abstract construct of "stress," a term that means different things to different people because of the many different levels of abstraction it represents.

There are at least four specific fears that motivate the stuttering reaction pattern:

1. Fear of the stigma involved in being found out to be a "stutterer." Evaluation of the nature of the stigma will vary from stutterer to stutterer. It will range from "What will the listener think of me?" to "What I have to say [the message] will not be considered to be important."

2. Once a person begins to stutter, he fears that he will be unable to finish the word — or, at least he experiences fear about how long it will take to "get out the word." This fear motivates people to do everything possible first to avoid stuttering; if they are unsuccessful, they begin to stutter, "to get out of it" as quickly as possible.

3. Fear that, if stuttering occurs once, it may precipitate an avalanche of stuttering, and hence make finishing the message impossible. This is reflected in statements such as, "Can I ask the question?" or, "Can I tell the story?" This motivates a behavioral reaction in which, when stuttering occurs, a person finishes the word with a "tense push" and continues with a burst of speed, tension, and relatively rapid exhalation of breath in an effort to "get it said."

4. Fear of "feeling out of control of one's behavior" — of behavioral disintegration or a loss of behavioral integrity. For most people, stutterers and nonstutterers, this is an embarrassing and even a humiliating experience.

The intensity and importance of each fear described above will vary from person to person and, furthermore, will obviously change during the course of therapy. Moreover, the several fears are affected differently by the structure of the particular therapy program employed.

Assumption 7

While talking or while preparing to talk, stutterers do not attend to what they are *doing*. They attend to what they are *feeling*. This may appear to be similar to assumption 5, but the implications are different.

The assumption involves the concept of *time*. We ordinarily divide time arbitrarily into three categories — future, present, and past. However, one must be aware that these three categories are continuously changing. People can think about the future and the past, but the only one that they can change or modify is what they are doing right *now* — and *now* — and *now*, ad infinitum — or, in other words, the continuously moving present.

One of the generally recognized components of the stuttering response pattern is anticipation. Considerable research has been done to determine the accuracy with which stutterers can predict (anticipate) correctly when they are going to stutter. By definition, "anticipation" refers to future events or occurrences. One usually anticipates future events in relation to past experiences that had certain similarities. If a child, for example, anticipates receiving some candy that in the past he liked very much, he may jump up and down, shake his hands, double his fists and yet not be aware of what he is doing (in the present). His attention is directed toward thoughts of "future" (expected candy) and "past" (how good it was). This represents an example of the effects of positive anticipation. Negative anticipation can have much more serious effects on our lives than does positive anticipation and, at times, can be debilitating. When anticipated occurrences are feared and similar past occurrences have led to reactions of embarrassment and shame, a person becomes caught up in a spiral of feelings, of emotion. These building emotions are fueled by the person's concentration on "future" and "past." The "present" is filled with emotional awareness and is a vacuum of behavioral awareness. In such situations, people can tense or scream or run or freeze and not be aware of what they are *doing*. The same behavior pattern occurs in stuttering. Stutterers attend to their feelings and are only vaguely aware of what they are *doing*. It is no wonder that the stutterer considers that the stutter just "happens" (animism). Consequently, there develops a form of learned helplessness.

The issues in stuttering therapy that Gregory presents in Chapter One are now discussed below against the background of the assumptions described above. In my discussion, referencing of viewpoints is minimal because, unless otherwise indicated, I refer to those that are documented so well by Gregory.

TEACHING THE STUTTERER TO "STUTTER MORE FLUENTLY" VERSUS TEACHING THE STUTTERER TO "SPEAK MORE FLUENTLY"

"Teaching stutterers to stutter more fluently" and "teaching stutterers to speak more fluently" represent two different therapy models that the beginning clinician should examine for philosophical similarities and differences. Of particular importance is the need to examine them in order to arrive at a reasonable rationale for the reported success obtained by each and for the possible problems encountered in the use of each. Gregory indicates in Chapter One that certain clinicians use combinations of both models. My discussion is limited, however, to the two distinct models. This approach should enable the reader to evaluate the degree to which clinician A is using a combination of therapy models or is, in fact, emphasizing certain aspects of a particular model, whereas clinician B is using the same model as clinician A but emphasizing different aspects of it. After this discussion, a third therapy model is presented that contains certain elements of the two models mentioned above but seems sufficiently different from the other two to warrant separate discussion.

Stutter More Fluently Approach

The stutter more fluently therapy model is based essentially on an orientation toward behavior reduction. That is, the stutterer's goal is to reduce emotion (desensitization), reduce avoidance (go ahead and stutter), and reduce the complexity of the stuttering pattern (simplification).

The therapy approach is instrumental in facilitating behavior change because 1) it requires that the stutterer practice staying in the time framework of the present, and 2) it offers the stutterer the opportunity to test and resolve the fears associated with stuttering.

Staying in the Present   When stutterers study what they are doing as they stutter (identification), when they study what they are experiencing (emotionally) as they stutter, when they vary their stuttering patterns, when they use "pull-outs," and when they simplify and smooth out an instance of stuttering, they must, by operational definition, be attending to what they are *doing* (present) and not be attending to future or past.

Fears Associated with Stuttering   Fears of stuttering are confronted directly in the stutter more fluently model.

The fear or stigma discussed in assumption 6 is met by counseling and by experiences. Procedures will vary among clinicians, but usually they involve two major strategies. The first one includes a confrontation with the stuttering the person is doing. The person observes his own stuttering. He discusses what he does when he stutters and how he feels when he stutters. He is informed that he must face his stuttering because attempts to avoid or conceal it only make it worse. He is advised that he probably will continue to stutter but that he can learn to control the stuttering. The second strategy involves urging the person to be willing to stutter openly on a temporary basis and accept any resultant stigma so that he can learn ways to control his stuttering. Insofar as stutterers are successful in accepting this approach, they experience a certain degree of fear reduction (desensitization). They perceive that they are facing the feared stuttering instead of denying it and attempting to hide from it. There is a reduction in avoidance behavior.

The fear of the length of time it will take to "get the word out" is met by working on ways to "terminate the stutter," or, said in a different way, "to ease out of the block and say the word." These procedures help reduce fear considerably because they eliminate the helpless feeling a person has that when he begins to stutter he just has to wait — and heaven only knows how long it will take — for the word to come out. As stutterers learn they can control the duration of the stuttering block, the fear of not being able to complete the message decreases.

The fear of behavior disintegration or of loss of behavioral integrity is met when stutterers work to modify and simplify the stuttering response pattern. The fear of helplessness during an instance of stuttering is reduced because stutterers stay in control of their behavior when they stutter and smooth out the stutter so that it is barely, if at all, perceptible to the listener.

Each aspect of therapy is introduced and practiced within the confines of the clinic, but the essential part of the therapy process takes place in various social situations where the fears are experienced.

Speak More Fluently Approach

The speak more fluently therapy model is based on teaching stutterers to use a particular technique to obtain immediate fluency, albeit not normal speech. An attempt is then made to shape the speech pattern so that, insofar as possible, it approximates normal sounding speech.

The special techniques used to "obtain fluency" differ from clinician to clinician. Even though clinicians may argue about which technique is "best," the techniques are all remarkably similar. To understand the similarity among them, we must first consider the behavioral parameters we must use to talk. These parameters are presented not as a means of discussing speech production per se but because they represent the parameters of speaking behavior with which stutterers usually interfere when they do what we call "stuttering." There are five general ways that stutterers interfere with talking. These are:

1. The airstream is stopped or is used inappropriately
2. Movement and placement of articulators is either stopped or is inappropriate

3. Timing is inappropriate
4. The degree of muscular tensing for breath support, vocalization, or articulation is inappropriate
5. Voicing ceases or is distorted, usually because of inappropriate use of the first four parameters

If stutterers exaggerate behavior on any one of these parameters, they usually speak fluently, or at least with much improved fluency. Consequently, various therapy techniques have been adopted that include exaggeration of one speech parameter. Indeed, for centuries persons have advocated the exaggeration of one of the parameters as "the cure" for stuttering. For example, if stutterers attend to and use continuous and exaggerated airflow, fluency increases dramatically. So are they usually fluent if they attend to and use exaggerated timing, as with a metronome, if they attend to and use slow movement and continuous vocalization, as in speaking 30 words per minute, or if they attend to their tensing level (biofeedback) and use techniques of relaxation.

Those who utilize the speak more fluently approach most often use techniques similar to those described above to "replace" stuttering with fluent speech. Then they use strict programming of contingencies for success or failure as the stutterers move from simple to more complex verbal responses, i.e., single word to several sentence response. Also, most use massed practice procedures. No specific attention is directed to the fears associated with stuttering.

The therapy approach is instrumental in facilitating behavior change because 1) when stutterers utilize the special techniques they must attend to the special way they are talking, and when they do this they are staying in the present, and 2) the approach utilizes strict and consistent contingencies for responses in massed practice situations.

Evaluation of the Two Therapy Models

Perhaps one of the most perplexing aspects of the stuttering problem is the relative ease with which most stutterers can become temporarily fluent. Such fluency is often attributed to the use of distractions. Bloodstein (1975b) discusses distractions in terms of attending behavior. Distraction is said to occur when stutterers' attention is directed away from their speech and feelings. This most certainly is true in instances when stutterers talk in the presence of loud noises or flashing lights. But there are other dimensions of attending behavior. These involve not only what the attention of the person is directed *from* but what his attention is directed *to*. Left to themselves, stutterers focus their attention not on what they are doing but on feelings about the present and concern for the future generated by remembrance of the past.

Both therapy models emphasize, although not with the same purpose, directing attention to what stutterers are doing as they talk. In the stutter more fluently model, stutterers attend to the "nowness" of what they are doing in order to modify an instance of stuttering. In the speak more fluently model, stutterers have to attend to the nowness in order, for example, to talk in the presence of delayed auditory feedback (DAF), or to talk with an exceedingly slow rate.

In fact, it is my opinion that directing attention to the present is a common aspect of most stuttering therapies.

The fears associated with stuttering are met quite differently by the two therapy models. There are two generally recognized ways to reduce or eliminate fear reactions. One way is to face the fear and, through observation and experience, learn that the fears are groundless — in the sense that the person can cope constructively with events in the presence of, and in spite of, the fear reaction. This is the way the stutter more fluently model meets the fear reactions. The other way to cope with fear reactions is to make sure the events producing them will never occur again. This is the method used by people with an abnormal fear of flying who resolve never to fly again. By so doing, they assure themselves they never again will have to experience a lead-in-the-stomach sensation, cold perspiration, and clenched fists as the plane moves out on the runway. The speak more fluently model utilizes this approach to fear. By reinforcement of fluency, it is intended that a speaking behavior will be established in which stuttering will never occur again.

It is difficult to evaluate the effects of a therapy model without examining the procedures used. Certainly, clinicians differ considerably in the procedures they use even though their therapy models may be similar. Evaluation is complicated by the fact that certain clinicians may report they use such and such a model when, indeed, they use a little bit of this and a little bit of that. Nonetheless, we can examine certain problems that are likely to surface in conjunction with the use of either of the two therapy models.

Stutter More Fluently Model   The stutter more fluently model requires that the person focus attention on an instance of stuttering and progressively reduce the complexity of the stuttering until it is barely noticeable. Fundamental to this approach is the assumption that "it" (the stutter) remains some place within the person even though it cannot be detected in the speaking behavior — hence, the term "stutter fluently." Such a philosophy is likely to be, and often is, confusing to student clinicians and to stutterers themselves because it tends to promote beliefs that the stuttering problem is very mysterious and incomprehensible. Furthermore, the practices of attending to and working to control each instance of stuttering place little or no direct emphasis on the things one has to do to talk normally. It is almost as if the assumption is made that if the person can control the stutter, the nonstuttered speech will continue by itself. At times, this approach results in speech that lacks spontaneity and is labored and cautious sounding because the person is set to control the stutter whenever and wherever it occurs. On the positive side, many persons react to this approach by relaxing and enjoying speech because they have learned they can control the severity of their stuttering. The fact that they have coped with fears of stuttering and that they knowingly have reduced the complexity of their stuttering pattern results often in fairly stable speaking behavior in all speech situations.

If "relapse" occurs within this therapy model, it is most often attributable to the principle of therapy whereby fluency is not achieved directly but instead comes as a by-product of controlling the stutterings. People are taught to approach openly (not avoid) a possible instance of stuttering and to stutter smoothly. As a result of doing this, fluency increases. As fluency increases, however, they have fewer and fewer opportunities to practice "stuttering fluently." They enjoy the fluency they have attained. Unless they fully understand the process by which they become fluent, they switch from being willing to stutter fluently to doing things to "maintain" the fluency they have accomplished. This can involve, operationally, little more than an attempt to "keep the stutter out" of their speech — they may begin pausing momentarily or tensing slightly for example. Unfortunately, these avoidance behaviors too often appear initially to be successful, yet they are similar to the behavior that caused the problem to start with. As is to be expected, the speakers soon begin to avoid more and more and then they report that their stuttering "is coming back."

The stutter more fluently therapy model has been used effectively for years. In spite of the fact that mild stuttering is often noticeable at times in the speech of those who have approached their problem in this way, they have usually resolved their fears and emotional reactions to such an extent that their speech is only a minimal handicap. They communicate their ideas and feelings honestly, and hence, effectively. They pursue their life goals in terms of their desires and not in terms of the constraints imposed by the internal feelings of stuttering helplessness.

Speak More Fluently Model   The objectives of the model involve replacing the stuttering behavior with fluency by the use of special techniques similar to those mentioned earlier. This is first accomplished with the clinician in the clinical room. Then, by the use of various strategies, attempts are made to transfer and to maintain the fluency in outside speaking situations. Usually no problems arise in establishing fluent speech within the confines of the clinic — clinicians have been able to do this for years — but the obtained fluency is meaningless in terms of solving a speech problem unless satisfactory transfer and maintenance can be accomplished. This is obvious to most clinicians who are knowledgeable both in the principles of behavior modification and in the nature of the stuttering problem. The point is emphasized here, however, because it is not so obvious to persons new to the field or to those with limited experience in the area of stuttering. Recently, for example, a clinician told me she was very successful in working with stutterers by the use of the metronome and time-out procedures. I asked her the degree to which the stutterers were able to transfer and maintain their fluency. She answered, "Most had a lot of trouble, but that's their problem. I get them fluent. It's their responsibility to stay that way." This clinician is confused about the basic, and actually the unique, nature of stuttering therapy. Most problems of speech and language other than stuttering are such that the clinician's major task is to assist the client in producing the correct response pattern in the clinic. Once this is done, transfer of the correct pattern to other situations is ordinarily accomplished relatively easily. In stuttering, fluent speech is accomplished in the clinic relatively easily. The major task is in the transfer and maintenance.

In fact, from the first day of therapy the basic goal of any program should be to prepare the person to talk better in social situations (transfer). Before the thoughtful clinician introduces the first therapy principle and implements the first procedure, he should have a clear idea of how it will assist transfer. In short, the essence of stuttering therapy is the transfer and maintenance of a desired response pattern; obtaining fluency is not the major goal. The problem that occurs more often than any other for those who use the speak more fluently model is transfer. In my opinion, this problem occurs because those persons who stutter receive little or no direct experience with the fears of stuttering. They obtain fluency in the clinical environment where the emotional reactions are stable and where they can cope with them. When they enter a new speaking situation, the old behavior pattern of anticipatory fear (future) begins spiraling with remembrances of past stuttering and embarrassment, and their attention is directed to the resulting emotions. They experience difficulty in coping positively with these emotions if none of the training in the clinic is directed toward constructive ways of dealing with them.

Gregory, in Chapter One, discusses certain clinicians who do more in establishing fluency than just replacing stuttering with a single technique, e.g., breath flow. These clinicians emphasize the multiple parameters of talking and provide considerable practice in monitoring and feeling motorically the *process* of fluency. This approach seems to have advantages over an approach whereby fluency is obtained by a single technique exaggerating one parameter of speech, e.g., airflow, or rate, or relaxation. It seems reasonable to assume that when the process of fluency is emphasized and followed by massed practice stutterers learn what to do and the motoric feeling of doing it, and, hence, the probability of fluency in new situations that promote negative emotional responses is increased.

The possible problems involved in maintenance (avoiding a relapse) in the speak more fluently model are different from those encountered in the stutter more fluently model. Whereas in the stutter more fluently model, the person practices stuttering smoothly less and less as fluency increases, in the speak more fluently model the person can practice speaking fluently as much or more after being dismissed from therapy as during it. This therapy model provides a means for maintaining the fluency — if the person will continue practicing on a regular basis. On the other hand, problems develop with some persons because they never have had experience understanding or coping with fears of stuttering. Life is full of situations that provide cues that can trigger the old response pattern called stuttering. Persons can find themselves once more in the claws of helplessness. If the person has had no experience coping with fears of stuttering, a relapse of rather great proportions can occur.

The speak more fluently therapy model is relatively new when compared to the stutter more fluently approach. Therefore, it is difficult to assess its long-term effects on a large group of people as to personal adjustment, communication ability and vocational choice, as well as fluency of speech. On the surface, it seems to result in two dichotomous groups: 1) those who retain fluency to a large extent and who adjust to it in ways that permit relatively normal interactions in our talking world, and 2) those who continue to stutter as much or more than they did before therapy and who present concomitant problems of adjustment to interacting in our society. Because of the conflicting reports of "success" and the differing criteria used in defining success, the proportion who fall into each category cannot, at this point, be ascertained.

NORMAL TALKING THERAPY MODEL

A therapy model for helping stutterers learn to use their normal capabilities to talk was introduced by Williams (1957). The interested reader should review that article to obtain a perspective about the philosophy that undergirds the "normal talking" therapy model. The model differs from the basic premises of the two previously discussed in that instead of focusing on "reducing undesirable behavior" or on "replacing undesirable behavior," it focuses on "increasing desirable behavior."

This therapy approach emphasizes the normal speech process. To state the obvious: if a person is to talk normally, all major behavioral parameters of speech must function appropriately. These include airstream, movement and placement of articulators, timing, proper tensing levels, and voicing. When a person superimposes on this process the behavioral correlates of a fear-motivated reaction pattern, the smooth process is disrupted. This is the problem in stuttering. The process may be disrupted to varying degrees. For example, the person may partially disrupt the process by tensing abdominal muscles more than necessary and using excessive airflow, yet the process continues even though certain characteristics of the parameters have been changed. He probably will evaluate this as, "I almost stuttered." Or, he may tense sufficiently in the laryngeal area that he blocks the airstream and he stops articulatory movement. Then, he is likely to evaluate this as, "I'm having a block." It is necessary to direct his attention from what he *evaluates* is happening to him toward 1) those things he is *doing* to interfere with talking, and 2) those things he is *doing* to facilitate it.

The goals and procedures of therapy are directed toward the beliefs, emotions, and motoric behavior that will facilitate the normal talking process and toward comparing and contrasting them with those that motivate and perpetuate disruptions in the talking process. The purpose of any therapy is *change*. To change efficiently, people need not only to know specifically what to change *from*, but also, and more important, they need a vivid, clear picture of what to change *to*.

It is not my purpose to present in detail the principles and procedures of therapy within the "normal talking" model. Only those are mentioned that will, it is hoped, capsulate the model.

Learning to Learn

Stutterers need to learn that they can learn to change what they are doing as they are talking. It is not a problem of controlling the stutter or of using some special technique so that the stutter will not occur. Three major concepts are involved in learning to change what one does in talking: emotions and fear, behavioral awareness, and the positive aspects of change and of talking.

Emotions and Fears

The principles and procedures of therapy should be structured to help stutterers develop a realistic perspective on their emotions and the relation of feelings to an occurrence of stuttering. Stutterers should learn by experience that their emotions need not determine whether they will stutter. The clinician should keep in mind that, to those who stutter, feelings are an integral part of the stutter. To them, these feelings represent the internal beginning of stuttering. What a listener observes as stuttering is, to those who are speaking, that part of the stutter they could not "hide."[1]

They need to learn that their emotions are just that — feelings — and that they can learn to initiate the normal speaking process by attending to what they are doing even though emotions are present. Operationally, they learn this as they enter situations outside the clinic and familiarize themselves with the ebb and flow of emotion that is such a normal part of human interaction.

---

[1]The concept of emotion and anticipation is discussed in considerable detail elsewhere (Williams, 1957).

In addition to the general concept of emotion, the specific stuttering fears discussed at the beginning of the chapter in assumption 6 need to be dealt with. These fears can be tested and resolved as a part of the program to be discussed next.

Behavioral Awareness

The first phase of therapy involves assisting persons who stutter to attend to what they are doing[2] as they are stuttering. The observations are organized to include each of the major parameters of speech discussed earlier. The stutterers study each behavioral parameter to assess what they are doing with that aspect of speech. They practice varying their behavior on each parameter. For example, for the parameter of tensing, they increase and decrease their tensing levels. Other procedures may include speeding and slowing rate of jaw movement or stopping and starting airflow. From this they learn 1) that various parameters of behavior interfere with talking, 2) that when they attend to what they are doing (not feeling) they can change what they do, and 3) that changing what they are doing changes their emotions and reduces or even eliminates the feelings of helplessness.

Changing and Talking

As persons who stutter practice changing what they are doing on planned speech parameters, they learn that their speaking behavior is governed by what they do and not by what they are feeling.

The next goal of therapy is to assist stutterers to learn the normal behavioral process of speaking. This involves experiencing the normal functioning of each of the speech parameters. For example, they experience the degree of tensing of the abdominal area, the laryngeal area, the jaw area, as they are talking normally. This same experience is provided for movement, placement of articulators, airflow, and voicing. Following a study of each speech parameter, attention is directed toward the interaction of two or more parameters, i.e., the way movement and tensing blend together, and airflow and voicing, etc. People cannot verbalize what they do on each speech parameter. A person leaves the level of words and enters the world of doing. No one can explain to me in words how to bend my arm "normally" at the elbow. Yet, as I stand and attend to doing it, I can learn at a "doing" level what it's like. Then, I can

---

[2]Hereafter, when I use the word "doing," I am referring to the "nowness," the time frame of the present — the sensation of the motoric feedback of "doingness."

reproduce it. Or, said in a different way, then I know what to do to do it. So it is with talking.

With an increased awareness of behavior during the normal talking process, stutterers can begin to compare what they can do to interfere with talking with what they can do to facilitate it. This provides the framework for constructive behavior change. They practice interfering on each speech parameter and then changing what they are doing to normal functioning on the parameter. Following this, they can practice interfering on combinations of speech parameters and then changing to normal talking behavior. As they practice in different speaking situations, they learn that they can be in charge of what they are doing. This reduces or eliminates most of the fears of stuttering.

The final phase of therapy is an obvious one. If they know they are in charge of what they are doing and can change what they do, then they can practice initiating the normal speaking process when they begin and as they continue talking. If they begin to interfere with talking on one or more parameters, they can change what they are doing in the direction of facilitating the talking process. It should be emphasized that the normal talking process involves the continuous changing of many behavioral parameters of speech as they relate to lips, tongue, jaw, etc. It is only the nature of the changing that is at issue in therapy.

In working toward all of the goals discussed above, there is a need to structure the experiences and to reinforce systematically the appropriate responses.

ATTITUDE CHANGE: WHAT IS IT? IS IT NEEDED?

People's beliefs affect the way they behave, and conversely, the ways they behave affect their beliefs. There is an interaction. This is obvious. In stuttering therapy, it is not a question of whether one works on both; it is a question of the ways it is done. As Gregory points out in Chapter One, clinicians emphasize different attitudes and beliefs they see as needing to be changed, and, furthermore, they advocate different ways by which the changes can be accomplished. In general, the attitudes and beliefs the clinician seeks to change and the means used to change them correspond to the assumptions the clinician makes about the nature of stuttering and to the model of therapy used. My discussion in this section is limited to the more important attitudes and beliefs that I think must be considered in relation to the normal talking therapy model presented in the previous section.

Presenting Information

When stutterers come for therapy, they bring with them a certain body of information. The degree to which the information is accurate or inaccurate varies from person to person. In any event, it is from this information that people mold their beliefs about the nature of the problem, their place in it, and the options they have in solving it. Ordinarily, we think that increased information serves to broaden the range of one's choices for problem solving. However, some kinds of information — and some ways it is presented — may serve to restrict, even severely limit, the choices people believe are open to them. If new information is about something they "never knew before," they are likely to accept it and to integrate it into their belief systems. On the other hand, if new information conflicts with beliefs already held, it is likely either to be rejected (although they may say that they "understood") or to be distorted in such a way that it is compatible with the person's current belief system. Inasmuch as adults who stutter have developed over a period of years an elaborate belief system about stuttering, a clinician who attempts to work on beliefs solely by "telling them" or by "explaining to them" or by "talking through" with them their faulty beliefs, is likely to effect little, if any, constructive behavior change.

To be clinically effective, information should be presented in conjunction with structured experiences. The purpose of the information is to direct observations made during the *experiencing* of the event. Thus, people can assess the possibility of a previously unrecognized relationship between the ways they are behaving and their beliefs of why they have, in the past, behaved that way. This procedure provides congruity between beliefs and behavior. Without providing new information that can be tested by observation and experience, people are likely to reconfirm continually old beliefs by repetitions of similar experiences.

One of the problems that may result from forced behavior change, as in behavior modification procedures with strict contingencies, is that one is never certain of what is "learned" even though behavior alters. What we, as clinicians, think we are "teaching" and what the person is "learning" can be two quite different things. The following example is presented to illustrate the point.

A young lady had received therapy based on the speak more fluently model. She had practiced a slow rate of speech (30 words per minute) and continuous vocalization. She had increased the rate to approximately 100 words per minute by the termination of therapy. When I asked her what she was instructing herself to do now (3 months later) when she talked, she replied, "Take a full breath and keep the air flowing." I asked her whether that had been included as part of her therapy program. She said, "No, but I think that's what helps me the most." I then asked her the degree to which that technique helped her. She thought for a moment and said, "Sometimes, when I do it, it helps make the feeling of stuttering go away, but if the feeling gets very strong, it doesn't help much."

In my opinion, her verbal report indicated that what had been "taught" was not what was "learned." Furthermore, she still maintained her own private interpretation of the reasons for the technique. She used the technique not to help her talk but as a means of reducing or eliminating her "feelings of stuttering."

The Problem with Beliefs

The major belief system that should be examined with adults who stutter concerns where the responsibility lies for the ways they talk. Many clinicians have recognized this and have included in their therapy programs the goal of "helping the stutterers accept the responsibility for the way they talk." Certain clinicians have attempted to solve the problem by castigating stutterers for their irresponsibility. Others have attempted to meet it by informing and then reminding stutterers of how uncomfortable they make their listeners when they stutter. Still other clinicians assist stutterers to accept responsibility for their own behavior by integrating into the therapy program principles and procedures for altering beliefs.

Three major belief systems can either deter or facilitate accepting responsibility for one's behavior: external control, internal control, and animism.

External versus Internal Control   There are people who believe their behavior is controlled largely by external forces. These people believe in "astrology," "luck," "good days," and "bad days." They look to external things or other people to solve problems for them. This general belief system is evident with stutterers who say that their bosses make them stutter, or that classrooms, telephones, and ever certain words *cause* them to stutter. The clinician's task is to help stutterers alter their belief systems so that they recognize they are dependent on internal control and learn that they can determine the way they talk by what they do regardless of what words they use, where they talk, or with whom they talk.

Animism and Behavior Control Elsewhere (Williams, 1957) I have discussed the effect of animistic belief on one's behavior. In brief, it is the belief that people possess certain attributes that explain why they act the way they do. If, for example, a man considers himself to be "shy," then obviously he cannot meet people very well. Furthermore, if he possesses this attribute — this thing called "shyness" — people (and he) cannot expect him to change his behavior until the "shyness" is removed. This belief involves little more than relinquishing responsibility for the way one behaves. This thing inside him called "shyness" is responsible. He is not. Similar animistic beliefs can be found among stutterers. Stuttering is something that happens when stutterers talk, and, furthermore, it happens *because* they are stutterers. Consequently, the person involved attends very little to the cause and effect of behavior because, to him, stuttering is both cause and effect.

A clinician can work to alter this belief system by encouraging stutterers to use a language that is descriptive and process-like. The clinician may give directions such as these: Instead of saying "my jaw tensed," say, "I tensed my jaw muscles." Or, instead of saying "the word got stuck in my throat," say, "I shut off the airflow by tensing my throat muscles." This type of language assists stutterers to direct their attention to what they are doing and hence introduces the possibility of alternative ways of behaving. It is a language that fosters responsibility, not excuses, for one's behavior.

Emotions and Control

The emotional aspects of stuttering are so obvious that they receive most of the attention in discussions about the attitudes and beliefs of stutterers. Because they cannot be quantified or described objectively, their role in the stuttering response is subject to more speculation and conjecture than any other aspect of the problem. In fact, it is probably accurate to state the emotional responses in stuttering and the ways people advocate they be met in therapy are at the heart of most of the controversies about stuttering therapy.

I discussed in the previous section my opinion about the role of emotion and fears in the stuttering response pattern. My discussion here is limited to the clinician's role in helping stutterers explore their beliefs about and reactions to their emotional responses.

The clinician-client relationship should be such that stutterers feel free not only to verbalize their fears but also to experience negative emotions and fears in the presence of the clinician. This takes courage. So, the clinician's role is to 1) provide support and acceptance of the person's feelings, and 2) assist the stutterer in identifying and exploring the behavioral correlates of fear. People want to avoid or to escape quickly the unpleasantness of fear, yet only by experiencing and studying the behavioral correlates of emotion can people begin to explore what they are doing and what might be alternative ways of responding. The behavioral correlates of fear are often things such as tensing of abdominal muscles, momentary shutting off the air at the glottis, and speeding up or freezing of movement. As people become increasingly willing to experience the feelings of fear and attend to what they are doing, they find they can change their behavioral responses. This discovery does not eliminate the feelings of fear. That is not the goal. But it does reduce feelings of helplessness and of "being out of control" and therefore serves to reduce fear. As I stated previously, this experience helps the person accept the feelings for what they are — emotions — and recognize that the ways they react to them are a matter of choice.

PSYCHOTHERAPY FOR STUTTERERS: WHAT IS IT, IS IT NEEDED, AND IF SO, HOW SHOULD IT BE DONE?

Many new clinicians in the field of speech pathology are frightened and confused by the word "psychotherapy." During discussions of principles and procedures of stuttering therapy, clinicians have asked me whether a particular aspect of therapy is still therapy or whether it is getting over into psychotherapy. Gregory in Chapter One presents an excellent discussion of the issues involved. His present point of view, as stated in that chapter, is so close to mine that there is no need to repeat it here.

It is important for the new clinician to realize that psychotherapists or psychiatrists use many of the same clinical techniques that speech-language pathologists use. These techniques include providing information, bibliotherapy, behavior modification, relaxation, systematic desensitization, and reality testing. There are others, of course. However, the point to be made is that "psychotherapy" is not a prescribed unitary procedure. Psychotherapists' major goal is to help resolve human interpersonal and intrapersonal difficulties by assisting the person to perceive expanded alternative ways of behaving in order to reduce feelings of being trapped and helpless. This goal is not too different from ours. The difference, as Gregory pointed out, is in the nature of the problem areas.

In view of the above, a speech-language pathologist is justified in referring a person who stutters for psychotherapy. If a person has certain personal problems that are of such concern that the stuttering problem is of secondary importance, it makes sense for the person to resolve the problem of primary concern so that his motivation for stuttering therapy becomes the number one priority. In several instances during my professional years I have accepted someone into stuttering therapy at the same time he was receiving psychiatric assistance for a problem that had little connection with stuttering. There have been more instances in which I referred a person for psychotherapy following a period of stuttering therapy. In these cases, the most common reason for referral was the fact that, even though fluency increased, all other problems of interaction did not automatically disappear, as the stutterer had assumed they would.

There is one additional point to be made with regard to referral to a clinical psychologist or a psychiatrist. A clinician must feel free to discuss all behavioral problems openly and frankly with a stutterer, although the discussions do not need to be directed toward arriving at solutions. The purpose is to identify problems that may justify referral so that, if referral is made, the stutterer understands and accepts the reasons for it. Under no circumstances is a clinician justified in referring clients simply because they are not making satisfactory progress on their speech by the use of the therapy program the clinician is using. Too often, this is done. Instead of re-examining their own clinical rationale, the clinicians assume that the stutterers "must need" psychiatric help. This can be injurious and at times devastating to the person who stutters.

STUTTERING THERAPY FOR CHILDREN

In providing stuttering therapy for children, and in conferences with parents relating to the prevention of stuttering, a clinician should act in accordance with the assumptions he makes about the nature of stuttering and the therapy model that evolves from those assumptions.

My rationale for early intervention with parents whose children seem to be starting to stutter is contained in assumption 1, presented at the start of this chapter. Although the statement of this assumption is brief, the implications of the assumption itself are extensive and far reaching. The more disfluent a child becomes, the more likely someone will evaluate his speaking behavior as "stuttering" or as "something wrong." This evaluation is likely to be communicated to the child in a variety of ways, both verbally and nonverbally. Hence, early intevention involves providing parents with information 1) about the ways that children learn to talk, and 2) about the ways they can bring about a reduction in disfluencies by modifying home conditions, their reactions to the child, and their listening habits. In addition:

> Everything possible is done to encourage an environment and a speaking atmosphere in which children will not develop negative reactions toward the ways they are talking or to themselves as speakers. On the contrary, we do what we can to help the child develop more positive feelings toward talking. We encourage parents to talk a great deal with their child in relaxed situations, and to listen attentively to the answers. We encourage them to share verbally with the child the things they do, their feelings and hopes and frustrations. Good verbal interaction consists of one person reaching toward another with words and the other person reaching back — and touching softly. The more parents can encourage a warm verbal-sharing relationship, the easier it will be for the child to react toward other listeners in increasingly positive ways and hence with increasing speech fluency. (Williams, 1978a, p. 199)

In the following publications, I have discussed the development of disfluencies in the speech of children (Williams, 1978a, d), the development of the stuttering response pattern (Williams, 1978a), the nature of the information to be obtained from parents (Williams, 1978b, c), and suggestions to parents about things they can do to help normal speech development (Williams, 1978a). In this section of the chapter I discuss stuttering therapy for elementary-school age children based on the normal talking model presented earlier as applied to the treatment of adult stutterers. In using the normal talking model with children the principles and procedures of therapy are adapted to fit the child's developing problems, which are somewhat different from those of an adult. In general, the problems described in assumptions 4, 5, and 6 are just in the beginning stages of development among elementary school children. On the other hand, the concept of "time" discussed in assumption 7 is just as applicable with children as it is with adults and is blended into the entire therapy approach with children.

The Structure of Therapy

As with the adult, the goals and procedures of therapy for children are directed toward the beliefs, emotions, and motoric behavior that will facilitate the normal speaking process. Unlike stuttering therapy for adults, however, treatment for stuttering children devotes minimal attention to the factors that can motivate and perpetuate disruptions in speaking. Children, compared to adults, have had relatively little experience with stuttering. Often they can tell you little of what they are doing, the ways they are feeling, or their beliefs about what is occurring.

The emphasis in therapy is placed on normal processes — the normal process of speaking, the normal process of behaving, and the normal emotions that everyone experiences. Presenting information about the normal aspects of these activities and giving opportunities for experiencing them prevent development of the faulty beliefs and evaluations that are such a part of the adult stuttering problem.

Whereas adults often have to learn that they *can* learn to change the ways they talk, children need primarily to learn *how* to learn to do it. For this, they are helped by having an informational context within which to work. For example, the concepts of emotion, behavior, and even stuttering are vague and abstract to a child. It is helpful to present each concept within a context that is known to them or that they can experience. The three concepts discussed below are similar to those outlined earlier for the adult. They include: emotions and fear, behavioral awareness, and positive aspects of change and of talking; the discussions here, however, take into account the perspectives of a child.

Discuss-Observe-Model-Experience Emotions and Reactions to Them in Various Situations Where These Feelings and Reactions Are Normal and Healthy A context of normalcy is provided within which children can explore their feelings while talking. Children will vary considerably in the degree to which this aspect of therapy needs to be explored. Some children will need to learn little about their emotional reactions and how to cope with them and others will need considerable experience in coping with them. The extent to which children need such experiences is determined by the degree to which emotional reactions such as increasing tension or increasing speed of movement interfere with making positive changes in their talking behavior and in their ability to integrate these changes into social situations.

Discuss-Observe-Model-Experience Speaking Behavior in the Context of General Behavior Involving Motor Systems Other Than Those Related to Speaking, e.g., Limb Movement A context of behaving is provided by comparing the process of talking with the process of, for example, playing the piano, typing, or throwing a ball. This comparison provides a basis not only for gaining a perspective on a behavioral process but also for studying ways a person can interfere with the process. For example, while studying the process of catching a ball, we can also study the ways we can interfere with catching it — by tensing, by quickly grabbing at it, or by jumping out of the way as the ball approaches. These experiences in behavioral awareness provide children with a meaningful context for viewing the third concept.

Discuss-Observe-Model-Experience the Process of Interrupting Speaking Behavior Within the Context of Ongoing, Forward Moving Speech The clinician utilizes the parameters of speech described previously for the adult in exploring the ways people can interfere with smooth talking. The disrupted speech is, however, compared with the easy speaking we do normally. The easy, forward moving speaking behavior is emphasized and serves as "home base." It should be emphasized that, in practice, the three concepts are not handled separately. They are all integrated so that there is one focal point: the behavior of talking easily.

Attitudes and Beliefs

Whereas there may be considerable need to emphasize attitudes and beliefs in a therapy program for adults who stutter, there is usually little need for such emphasis with children.

Through the process of therapy just described, faulty beliefs can be altered if necessary or, in many instances, can be prevented from developing. As children learn how we make sound, how we need air and the movement of many structures to create words, it is easy for them to see the fallacy of the belief, for example, that "words get stuck in my throat," or of the notion that it helps to "tense and push hard to get words out." As they experience the "doingness" of talking, and learn the ways they can change what they are doing, they are also learning that they, not external forces, control what they do. As they learn the normalcy of emotions and the ways we can do things even though we are scared, they are preventing the development of the faulty belief that there is a unique "feeling of stuttering" that "tells" whether they will stutter or will be fluent.

A Final Note

Even though the emphasis in this section is on a therapy model, a point should be made with regard to procedures. In the early stages of the development of this therapy program (Williams, 1971) both discussion and direct behavior change procedures were utilized, but greater emphasis was placed on discussion than on structured behavior change. In recent years, discussion has been incorporated into direct experiencing and modeling of behavior and behavior change. Once children know by experience the difference between doing positive things to talk and doing negative things to "try not to have trouble," the desired behavior changes are practiced in structured situations, first with consistent reinforcement given by the clinician for appropriate responses and then with reinforcement through the children's own self-evaluation.

TRANSFER OF CHANGES TO THE NATURAL ENVIRONMENT AND THE PROBLEM OF RELAPSE

The fundamental objective of therapy is contained in the concept of transfer. The major problems involved in transfer are inherent in the therapy model used. These problems have been mentioned earlier in this chapter during the discussion of different models of therapy. It is difficult to discuss meaningfully general problems of transfer applicable to all models of therapy.

Within the normal talking therapy model stutterers integrate desired behavior changes into social speaking situations as they progress through the therapy program. The major purpose of this procedure is to enable them to learn that they *can* cope constructively with their talking behavior in the presence of the feelings generated by their past experiences with similar speaking situations. Once they learn this, they are able to plan and practice the kinds of changes they *want* to make in everyday conversations. Enabling these changes is the purpose of transfer and it is the essence of therapy.

CRITERIA FOR THE SUCCESS OF STUTTERING THERAPY: THE RESULTS OF STUTTERING THERAPY

Clinicians are continually faced with the problem of evaluating the successes reportedly obtained by the use of different therapy approaches to stuttering. It is not easy to do. In fact, such evaluation can be, and often is, confusing. At least part of the confusion can be resolved by recognizing the differing meanings of "improvement" and of "success." These are not *descriptive* terms. They are *evaluative*. Their use depends upon a judgment made by someone of the significance of a change in behavior. This "someone" may be the clinician, it may be the person who stutters, or it may be an acquaintance at the corner drug store. In any event, it is worthwhile to examine questions that arise in evaluating therapy approaches.

To assess the effects of therapy procedures, we describe, either by the use of quantitative measures or by the self-reports of the client, the behavioral changes. Depending upon who is doing the evaluating, changes may or may not be seen as "improvement." Two rather extreme examples make the point.

A man who stutters may achieve considerable fluency but talks with an excessive amount of breathiness and with a substantial increase in anxiety. Therefore, he may deem his speech behavior to be very undesirable. On the other hand, the clinician and other listeners may think it represents "tremendous" improvement. Conversely, a man who stutters may cease substituting words and circumlocuting and, by so doing, experience a great reduction in anxiety. Even though he is stuttering a good bit, he is greatly impressed by the fact that he is saying what he wants to say. He and his clinician may consider this to be great improvement. Listeners may consider that not only has no improvement taken place but that he has become worse. Behavioral changes and improvement are not necessarily synonymous, yet, it seems to me, this is not always obvious. Gregory discusses in Chapter One the concern for improved reliability in assessing behavior change. Little is said, however, about the validity of such measurements. Most certainly reliability of measurement is important, but it should not be confused with the validity of improvement.

A question also arises when clinical researchers either implicitly or explicitly equate statistically significant change with improvement. Through their clinical program they obtain a reduction in stuttering frequency that is statistically significant but may or may not represent meaningful improvement. It is left to one's judgment as to whether statistical significance is also clinical significance. Another question may arise when a clinician obtains a reduction in stuttering frequency during individual and group sessions in a clinic and reports that the stutterers "improved" by a specified amount as a result of a particular therapy approach. Unless the people have integrated the desired speaking behavior into their everyday speaking activities, the reader must judge for himself the degree to which such reductions in stuttering frequency really constitute improvement.

These examples most certainly do not exhaust the possibilities for confusion in assessing improvement, nor do they resolve the problems; but it is hoped they serve to clarify some points that must be given thought. For the most part, controversies surrounding the effectiveness of stuttering therapy do not involve the assessment of behavioral changes, per se. Instead, they cluster around the question of which specific changes or which combination of changes people agree constitute "improvement." A similar question is involved in a person's evaluation of what constitutes "success."

Fluency is the criterion of success for the speak more fluently therapy model. By definition, therefore, 100% fluency in all speaking situations represents "success." I am unaware of a provision within the model that permits modifications of procedures for persons who fall short of "success." Perhaps such a provision would be useful, or perhaps, within the concept of the model, there is no need for such a provision. The question is a provocative one that is seldom, if ever, addressed. It is recognized that the emphasis in this therapy model is on establishing fluency. The results of a therapy program, however, are reported in terms of the *degree* of fluency attained, e.g., 98%; nothing is mentioned about the severity of, and emotional reactions to, the instances of stuttering that still occur, e.g., 2%. Data about severity and emotional reactions would, it seems to me, be meaningful for one who is attempting to evaluate the relative effectiveness of different therapy approaches within the model.

Within the stutter more fluently therapy model, a person's ability to control instances of stuttering is the criterion of success. Stuttering smoothly and minimal interference with the ongoing speaking behavior whenever one speaks represent 100% success. Inasmuch as the therapy procedures emphasize a gradual modification of stuttering, there is built into the program a means whereby the person can deal constructively, not destructively, with times when the 100% criterion is not attained.

There is an additional point I want to discuss with regard to the concept of "success." This point is pertinent regardless of which model of therapy one uses. "Success" or "failure" are evaluations made by someone with reference to whether a person reaches or does not reach a stated goal. Who sets the goal and establishes criteria to measure whether it has been attained? Clinicians should guard against adopting their own criteria for success without giving due thought, respect, and understanding to the goals of the client. If there is a conflict between the clinician's and client's criteria for success, it has been my observation that ultimately the client's criteria will prevail. This observation may be more closely related to the problem of maintenance than some of us would like to admit.

With due consideration given to the viewpoint expressed throughout this chapter, it seems reasonable and consistent to conclude that the most important thing for stutterers to learn as a result of therapy is "copability." They do not learn this by attending solely to their stuttering or to their fluency. Rather, they learn it by attending to, and experiencing, the total process of talking and the many ways that they can vary the process. As a part of experiencing this, they develop the knowledge that they have the freedom to change different aspects of the process as the need arises to do so. As I stated elsewhere (Williams, 1978a), until persons who have stuttered "can interact with people and talk the way *they want* to talk, at any time, to any one, *they* still have a problem of stuttering." This, to me, is a realistic appraisal of "success." Quantitative analysis of their speaking behavior when compared to self-reports can assist the clinician in determining how well they achieve their goals.

chapter EIGHT

The Controversies: Analysis and Current Status

Hugo H. Gregory, Ph.D.

All of the contributors, in describing their therapy and dealing with the controversies, considered it important to set forth their assumptions and beliefs about the problem of stuttering. Perkins[1] focuses his chapter on a description of the evolution of his ideas about stuttering and its treatments, showing the development from a psychoanalytic orientation to a point of view that stuttering is a discoordination problem. Cooper lists four assumptions about the problem of stuttering in young children ranging from ones concerning etiology of the problem to what stuttering children can learn in therapy. Williams bases his chapter on a list of seven assumptions about the nature of stuttering that is the frame of reference for his approach. At the beginning of his comments, Webster states that his work was based on a belief that it was time for a strong empirical approach based on observable aspects of speech. To prepare the reader for his contribution, Ryan reviews the behavior analysis/behavior modification frame of reference and says he views stuttering as learned behavior. Sheehan cites the many puzzling problems

---

[1] In this chapter, when no bibliographic date is given, the reference is to the author's chapter in this book. Page numbers accompanying quotes with no date of reference refer to page numbers in this volume.

about stuttering that still exist, but in spite of these, refers to his understanding of treatment with reference to self-role and approach-avoidance conflict.

Several years ago, Williams (1968) discussed the way in which a clinician's work is influenced by his knowledge and resulting evaluations. Perhaps the first conclusion we can draw from reading the foregoing chapters is that controversies arise not only from our collective lack of knowledge, but from differing frames of reference and variations in experience. Like our contributors, every clinician beginning as a student and evolving through a professional career develops ideas about stuttering and stuttering therapy. Books such as the present one throw light upon issues, but each individual clinician must decide what approaches and methods to use. The better the issues involved are understood, the wiser will be the clinician's decisions. Hopefully, our belief in objective, rational thought and the scientific method will motivate us all to remain open to new information and in turn to re-evaluate our ideas and to modify our approaches to the management of stuttering as it seems reasonable to do so.

The remainder of this chapter is a comparative analysis of the authors' responses to the controversial issues, highlighting areas of agreement and disagreement as perceived by this writer. A related objective is to speculate about ways in which certain controversies might be resolved.

STUTTER MORE FLUENTLY VERSUS SPEAK MORE FLUENTLY

Williams, in his analysis of the stutter more fluently vs. speak more fluently issue, points out that both of these therapy models direct the stutterer's attention to his behavior at the moment, "to the 'nowness' of what they are doing." In this way, he does not see the change brought about by either approach as being attributable to any great extent to distraction defined as attention being directed away from speech. In both cases attention is directed to speech, although in different ways. We see that Sheehan, with reference to distraction, continues to classify the speak more fluently approaches as methods that cultivate avoidance and as being based on distraction. Williams believes that the stutter more fluently method is more responsive to the fear component of stuttering, and Sheehan is very critical of the speak more fluently model because he says the stutterer is not given a method for meeting future difficulty.

Both Cooper and Williams draw our attention to the observation that as a stutterer learning to stutter more fluently actually becomes more fluent, he has fewer opportunities to practice "stuttering fluently." According to Williams, this can lead to an increased desire to maintain fluency and subsequently an increased avoidance of stuttering. Interestingly, Williams points out that "in the speak fluently model the person can practice speaking fluently as much or more after being dismissed from therapy as during it" (p. 252). He believes that problems can develop, however, if the person has had no experience understanding and coping with fears of stuttering. Williams briefly discusses his "normal talking therapy model," in which he says the emphasis is on increasing desirable behavior instead of focusing on reducing undesirable behavior (stutter more fluently model) and replacing undesirable behavior (speak more fluently model).

Several of the authors mention that the specific procedures utilized by clinicians associated with either of the two main ways of viewing therapy differ in a number of ways.

Webster, while saying that his personal preference is for the concept of speaking more fluently, points out that all of the therapies ordinarily identified in this way are not equally as powerful or desirable. He refers to the difficulty of accomplishing transfer and retention with "fluency-forcing procedures" such as delayed auditory feedback, masking, and rhythm and cites as the probable reason for this that the stutterer does not learn enough about the specific movement patterns that generate fluent speech.

Although Webster's specific techniques in his fluency-shaping program differ from the normal talking therapy used by Williams, it seems both have the same general objectives. Both stress learning to change and both emphasize what the person can do to facilitate normal talking.

Differences are important to clarify also, and in the case of Williams and Webster we find that Williams sees a need for the stutterer to become aware to some extent of what he is doing as he stutters. On the other hand, Webster has not found this to be a profitable way to utilize therapy time in terms of the benefit derived. Williams helps stutterers develop an understanding of the relation of feelings to the occurrence of stuttering and speaking normally.

Webster indicates that when the client achieves definitive control of fluency-generating targets, he can ordinarily speak fluently in spite of fears, anxieties, and life stresses. This may be viewed as helping the stutterer to deal with fear by developing considerable skill in his ability to make responses that are incompatible to stuttering. Webster further states that reduction in fear normally occurs as competency is developed in the production of normally fluent speech.

Cooper describes how he re-evaluated the approach of teaching more fluent stuttering in view of the frequently noted observation that almost all stutterers are fluent most of the time and that most stutterers when instructed are able to increase their fluency. He now helps stutterers identify and practice fluency-increasing gestures. Cooper acknowledges the similarity of this approach to that of Webster, but unlike Webster he integrates attention to the client's feelings and attitudes with attention to disfluencies. In Cooper's contributions, we can trace an evolution from a stutter more fluently procedure to one that in its approach to speech change includes analysis of stuttering behavior but also fluency-increasing techniques similar to those used by Perkins and Webster. Even though Cooper does not describe what he is doing in the same way as does Williams, a normal talking model is apparent in the latter stages of his therapy.

In his chapter, which describes how he came to favor a discoordination hypothesis to explain stuttering, Perkins points out that both retarded phonetic rate and simplification of phonatory complexity facilitate speech coordination and contribute to increased fluency. In therapy, rate control and a soft breathy attack are used initially to help the stutterer learn to manage the breath stream throughout a phrase unit. In contrast to Webster, who begins by teaching monitoring and change at the syllable level, Perkins states that information about our ability to control speech indicates that we cannot monitor and control speech at the speed that sounds and syllables are normally produced. Hence, the stutterer should learn to monitor change at the phrase level. In comparing Perkins with Webster, the clinician must decide, for one thing, whether working at the syllable level is valuable. Thus Perkins, like Cooper and Webster, has stutterers practice certain skills that take into consideration the various parameters of speaking: airflow, phonation, and articulation. The word "practicing" is used here rather than "learning" since some may argue that the person already has the skill in his repertoire. Also, those who use these procedures imply that they realize this and that they are conditioning the stutterer to be able to modify his behavior when speaking in situations where he has previously emitted behavior that interfered with normal fluency. Williams comments that these techniques, which go further than merely replacing stuttering with fluency using a single technique, focus on the multiple parameters of speech and provide considerable practice in monitoring and feeling motorically the process of fluency using massed practice and therefore have a better chance of being effective. Finally, there is considerable similarity in what Cooper, Perkins, Williams, and Webster do in teaching more normally fluent speech, although Cooper and Williams place more emphasis on having the person contrast specific behavior that interferes with talking with ways in which talking can be facilitated. All four emphasize stutterers gaining confidence in their ability to modify their speech.

Ryan emphasizes that most therapies give attention to the speech act and that the core of all successful therapy is the improvement of fluency, whether it be called controlled stuttering or fluency shaping. He believes it would be constructive to focus more definitively on how we do this effectively and efficiently. Therapy evaluation demands explicit description of what we do and definitive measures of speech change. The goal should be normal speech operationally defined as a stuttering rate of 0.5 SW/M (stuttered words per minute) or less. Ryan presents data to indicate that the average rate of stuttering is mild to moderately severe. Thus, on the average, stutterers exhibit 92% fluency when therapy begins. In pointing this out, Ryan implies that his establishment program is actually a program for increasing, and perhaps modifying to some extent, speech behavior that is already in the repertoire of stutterers. Currently, two programs, DAF (Delayed Auditory Feedback) and GILCU (Gradual Increase in Length and Complexity of Utterance), are used most often in the establishment phase to increase fluency. Transfer and maintenance programs follow. Ryan is impatient with what he views as the inefficiency of "more totalistic" treatment that may not concentrate on the systematic practice of fluency. He does not refer to the parameters of speech attended to in therapy and it is assumed that a client would not focus on these as he does in Cooper, Perkins, Webster, or Williams' therapy. Since one of Ryan's programs, the Traditional, is an adaptation of Van Riper's method of analyzing and modifying stuttering behavior, he apparently believes that increased fluency can be accomplished in several ways. Again, the essential point is objective evaluation to discover the most effective and efficient method to increase fluency and then maintain it.

Sheehan directs attention to the possibility that the issue of stuttering fluently vs. speaking fluently is often misleadingly stated by writers and lecturers contrasting the two. As we saw in the review of the literature in Chapter One, Sheehan stresses that it is the *role* the stutterer is being asked to accept, not the *speech behavior*. He says, "Most of the original behaviors are destined to go. Otherwise, there would be no point to the therapy" (p. 177). More realistic acceptance of role as it shifts over time is the central concept. For example, when the stutterer begins therapy he must develop sufficient acceptance of himself as a stutterer to begin monitoring and modifying the behavior. Furthermore, he must understand that normal speech does not mean perfect fluency. Increased fluency is a by-product of changed attitudes, and the changed attitude of increased acceptance on the part of the stutterer is modeled by the clinician's acceptance. The stutterer then goes on to learn to stutter more easily, openly, and simply when the old fear cues are present.

Along the "Great Divide" of avoidance vs. acceptance, Sheehan does not differentiate among the various therapies reviewed in Chapter One as speak more fluently approaches. He sees them all as counterproductive: "Aiming for perfect fluency and encouraging denial of the stutterer role is merely a way of ensuring that the behaviors will continue" (p. 183). In this connection, Ryan and Webster, with their emphasis on quantifying behavior, both observe in their chapters that speech fluency involving some normal disfluency is the goal. This probably helps to clear the air somewhat. "Normally fluent speech" as opposed to "fluent speech" is a better way to describe the objective of therapy. Perkins refers to "normal sounding speech."

An important aspect of Sheehan's therapy related to the issue being discussed is the recommended activities aimed toward "Improving general speaking skills: Making up for lost time" (1975, p. 171). As therapy progresses, Sheehan says that monitoring "can be expanded to the speaking pattern, not just the stuttering pattern" (1975, p. 171). He mentions work on pausing, phrasing, appropriate stress, and suitable inflection. Therefore, we see that what Sheehan criticizes as potentially harmful during the beginning stages of therapy is useful when placed appropriately in the context of role acceptance and avoidance-reduction activities.

Having worked with combinations of the two methods, I am of the opinion that the stutter more fluently procedure is more difficult for the client in the early stages and obviously requires the clinician to give the client more emotional support. Students and practicing clinicians report frequently that, compared to speak more fluently procedures, stutter more fluently methods are somewhat more abstract. As a group, those who adhere to speak more fluently methods have been more devoted to operant conditioning and programmed learning, and perhaps this frame of reference has given a specificity or concreteness to their therapy. Related to this, Sheehan observes that in spite of the wide use of his and Van Riper's publications, retrospective recovery studies (Wingate, 1964b; Shearer and Williams, 1965; Sheehan and Martyn, 1966; Dickson, 1971; Cooper, 1972) revealed that practicing clinicians have made minimal use of methods they advocate. Gregory (1969, 1972) and Prins (1970) suggested, based on outcome therapy studies, that procedures based on the work of Bryngelson, Johnson, Sheehan, and Van Riper would be more effective if structured and programmed more definitively.

A question asked in Chapter One pertained to the possibility that secondary stutterers need different approaches to speech modification depending on the types of behavior emitted, the severity of their speech difficulty, and their reaction to their speech. Webster implies the recognition of individual differences and says these can be dealt with by spending increased time on a particular stage of fluency shaping. Perkins and Ryan observe that differences in stuttering behavior do not have a noticeable effect on the results of behavior modification, but Perkins notes that more severe stutterers tend to have more difficulty maintaining improvement. Overall, the authors indicate very little change in approach based on characteristics of stuttering behavior, but all mentioned or implied that certain individual differences in attitudes or personal reactions influenced therapy outcome.

In this discussion, I have attempted to show more precisely how the methods discussed in the preceding chapters have common elements and differences. None of these prominent contributors agrees precisely. Therefore, as was said earlier, we will all differ somewhat in our understanding of specific problems and what we do. Nevertheless, this analysis should reduce the confusion and help us clarify our point of view. Some clinicians may gravitate one way or the other, some may combine the two methods in unique and successful ways, and others may originate approaches that are not closely related to either school of thought as presently described.

Shames and Egolf's (1976) description of ways in which adaptations of therapeutic procedures advocated by clinicians with different ideas about therapy can be implemented utilizing operant conditioning procedures may be helpful in resolving some of the issues discussed. Gregory's example (1968, 1973a), reviewed in Chapter One, of the way in which approaches similar to those advocated by Sheehan and Van Riper are used earlier in therapy and procedures to practice normal fluency and fluency variations are used in later phases of treatment may prove to be a meaningful model. Whatever is done, it is important that it be done with greater understanding of the issues involved.

ATTITUDE CHANGE

In one way or another, all of the contributors referred to the relationship between attitudes (cognitive and affective responses) and overt behavioral responses in stuttering therapy.

Ryan and Webster seem to agree that by far the most effective way to change attitudes is to alter speech behavior. Ryan reports some preliminary research indicating that attitude change accompanies speech change. He gives examples of cases in which attitudes interfered with therapy and suggests that attitudinal therapy like that suggested by Shames and Egolf (1976), in which the thematic content of the client's verbalization is shaped, can be useful. Webster refers to the personal reactions of stutterers and states that these are most likely tangential to disruptions in the stutterer's speech. He cites changes in perceptual scales and inventories that demonstrate marked attitudinal and emotional changes accompanying improved speech fluency. Webster has observed that, in a few cases, negative attitudes thwarted a client's positive response to speech change. Although Ryan and Webster do not refer to systematic attempts to modify attitudes, they no doubt do influence attitudes to some extent by communicating their assumptions about stuttering and therapy to their clients. In fact, Ryan calls our attention to the importance of the clinician's attitude toward the person who stutters in determining what the clinician does in therapy and how the client, in turn, views therapy. In addition, Ryan counters the assertion that those using a programmed learning format do not form an appropriate client-clinician relationship. His experience and observation indicate that most clinicians using this frame of reference are warm, empathetic, and understanding.

Cooper, Sheehan, and Williams describe in greater detail verbalizations between clinician and client that are fairly similar in purpose, although there are, of course, variations in specific objectives and methods.

Cooper tells how the parents' stereotypes of stuttering children's behavior, e.g., "the child is nervous," may lead them to incorrect perceptions and subsequent reactions that require clarification. He discusses fluency-enhancing perceptions and attitudes that the clinician may convey to the child and parents. This is done in a therapeutic situation in which time is taken to understand the parents' and child's attitudes. Cooper concludes that comprehensive therapy programs must include procedures for clarifying attitudes about stuttering and fluency control as well as procedures for actually increasing normal fluency. Just as Ryan is apprehensive that clinicians are not being adequately trained to analyze and modify speech behavior systematically, Cooper is concerned that they are not learning sufficient skills to cope effectively with beliefs and affective responses.

Sheehan's and Williams' attention to the stutterers' attitudes is closely associated with their points of view about the way in which stutterers monitor and modify their speech. The client's belief system must be explored and modified to be more in harmony with, in Sheehan's case, the role acceptance/avoidance-reduction conceptualization of therapy, and, in Williams' approach, the normal talking model. Sheehan, Williams, and Cooper emphasize that discussions of attitudes must accompany and grow out of the experiencing of events in therapy. In other words, the changing of beliefs and affective responses and the analysis and modification of speech behavior are integrated and simultaneous. Finally, William states that the nature of emotional responses in stuttering and the way this is dealt with in therapy are at the heart of most of the controversies about stuttering therapy.

Perkins believes, although he states he has little supporting research information, that the gap between sounding normal in speech and feeling normal about it, is a matter of attitude. Accepting change is seen as one objective of therapy in a way very similar to the way it is described by Sheehan. Perkins joins Cooper,

Sheehan, and Williams in using group therapy as an environment for attitudinal modification in the context of speech change.

The substance of this controversy can be reduced to the specialization and extensiveness of procedures used to bring about change. The clinician should decide whether he is going to rely mainly on change in speech to bring about sufficient attitude shift to ensure long-term success or how attitudes will be handled if speech change is the main objective, with incidental attention given to attitudes as needed. Another option for the clinician is to choose a method in which speech modification and specific attitude change activities are related and considered necessary to one another.

All of the contributors agree that we need better attitude assessment procedures and research aimed toward clarifying this variable and its change during treatment. Webster says, "It is incumbent upon those who stress the importance of attitude change procedures to demonstrate the relationship of such procedures to the efficacy of therapeutic practice" (p. 221).

PSYCHOTHERAPY AND THE PROBLEM OF STUTTERING

Williams agrees with Gregory's analysis in Chapter One that psychotherapists, counselors, and speech pathologists share the use of techniques aimed toward insight, affective change, and behavior modification, but that the difference between these specialists is the nature of the problem areas with which they are concerned. The speech-language pathologist's role is specific to speech and language problems. A counselor's goals are specified by designations such as marriage, vocational, educational, and rehabilitation. A psychotherapist usually deals with emotional distress and unadaptive behavior that is less specifically focused or more pervasive than that with which a speech pathologist would work. Some speech-language pathologists may specialize with stutterers, but some may not work with them. Also, a few psychotherapists have specialized in stuttering therapy.

This goes a long way toward solving the student and practicing clinician's questions about how much of a psychotherapist the speech-language pathologist needs to be to work with stutterers. The question is reduced to specifying the skills that should be acquired by speech-language clinicians who work with stutterers in carrying out stuttering therapy and in recognizing clients who need the help of other professionals, a topic related to all of the issues discussed in this book.

The authors agree that psychotherapy, taking into consideration the broad differences in methods used, has not been effective with stutterers. This conclusion is stated making allowance for the work of psychotherapists (psychologists and psychiatrists) who have specialized in stuttering therapy using speech modification procedures combined in varying degrees with other cognitive and affective change techniques. The treatment of stuttering involves the use of techniques that are specialized in terms of the nature of the speech problem. A clinician should not be working with stuttering in children and adults without an understanding of the problem and the decisions involved in therapy.

There is agreement that clinicians working with stutterers should be able to recognize personality characteristics that may interfere with success in therapy and with which a psychotherapist may be of assistance. Cooper refers to instruments within his Personalized Fluency Control Therapy program that provide the clinician with indications concerning the general psychological state of the client and thus alert the clinician to more pervasive needs that may exist.

Perkins and Ryan report becoming aware that some clients need more general psychotherapeutic help as therapy gets underway. Perkins observes that the modification of stuttering requires "self-directed diligence." Therefore, in his work he gives attention to attitudes of stutterers that may be related to their ability to exert the effort required. The focus of group work, mentioned in the preceding section, is on certain common attitudinal problems such as the person's dependence upon stuttering as it functions in his general pattern of adjustment. Referral is made if a greater commitment to solving adjustment problems is needed. Ryan has found that a very small number of stutterers show psychosocial problems requiring a referral for psychotherapy, and that this can be recognized during therapy. He points out that fluency is an important social-vocational skill and implies that we can be certain the person needs additional help only after improvement in speech is accomplished.

In keeping with his belief that speech reconstruction procedures may not be applied effectively, Webster cautions that we not make a referral for psychotherapy until we are certain we have sufficiently explored the avenues of treatment that have a direct impact on speech production.

Williams' most common reason for referral has been that, even though fluency increased, all of the other problems of interpersonal relations did not disappear, as the stutterer often assumed they would. He emphasizes that a referral must not be made for psychotherapy just because progress in speech change has not been satisfactory. Rather, the clinician must first re-evaluate his own clinical rationale and procedures.

Finally, when clinicians working with stutterers consider a referral, they must make a choice taking into consideration the particular psychotherapist's philosophy and experience. In terms of his work as a speech pathologist and a psychotherapist, Sheehan advises that insight-directed therapies are not sufficient for stutterers who have a well developed instrumental stuttering pattern. He recommends an action-oriented, avoidance-reduction therapy using the stutterer's response to this therapeutic opportunity as an index of his need for more specific psychotherapy. A psychotherapist with knowledge and expertise on the problem of stuttering is best suited to offer such help.

EVALUATION OF CHILDREN AND APPROPRIATE INTERVENTION

Evaluation

As research and clinical observation have resulted in more information about the nature of disfluency in children's speech (see review in Chapter One), we have acquired greater confidence in our ability to make judgments about the status of a child's speech fluency similar to evaluations of language and articulation. This knowledge, along with his own experience, has given Ryan considerable confidence in the criteria of 3 SW/M as the definition of a problem when stuttered words are defined as whole word repetitions, part-word repetitions, prolongations, and struggle behaviors. Ryan says his most difficult decisions have been with children between 3 and 5 years of age who demonstrated a rate of 3 SW/M with a topography of entirely whole or part-word repetitions, the repetitions being short and effortless. In cases where the decision was questionable, Ryan did parent counseling and re-evaluated the child 3 months later. Thus, he acknowledges that clincians must be flexible at what I call the "cross-over points" between more usual and more unusual disfluency.

Evaluating disfluency requires that attention be given to the circumstances in which the sample is made. To standardize this speech sample, Ryan developed The Fluency Interview (Ryan, 1974) that taps speaking in a broad range of tasks from rote counting or repeating after the examiner to conversational speech in a natural setting.

Other clinicians, for example Van Riper (1971a) and myself, prefer counting the number of disfluency types per 100 words rather than stuttered words per minute. Van Riper speaks of being concerned about a child's speech if he is showing two or more syllable repetitions (containing more than two repetitions per instance) per 100 words and one or more prolongations (1 second or more in duration) per 100 words. Of course, the speech sample should be sufficient in length, at least 500 words, to be representative. Van Riper mentions several other qualitative guidelines for differentiating normal disfluency from stuttering.

As for assessing a child's perception of his speech, and his possible awareness of difficulty, Ryan says his attempts to evaluate this were frustrating, resulting in his adhering to the objective observation of speech behavior. In a related way — although Williams (1969, 1971) has shown how we can gain an impression of the child's awareness by talking with him about talking, not stuttering — statements in his chapter imply that behavioral observations are the best indicators of a child's attitude about speaking.

Cooper refers to his Chronicity Prediction Checklist, which includes questions about the history of the child's speech development including stuttering, attitudinal indications based on questions about both child reactions to his speech and the parent reactions, and specific questions about the child's speech behavior.

Suggestions and specific procedures offered by Cooper, Ryan, and Williams in their chapters and by Van Riper (1971a) should enable practicing clinicians to put together a speech analysis procedure that, with reference to the best information now available, enables them to be more objective and to have more confidence in their judgments.

As was noted in Chapter One, those who have written about the evaluation of a child to determine whether a problem exists or to decide the nature of an existing problem have also described an evaluation of factors that may contribute to the development of stuttering. Several of the contributors have made statements that have a bearing upon the clinical examination including variables, about which we need research data. Ryan advocates research exploring fluency patterns of parents' speech (Knepflar, 1964), parent-child interactions, and the child's language competency as contributing factors in the development of stuttering. Perkins implies that we should refine procedures for evaluating the coordination of phonation and articulation in children's speech as related to the child's speech rate and response to environmental pressures. He hypothesizes that stuttering in children is related to a discoordination of speech coupled with the children's desire to speak at rates in excess of those they can manage or to speak when experiencing stress. Webster believes it is reasonable to hypothesize that "organismic properties figure heavily in the determination of stuttered speech" (p. 216), presumably the onset and development of stuttering. Sheehan questions that stuttering is a unitary disorder and refers to the pattern of familial incidence "12% or 13% when first-order relatives only are counted, and twice that when all known relatives are considered" (p. 176). Sheehan and Costley (1977), in a critical evaluation of the role of heredity in stuttering, raise the possibility of a "familial stutterer who differs in his history of onset and development . . ." (p. 57). As Bloodstein (1975b) says, the difficult question is *what* is inherited. Rutherford (1977) has noted the possibility that some specific language problems are inherited, and this may be related to Ryan's and others' (Gregory, 1973a; Bloodstein, 1975a) interest in the language competency of children as related to the development of stuttering. Moreover, the motolinguistic conditions about which Perkins, Wingate (1976), and Webster hypothesize may have a genetic basis. Cooper believes it is important to assume for treatment purposes that stuttering behavior is the result of multiple co-existing factors including both physiological and psychological variables. He is explicit about psychological influences but does not speculate about the specific physiological variables involved.

Based on the interest shown by contributors in both subject variables and environmental variables related to the development of stuttering, it is concluded that clinicians should use a differential evaluation procedure of the type discussed by Gregory (1973a). In addition to the speech analysis, the examiner looks for various patterns of contributing factors (characteristics of the child and environmental variables) that may occasion increased disfluency or stuttering. As exemplified by Shames and Egolf (1976) we should search for more efficient ways to evaluate environmental variables. Evaluation results should be profiled to look for patterns. We should not just stockpile data, but strive to relate information gathered to what is done in therapy and to eliminate case history information and measurements that are not therapeutically useful, unless of course there is some longer range research rationale that may not be immediately practical.

Intervention

Cooper summarizes some recent research findings on clinician attitudes toward stutterers and parental attitudes about their children who stutter to show that speech clinicians have attitudes toward children who stutter that might be evaluated as negative and predictive of failure, and that parents tend to stereotype these children as more anxious, sensitive, and insecure than do mothers of nonstuttering children. As for the latter finding about parental attitude, Cooper refers to the hypothesis of Woods and Williams (1976) that parents react to the momentary high "state anxiety" a child displays when stuttering and infer that the child has a high level of "trait anxiety." Cooper believes that clinicians' statements, as well as literature and films on stuttering, have led many parents to blame themselves unduly for their child's stuttering. In other words, in too many ways professionals may be reinforcing parental guilt. This analysis of research findings and Cooper's ideas reinforce some of the statements about the prevention of stuttering and reducing parental feelings of guilt made by others such as Williams (1971) and Gregory (1973a).

Finally, with reference to the findings on "spontaneous recoveries" from stuttering (Wingate, 1964b; Shearer and Williams, 1965; Sheehan and Martyn, 1966; Dickson, 1971; Cooper, 1972), Cooper believes that parents, through their early and active intervention procedures with their abnormally disfluent children, may be primarily responsible for the positive turn of events that apparently takes place in about two out of three cases (Cooper, 1973), rather than the other way around. In a provocative way, this speculation cuts across the current of much present thinking about what we do with young beginning stutterers. Cooper believes that clinicians should consider carefully the possibility that earlier and more active intervention may facilitate the reduction of stuttering and more recovery from stuttering.

The review of developmental intervention in Chapter One revealed that most writers advocate parent counseling, including the providing of information and steps to alter the interaction between parent and child. In addition, most advocate working with the child. Some such as Glasner (1970) and Sheehan (1970a) focus on interpersonal relations (between clinician and child, between parent and child). But we also saw that many contributors (Luper and Mulder, 1964; Bar, 1971, 1973; Gregory, 1973b; Van Riper, 1973; Bloodstein, 1975a; Hill and Gregory, 1975), in addition to the interpersonal aspect of therapy, include more direct procedures for facilitating the child's fluency.

In his chapter, Ryan states that clinicians are becoming less apprehensive about making the problems worse by working with children to increase their fluency. He reports that the use of his GILCU Program has been successful with children as young as age 4. Based on these results, he concludes that the unadaptive speech behavior and emotional responses are weaker in strength and therefore, considering stuttering as learned behavior, it is easier to treat children at the younger ages.

Cooper details the way in which the clinician explores the child's behavior and the parent's understanding of the child, including speech, as the clinician and parent decide jointly whether the child needs help with his fluency. Cooper suggests specific steps the clinician may follow in utilizing fluency-initiating gestures (FIGs) with children, including a cooperative relationship between the clinician and the parent.

Commenting on intervention with preschool children, Perkins tells us he teaches the parents to decrease their speaking rates and to model a smooth pattern for the child. The family is advised to improve their listening skills. In addition, the family is counseled to understand how attention to stuttering behavior may reinforce it. Perkins admits that his instruction of parents "... to attend selectively to their children when they speak smoothly and easily, and to be less attentive when speech becomes choppy and stuttered" (p. 118) is a controversial approach. Modeling for the child and training parents to model what we call "more easy relaxed speech with smooth movements" has also been used successfully at Northwestern University for several years.

For a more detailed description of what Williams recommends in the way of early intervention, the reader should see Williams (1978a). Comments in his chapter show that he emphasizes informing parents about children's speech development and helping them to create "a warm verbal-sharing relationship." More positive talking relations will have a positive effect on speech fluency.

In summing up on intervention for the preschool child for whom we have concern about the quantity and quality of his disfluency, it seems there is a trend toward the use of more specific fluency-enhancing procedures, ranging from modeling recommended by Gregory (1973b), Van Riper (1973), Hill and Gregory (1975), and Perkins in his chapter, to Ryan's gradual increase in length and complexity of normally fluent utterances, to Cooper's use of fluency-initiating gestures. No one takes lightly, however, the decision-making process involved in planning effective treatment that can include other procedures such as desensitization (Van Riper, 1954) and activities to facilitate speech and language development. Obviously, clinicians include the parents in ways that coincide with their evaluation of contributing factors and objectives of therapy.

The authors' statements in the preceding six chapters agree with an analysis in Chapter One that there is less controversy about therapy for school-age children having more confirmed stuttering problems than there is about the treatment of adults or preschool-age incipient stutterers just discussed. With the age group from 6 or 7 to around 14, who have experienced speech difficulty from perhaps 3 to 11 years, it is difficult to evaluate awareness, the consistency of avoidance and inhibitory tendencies, and the child's self-image as a person with a speech problem. Consequently, the issue of stutter more fluently vs. speak more fluently fades in importance. Cooper, Gregory, Perkins, Ryan, Webster and Williams in this book, and other clinicians elsewhere, such as Van Riper (1973) and Bloodstein (1975a), essentially agree that procedures should be used to enhance the child's confidence in his ability to speak easily and enjoy communication. Analysis of stuttering behavior is viewed as counterproductive. One aspect of Williams' program may include a comparison of "talking hard" or "talking easy." However, he cautions the clinician not to focus on stuttering but on the overall way of talking. I have found considerable success in using a less specific approach at first in which the clinician models "more easy relaxed speech with smooth movements" beginning with short utterances and working up to longer and more complex ones in more propositional situations. More specific analysis of the child's speech and work on modification is used only to the extent necessary.

With reference to attitudes, all clinicians are striving to prevent or to alter the belief that speech is difficult and to condition positive emotion to the act of speaking, and hence to countercondition negative emotion that may have developed. Most writers point to the importance of counseling with the parents to encourage and model changes in the parent-child relationship that may be deemed desirable and to inform them about therapy so that they may be supportive.

TRANSFER TO THE NATURAL ENVIRONMENT

Several factors are prominent in the authors' discusions of transfer of changes to the natural environment and the maintenance of change.

First, the approach to speech modification must be carried out effectively. There is no need at this point to review their approaches, but all of our contributors see a strong connection between how effectively the clinician executes the various therapeutic activities, how well the client responds, and the success of transfer of clinical change to extra-therapeutic environments. Webster reports research demonstrating the clinicians who were judged, using independent criteria, to be more effective in technical skills, were more successful in terms of the progress of their clients. We also see that the methods of measuring success are related to this point because we must assess change adequately in order to know whether speech or attitude modification procedures have been effective.

Self-monitoring and evaluation are emphasized in all systems of therapy, and proficiency in these skills is viewed as very important to carryover. In this regard, clinicians and clinical researchers should give additional attention to the study of self-regulation procedures including self-reinforcement as exemplified by the work of Kanfer and Phillips (1966) and Goldfried and Merbaum (1973) in clinicial psychology.

Second, all contributors agree that as therapy progresses specific attention is given to the planning of activities aimed toward enabling the client to change behavior in progressively more natural environmental situations. Ryan has been associated prominently with rather elaborate transfer and maintenance procedures. He describes these as coming after the establishment programs, and reports data gathered before and after transfer programs to show the positive effects of such methods. Sheehan, Webster, and Williams emphasize that change, as it takes place, should be integrated into social and nonclinic situations. Webster designates this as the "parallel transfer process." Sheehan comments that a transfer problem represents the clinician's failure to bring about assignment fulfillment outside of the therapy environment during the course of treatment. All of the writers state or imply that transfer activities should begin with easier situations and move gradually to more difficult ones. In passing, it should be noted that Ryan cautions that there is a danger in overtraining in the clinical situations.

The intensiveness of therapy is related to both the effectiveness of initial stages of behavior modification and specific procedures for transfer and carryover. Webster describes his success with a 3-week intensive program, but Cooper states a preference for nonintensive therapy over a longer period of time. However, Cooper believes that a combination of more intensive therapy at first, followed by less intensive, may be an optimal approach. Gregory (1968), with reference to behavioral concepts, suggested that one of the problems in treatment programs for stutterers in the public schools was that counterconditioning was not sufficiently intensive. With reference to school-based therapy, Cooper points to the many opportunities available for transfer activities in that setting.

Finally, the third factor related to the performance of modified speech behavior in the natural environment pertains to the personal adjustment and related motivation of the individual in therapy. Cooper, Perkins, and Webster describe individual differences in the amount of effort clients will devote to maintaining speech changes. Perkins observes that more severe stutterers are more likely to tire of using their controls and that what he calls "lucky-fluency" (fluent speech that comes quite easily) is less likely to be available to them. Also, according to Perkins, some people seem to have trouble changing their self-image as stutterers, and for these he recommends psychotherapy. Webster says that a few stutterers apparently derive social benefits from stuttering and therefore resist change. Cooper believes that one of the clinician's responsibilities is to help the client decide how much psychic energy he wishes to exert in continuing his improvement. Sheehan's lectures and writing over the years, including his contribution to this book, have elucidated the way in which the stutterer must adjust to a changing role and self-concept as he becomes a more fluent speaker. These adjustments are viewed as critical to long-term success.

It seems that our authors agree that attitudinal factors can influence stutterers' ability to take responsibility for their behavior, exercise self-control, and maintain change. Therefore, conclusions about the amount of emphasis to be placed upon specific attitude change procedures in the process of therapy, as summarized in the previous section on attitudes, are relevant here. The clinician chooses to stress certain attitude changes in keeping with the importance attached to these changes in bringing about effective transfer, stabilizing speech improvement, and expanding the change process into the natural environment over time.

As Williams says, transfer is the essence of therapy. As I said in Chapter One, transfer of change to the natural environment and preventing relapse is probably the most important topic in the contemporary study of stuttering therapy. Clinicians should be planning for transfer from the beginning of therapy. Specific procedures should be described explicitly, refined, and evaluated. A particularly important area of research is the utilization of parents, teachers, and peers or friends as carryover observers and reward agents. Self-modification activities (Watson and Tharp, 1972) should be utilized more extensively since, without doubt, this ability is important in the maintenance of improved fluency.

CRITERIA FOR SUCCESS: MEASURING THE RESULTS OF THERAPY

The overt speech behavior of stutterers can be observed and quantified with satisfactory reliability. Researchers have found stuttering a rewarding area of study, in part, because it can be analyzed and quantified so much more easily than many other maladaptive problem behaviors. Stuttering research throughout the 1940s and 1950s, for example, that on the adaptation and consistency effects, included counts of stuttered words and data showing acceptable reliability of observation. Johnson, Darley, and Spriestersbach (1963) reviewed rating scales of severity and methods of counting disfluencies and cited the value of these procedures in evaluating therapy. Yet, many articles and books describing stuttering therapy have been published, even in recent years, with very few or no objective data given about speech change.

This situation is changing rapidly. More clinicians and clinical researchers are charting progress in terms of carefully defined speech measures, and reports in journals reflect a growing opinion that a clinician cannot write about what he does unless he presents reliable data evaluating speech change. In addition to quantifying stuttering behavior, there is agreement that an assessment of speech rate should be included in a speech analysis and in a therapy report.

Perkins believes that the computation of percentages of syllables stuttered and rate in syllables per minute are the most valid basic measures to be made of the stutterer's speech. In addition, he mentions in his chapter what he has noted previously (Perkins, 1973a, b), that for measuring improvement more definitively in terms of normal sounding speech, ratings of phrasing and prosody should be included. Ryan has found stuttered words per minute and words spoken per minute to be very convenient measures for clinical uses, and although he implies that he would always include both and a percentage of stuttering derived from these two in research reports, he believes the "on-line" clinician can use only stuttered words per minute to follow a client's progress. But obviously, speaking is not acceptable unless the rate is within the normal range, and Ryan says the clinician should attend to this. Webster, like Perkins and Ryan, defines the disfluency types that he counts, what he terms the primary response measures, and includes a measure of speech rate. Webster, as do other writers, emphasizes that clinicians must be trained to be reliable observers. Moreover, he points out that we must have quantifiable knowledge of the consistency of behavior under the same or similar conditions, i.e., the reliability of the behavior. This is a significant point. Basic knowledge about the variability of stuttered speech, both before and after therapy, is essential for the accurate assessment of therapeutic effects.

Cooper describes the assessment of fluency and changes in fluency using several checklists and rating scales that he believes provide a more global picture of the client's speech as perceived by the client and the clinician. These procedures seem to add to, but not replace, the more precise measurements of stuttering.

With the emphasis upon the measurement of stuttering by counting disfluencies, it is important that more normal disfluencies be discriminated from disfluencies that the clinician has defined as stuttering. In the case of children with more confirmed problems, and with adults, it is often helpful for them to understand that certain types of disfluencies are expected to occur and that "successful speakers" are, to varying degrees, disfluent.

The validity of measures of transfer made in the natural environment continues to be a problem. The reactive measurement effect, i.e., the interaction of certain stimulus conditions involved in assessment with the behavioral response of stuttering, is difficult to eliminate. Reports on therapy must be honest about these effects. When a client knows that a tape recorder has been turned on in his home, this probably has a stimulus control influence upon his speech. Knowing about these effects and taking them into consideration does not mean that we should not make recordings in the natural environment. But, as Cooper, Perkins, Ryan, and Webster recommend, we should supplement these speech measurements with self-reports and reports from family and friends. The more agreement among these, the greater the confidence we can have in our evaluation of results.

Perkins described a Speech Performance Questionnaire used to obtain a subjective evaluation of improvement. Earlier Perkins et al. (1974) reported using a modification of the Iowa Stutterer's Self-Rating of Reactions to Speaking Situations to tap self-evaluations. Woolf's Perceptions of Stuttering Inventory (Woolf, 1967) is used frequently by clinicians to assess stutterers' changes in feelings of struggle, avoidance, and expectancy (Van Riper, 1973), and Webster discussed the value of this questionnaire. Cooper described the use of a Situation Avoidance Behavior Checklist for assessing change. There seems to be general agreement that self-report data on speech improvement should be obtained and compared to more objective information.

All of our authors, regardless of their points of view about the systematic use of approaches to modify attitudes in therapy, refer to the use of attitude measures as criteria of success. Perkins refers to a recent report by Guitar (1976) showing that of three pretreatment measures (stuttering behavior, attitudes about speaking, and personality), attitudes were most highly related to the outcome of therapy based on speech measures made a year following treatment. An abbreviated form of the Erickson Scale of Communication Attitudes (Erickson, 1969) and avoidance and reaction portions of the Stutterer's Self-Rating of Reactions to Speech Situations (Johnson, Darley, and Spriestersbach, 1963) were used to assess attitude. More recently, Guitar and Bass (1978) found that follow-up assessments of stutterers a year after therapy showed that those whose attitudes on the Erickson Scale had normalized by the end of transfer activities were stuttering significantly less than a group for whom attitude measures were not in the normal range. Guitar (1976) also reported that pretreatment attitude scores are independent of stuttering severity. This latter finding, along with the observation that pretreatment attitudes and the normalization of attitudes during therapy are important predictors of outcome measured a year following therapy, indicate that attitude change should be included in an assessment of therapy results. For evaluating attitudes, Cooper provides a Stuttering Attitudes Checklist, and in keeping with the widely accepted point of view that parents' attitudes are important in the case of a child, Cooper has developed a Parent Attitudes Toward Stuttering Checklist.

Even though we cannot deal as precisely with cognitive attitudes as we can with speech behavior, we should not omit evaluating changes in this variable as well as we can. In addition to Guitar's research (in press), other studies by Andrews and Cutler (1974) and Perkins et al. (1974), reviewed in Chapter One, and case observations mentioned by our contributors, all point to the importance of evaluating: 1) the relationship between attitudinal responses and speech behavior, 2) the relationship between attitudinal responses and the amount of speech change, 3) the effects of various procedures in therapy with reference to attitude change, and 4) the relationship between attitude shifts and speech changes. As mentioned earlier, we need better attitude assessment procedures. Changes in self-report personality measures such as the Adjective Check List (Gough and Heilbrun, 1965), which Webster has related to speech improvement, can be viewed as assessments of more general attitudes in terms of beliefs and verbal reports of affective and overt responses. There continues to be some interest in gathering personality data and comparing this information to more objective speech change results and other self-reports of progress (Gregory, 1969; Perkins et al., 1974; Guitar, 1976).

None of the authors reported using physiological measures of affective responding (e.g., palmar sweating, galvanic skin resistance, heart rate, blood pressure) to assess results. Apparently clinicians' awareness of research showing inconsistent relationships between these measures and stuttering and changes during therapy (Perkins, 1970; Van Riper, 1971a; Bloodstein, 1975b) has resulted in little use of these procedures to assess outcome.

Ryan and Webster place special emphasis on the number of hours of therapy required to reach success criteria. The less time involved by both client and clinician, the more efficient the therapy. However, this does not mean that long-term follow-up or maintenance procedures are curtailed, only that all of therapy is efficient. Ryan discusses efficiency with reference to the entire process of therapy including the permanence of change.

Williams cautions that even though speech change is obviously the goal of treatment, we must remember that criteria of "success" and "failure" represent evaluative statements. Cooper and Perkins agree with Williams that clinicians should be careful to give "due thought, respect, and understanding to the goals of the client" (Williams, p. 268). With reference to the efficiency of therapy and effectiveness as evaluated using objective measures, attention should be given to the need to adjust clinical goals depending upon the way the client's goals evolve. Cooper, Perkins, and Williams show how they give consideration to this in the attitudinal aspect of therapy.

Regarding all improvement measures, Sheehan believes increased consideration should be given to making provisions for judgments by independent observers to verify reported results of stuttering therapy.

In conclusion, a continuation of the present trend toward more precise definition and assessment of speech behavior and attitudinal responses before, during, and after therapy, along with more specific descriptions of treatment, should lead to an increased understanding of the results of various procedures, and in this way improve the outcome of stuttering therapy. This is probably the best way to reduce controversy.

References

Adamczyk, B. 1959. Use of instruments for the production of artificial feedback in the treatment of stuttering. Fol. Phoniatr., 11, 216–218.

Adamczyk, B. 1965. Die Ergebnisse der Behandlung des Stotterns durch das Telephonechosystem. XIII Congress. International Society of Logopedics and Phoniatrics, pp. 433–435.

Adamczyk, B., Sadowska, E., and Kuniszyk-Jozkowiak. 1975. Influence of reverberation on stuttering. Foli. Phoniatr., 27, 1–6.

Adams, M., Lewis, J., and Besozzi, T. 1973. The effect of reduced reading rate on stuttering frequency. J. Speech Hear. Res., 16, 671–675.

Adams, M., and Reis, R. 1971. The influence of the onset of phonation on the frequency of stuttering. J. Speech Hear. Res., 14, 639–644.

Adams, M., and Reis, R. 1974. The influence of the onset of phonation on the frequency of stuttering: a replication and evaluation. J. Speech Hear. Res., 17, 752–754.

Agnello, J. G. 1975. Laryngeal and articulatory dynamics of dysfluency interpreted within a vocal track model. In L. M. Webster and L. C. Furst (Eds.), Vocal Track Dynamics and Dysfluency. New York: Speech Institute.

Ainsworth, S. 1975. Stuttering: What It Is and What to Do About It. Lincoln, Neb.: Cliffs Notes, Inc.

Ainsworth, S. 1977. The relationship of theory and clinician characteristics to therapy for stutterers: a discussion of the Murphy and Wingate paper. Second Emil Froeschels conference on the problem of stuttering. Pace University, New York, 1975. J. Commun. Dis., 10, 53–59.

Allport, G. W. 1935. Attitude. In C. Murchison (Ed.), Handbook of Social Psychology. Worcester, Mass.: Clark University Press.

American Speech and Hearing Association. 1975. Code of Ethics. In Annual Directory. ASHA, Washington, D.C.

Anastasi, A. 1976. Psychological Testing. New York: Macmillan.

Andrews, G., and Cutler, J. 1974. Stuttering therapy: the relation between changes in symptom level and attitudes. J. Speech Hear. Dis., 39, 312–319.

Andrews, G., and Harris, M. 1964. The Syndrome of Stuttering. London: Levenham Press.

Andrews, G., and Ingham, R. J. 1971. Stuttering: considerations in the evaluation of treatment. Br. J. Dis. Commun., 6, 129–138.

Andrews, G., and Ingham, R. J. 1972a. An approach to the evaluation of stuttering therapy. J. Speech Hear. Res., 15, 296–302.

Andrews, G., and Ingham, R. J. 1972b. Stuttering: an evaluation of follow-up procedures for syllable-timed speech/token economy system therapy. J. Commun. Dis., 5, 307–319.

Azrin, N., and Nunn R. 1974. A rapid method of eliminating stuttering by a regulated breathing approach. Behav. Res. Ther., 12, 279–286.

Bandura, A. 1969. Principles of Behavior Modification. New York: Holt, Rinehart and Winston.

Bar, A. 1971. The shaping of fluency, not the modification of stuttering. J. Commun. Dis., 4, 1–8.

Bar, A. 1973. Increasing fluencies in young stutterers vs. decreasing stuttering: a clinical approach. J. Commun. Dis., 6, 247–258.

Beech, H. R., and Fransella, F. 1968. Research and Experiment in Stuttering. Oxford: Pergamon Press.

Beech, H. R., and Fransella, F. 1969. Explanations of the "rhythm effect" in stuttering. In G. Gray and G. England (Eds.), Stuttering and the Conditioning Therapies. Monterey, Cal.: Monterey Institute for Speech and Hearing.

Berry, M. F. 1938. Developmental history of stuttering children. J. Pediatr., 12, 209–217.

Berryman, J., and Kools, J. 1975. Disfluency of non-stuttering children in relation to specific measures of language, reading and mental maturity. J. Fluency Dis., 1, 18–24.

Biggs, B. E., and Sheehan, J. G. 1969. Punishment or distraction? Operant stuttering revisited. J. Abnorm. Psychol., 74, 256–262.

Blind, J., Shames, G., and Egolf, D. 1971. The combined use of operant procedures and theroretical concepts in the treatment of an adult female stutterer. J. Speech Hear. Dis., 36, 414–421.

Bloodstein, O. 1958. Stuttering as an anticipatory struggle reaction. In J. Eisenson (Ed.), Stuttering: A Symposium. New York: Harper & Row.

Bloodstein, O. 1975a. Stuttering as tension and fragmentation. In J. Eisenson (Ed.), Stuttering: A Second Symposium. New York: Harper & Row.

Bloodstein, O. 1975b. A Handbook on Stuttering. Chicago: National Easter Seal Society.

Bloodstein, O. 1977. Foreword. In R. W. Rieber (Ed.), The Problem of Stuttering: Theory and Therapy. New York: Elsevier/North-Holland.

Bloodstein, O., and Gantwerk, B. 1967. Grammatical function in relation to stuttering in young children. J. Speech Hear. Res., 10, 786–789.

Boberg, E. 1976. Intensive group therapy program for stutterers. Human Commun., 1, 29–42.

Boberg, E., and Sawyer, L. 1977. The maintenance of fluency following intensive therapy. Human Commun., 2, 21–28.

Boehmler, R. 1958. Listener responses to non-fluencies. J. Speech Hear. Res., 1, 132–141.

Boehmler, R. 1970. An evaluation of behavior modification in the treatment of stuttering. In W. Starkweather (Ed.), Conditioning in Stuttering Therapy. Memphis, Tenn.: Speech Foundation of America.

Boring, E. G. 1950. A History of Experimental Psychology. New York: Appleton-Century-Crofts.

Brady, J. P. 1968. A behavioral approach to the treatment of stuttering. J. Psychiatr., 125, 843–847.

Brady, J. P. 1969. Studies on the metronome effect on stuttering. Behav. Res. Ther., 7, 197–204.

Branscom, M., Hughes, J., and Oxtoby, E. 1955. Studies of nonfluency in the speech of preschool children. In W. Johnson and R. Leutenegger (Eds.), Stuttering in Children and Adults. Minneapolis: University of Minnesota Press.

Brenner, N., Perkins, W., and Soderberg, G. 1972. The effect of rehearsal on frequency of stuttering. J. Speech Hear. Res., 15, 483–486.

Brownell, W.1973. The relationship of sex, social class, and verbal planning to the disfluencies produced by non-stuttering pre-school children. Unpublished doctoral dissertation, State University of New York at Buffalo.

Brutten, G. J. 1975. Stuttering: topography, assessment, and behavior change strategies. In J. Eisenson (Ed.), Stuttering: A Second Symposium. New York: Harper & Row.

Brutten, G. J., and Shoemaker, D. 1967. The Modification of Stuttering. Englewood Cliffs, N.J.: Prentice-Hall.

Butterfield, H. 1957. The Origins of Modern Science. New York: The Free Press.

Cherry, E. C., and Sayers, B. M. 1956. Experiments upon the total inhibition of stammering by external control and some clinical results. J. Psychosom. Res., 1, 233–246.

Cherry, E. C., Sayers, B. M., and Marland, P. 1955. Experiments in the complete suppression of stuttering. Nature, 176, 874–875.

Combs, A., and Snygg, D. 1959. Individual Behavior: A Perceptual Approach to Behavior. New York: Harper & Row.

Connell, P., Spradlin, J., and McReynolds, L. 1977. Some suggested criteria for evaluation of language programs. J. Speech Hear. Dis., 42, 563–567.

Cooper, E. B. 1965. Structured therapy for therapist and stuttering child. J. Speech Hear. Dis., 30, 75–78.

Cooper, E. B. 1968. A therapy process for the adult stutterer. J. Speech Hear. Dis., 33, 246–260.

Cooper, E. B. 1971. Reflections on conceptulizing the stuttering therapy process from a single theoretical framework. J. Speech Hear. Dis., 36, 471–475.

Cooper, E.B. 1972. Recovery from stuttering in a junior and senior high school population. J. Speech Hear. Res., 15, 632–638.

Cooper, E. B. 1973. The development of a stuttering chronicity prediction checklist for school aged stutterers: a research inventory for clinicians. J. Speech Hear. Res., 38, 215–223.

Cooper, E. B. 1975. Clinician attitudes toward stutterers: a study of bigotry? Paper presented at the American Speech and Hearing Association Convention, Washington, D.C.

Cooper, E. B. 1976. Personalized Fluency Control Therapy: An Integrated Behavior and Relationship Therapy for Stutterers. Austin, Tex.: Learning Concepts.

Cooper, E.B. 1977. Controversies about stuttering behavior. J. Fluency Dis., 2, 75-86.

Cooper, E. B. Cady, B. B., and Robbins, C. J. 1970. The effect of the verbal stimulus words "Wrong," "Right," and "Tree," on the disfluency rates of stutterers and nonstutterers. J. Speech Hear. Res., 13, 239-244.

Cooper, E. B., Parris, R., and Wells, M. T. 1974. Prevalence of and recovery from speech disorders in a group of freshmen at the University of Alabama. Asha, 16, 359-360.

Costello, J. 1975. The establishment of fluency with time-out procedures: three case studies. J. Speech Hear. Dis., 40, 216-231.

Cross, D., and Cooper, E. B. 1976. Self versus investigator-administered presumed fluency reinforcing stimuli. J. Speech Hear. Res., 19, 241-246.

Crowe, T. A., and Cooper, E. B. 1977. Parental attitudes toward and knowledge of stuttering. J. Commun. Dis., 10, 343-357.

Culatta, R. A.1976. Fluency: the other side of the coin. Asha, 18, 795-799.

Curlee, R., and Perkins, W. 1969. Conversational rate control therapy for stuttering. J. Speech Hear. Dis., 34, 245-250.

Daly, D. A. 1977. Intervention procedures for the young stuttering child. Paper presented at the Council for Exceptional Children Convention, Atlanta.

Daly, D. A., and Cooper, E. B. 1967. Rate of stuttering adaptation under two electro-shock conditions. Behav. Res. Ther., 5, 49-54.

Damste, P. H. 1970. A behavioral analysis of a stuttering therapy. In W. Starkweather (Ed.), Conditioning in Stuttering Therapy. Memphis, Tenn.: Speech Foundation of America.

Davis, D. 1939. The relation of repetitions in the speech of young children to certain measures of language maturity and situational factors. Part I. J. Speech Dis., 4, 303-318.

DeFeo, T. 1975. A clinical investigation of procedures designed to facilitate generalization and carry over of treatment effects among five elementary school age children who stutter. Unpublished manuscript, Northwestern University, Evanston, Ill.

DeJoy, D. 1975. An investigation of the frequency of nine individual types of disfluency and total disfluency in relation to age and syntactic maturity in nonstuttering males, three and one half years of age and five years of age. Unpublished doctoral dissertation, Northwestern University, Evanston, Ill.

Dickson, S. 1971. Incipient stuttering and spontaneous remission of stuttered speech. J. Commun. Dis., 4, 99-110.

Ellis, A. 1962. Reason and Emotion in Psychotherapy. New York: Lyle Stuart.

Emerick, L. L. 1965. Therapy for young stutterers. Except. Child., 31, 398-402.

Emerick, L. L., and Hood, S. B. (Eds.). 1974. The Client-Clinician Relationship. Springfield, Ill.: Charles C Thomas.

Emrick, C. 1971. Language performance of stuttering and nonstuttering children. Unpublished doctoral dissertation, University of Iowa, Iowa City.

Erickson, R. 1969. Asssessing communication attitudes among stutterers. J. Speech Hear. Res., 12, 711–724.

Fowlie, G. M., and Cooper, E. B. 1978. Traits attributed to stuttering and non-stuttering children by their parents. Unpublished paper, University of Alabama, Tuscaloosa.

Freeman, F. 1975. Phonation and fluency. In L. M. Webster and L. C. Furst (Eds.), Vocal Tract Dynamics and Dysfluency. New York: Speech and Hearing Institute.

Frick, J. 1965. Evaluation of motor planning techniques for the treatment of stuttering. Pennsylvania State University, Office of Education Project 32-48-0720-5003, U.S. Department of Health, Education, and Welfare.

Gifford, M. 1956. Theory and therapy. In E. F. Hahn and E. S. Hahn (Eds.), Stuttering: Significant Theories and Therapies. Stanford, Cal.: Stanford University Press.

Gillespie, S., and Cooper, E. B. 1973. Prevalence of speech disorders in a junior and senior high school. J. Speech Hear. Dis., 16, 739–743.

Giolas, T., and Williams, D. 1958. Children's reaction to nonfluencies in adult speech. J. Speech Hear. Res., 1, 86–93.

Glasner, P. J. 1970. Developmental view. In J. Sheehan (Ed.), Stuttering: Research and Therapy. New York: Harper & Row.

Glauber, I. P. 1958. The psychoanalysis of stuttering. In J. Eisenson (Ed.), Stuttering: A Symposium. New York: Harper.

Goldfried, M., and Merbaum, M. 1973. Behavior Change Through Self-Control. New York: Holt, Rinehart and Winston.

Goldiamond, I. 1965. Stuttering and fluency as manipulatable operant response classes. In L. Krasner and L. Ullman (Eds.), Research in Behavior Modification. New York: Holt, Rinehart and Winston.

Goldiamond, I. 1974. Personal communication to Bruce Ryan.

Goldiamond, I. 1977. Personal communication to Hugo Gregory.

Goodstein, L. 1958. Functional speech disorders and personality: a survey of the research. J. Speech Hear. Res., 1, 359–376.

Gough, H. G., and Heilbrun, A. B. 1965. The Adjective Check List. Palo Alto, Cal.: Consulting Psychologists Press.

Gray, B., and England, G. 1969. Stuttering: the measurement of anxiety during reciprocal inhibition. In G. Gray and G. England (Eds.), Stuttering and the Conditioning Therapies. Monterey, Cal.: Monterey Institute for Speech and Hearing.

Gray, B., and England, G. 1972. Some effects of anxiety deconditioning upon stuttering frequency. J. Speech Hear. Res., 15, 114–122.

Gray, B., and Ryan, B. 1973. A Language Program for the Non-Language Child. Champaign, Ill.: Research Press.

Gregory, H. 1968. Applications of learning theory concepts in the management of stuttering. In H. Gregory (Ed.), Learning Theory and Stuttering Therapy. Evanston, Ill.: Northwestern University Press.

Gregory, H. 1969. An assessment of the results of stuttering therapy. Evanston, Ill.: Northwestern University. Final Report. Research and Demonstration Project 1725-S, Social and Rehabilitation Service, U.S. Department of Health, Education, and Welfare.

Gregory, H. 1972. An assessment of the results of stuttering therapy. J. Commun. Dis., 5, 320–334.

Gregory, H. 1973a. Stuttering: Differential Evaluation and Therapy. Indianapolis: Bobbs-Merrill.

Gregory, H. 1973b. Modeling procedures in the treatment of elementary school children who stutter. J. Fluency Dis., 1, 58–63.

Gregory, H. 1977. Review of Stuttering Solved by Martin F. Schwartz. Rehab. Lit., 38, 157–159.

Gregory, H., and Haerle, J. 1976. Some systematic approaches to working with elementary school age children who stutter. Unpublished paper, Northwestern University, Evanston, Ill.

Gregory, H., and Mordecai, D. 1977. Programs for identification, analysis, and modification of stuttering. Unpublished programs, Northwestern University, Evanston, Ill.

Guitar, B. 1975. Reduction of stuttering frequency using analog electromyographic feedback. J. Speech Hear. Res., 18, 672–685.

Guitar, B. 1976. Pretreatment factors associated with the outcome of stuttering therapy. J. Speech Hear. Res., 19, 590–600.

Guitar, B., and Bass, C. 1978. Stuttering therapy: the relation between attitude change and long-term outcome. J. Speech Hear. Dis., 43, 392–400.

Hanna, R., and Owen, N. 1977. Facilitating transfer and maintenance of fluency in stuttering. J. Speech Hear. Dis., 42, 65–76.

Haroldson, S., Martin, R., and Starr, C. 1968. Time-out as a punishment for stuttering. J. Speech Hear. Res., 11, 560–566.

Helmreich, H., and Bloodstein, O. 1973. The grammatical factor in childhood disfluency in relation to the continuity hypothesis. J. Speech Hear. Res., 16, 731–738.

Hersen, M., and Barlow, D. G. 1976. Single Case Experimental Designs: Strategies for Studying Behavior Change. New York: Pergamon Press.

Hessell, W. F. 1971. Anxiety level in relation to time delay and stuttering during self-formulated speech. Unpublished doctoral dissertation, University of Calfornia, Los Angeles.

Hill, D., and Gregory, H. 1975. Modeling procedures in stuttering therapy. Short course, Midwest Regional Conference, American Speech and Hearing Associaton, Minneapolis.

Hood, S. 1974. Clients, clinicians, and therapy. In L. Emerick and S. Hood (Eds.), The Client-Clinician Relationship. Springfield, Ill.: Charles C Thomas.

Ingham, R. J. 1975. A comparison of covert and overt assessment procedures in stuttering therapy outcome evaluation. J. Speech Hear. Res., 18, 346–354.

Ingham, R. J. 1976. Onset, prevalence, and recovery from stuttering: a reassessment of findings from the Andrews and Harris study. J. Speech Hear. Dis., 41, 280–281.

Ingham, R. J., and Andrews, G. 1971. Stuttering: the quality of fluency after treatment. J. Commun. Dis., 4, 279–288.

Ingham, R. J., and Andrews, G. 1973. Behavior therapy and stuttering: a review. J. Speech Hear. Dis., 38, 405–441.

Ingham, R. J., Martin, R., and Kuhl, P. 1974. Modification and control rate of speaking by stutterers. J. Speech Hear. Res., 17, 489–496.

Jackson, B. 1949. Cited by C. Van Riper (1973) in The Treatment of Stuttering. Englewood Cliffs, N.J.: Prentice-Hall.

Johnson, P. 1951. An exploratory study of certain aspects of the speech histories of 23 former stutterers. Unpublished masters thesis, Unversity of Pittsburgh.

Johnson, W. 1946. People in Quandries. New York: Harper & Row.

Johnson, W. et al. 1959. The Onset of Suttering. Minneapolis: University of Minnesota Press.

Johnson, W. 1961a. Measurement of oral reading and speaking rate and disfluency of adult male and female stutterers and nonstutters. J. Speech Hear. Dis., Monogr. Suppl. 7, 1–20.

Johnson, W. 1961b. Stuttering and What You Can Do About It. Minneapolis: University of Minnesota Press.

Johnson, W. 1967. Stuttering. In W. Johnson and D. Moeller (Eds.), Speech Handicapped School Children. New York: Harper & Row.

Johnson, W., Darley, F. L., and Spriestersbach, D.C. 1963. Diagnostic Methods in Speech Pathology. New York: Harper & Row.

Kanfer, F., and Phillips, J. 1966. Behavior therapy: a panacea for all ills or a passing fancy? Arch. Gen. Psychiatr. 15, 114–28.

Kanfer, F., and Phillips, J. 1970. Learning Foundations of Behavior Therapy. New York: John Wiley & Sons.

Katz, M. 1977. A survey of potential anti-stuttering devices. In R. W. Rieber (Ed.), The Problem of Stuttering: Theory and Therapy. New York: Elsevier/North-Holland.

Kimbarow, M. L., and Daly, D. A. 1977. Effects of "Wrong," "Right," and "Tree": replication with school age stutterers. Paper presented at the American Speech and Hearing Association Convention, Chicago.

Knepflar, K. J. 1964. A study of speaking fluency in the parents of stutterers and non-stutterers. Unpublished doctoral dissertation, University of California, Los Angeles.

Knepflar, K. J. 1973. Personal communication to Bruce Ryan.

Lankford, S. D., and Cooper, E. B. 1974. Recovery from stuttering as viewed by parents of self-diagnosed recovered stutterers. J. Commun. Dis., 7, 171–180.

Leach, E. 1969. Stuttering: clinical application of response contingent procedures. In B. Gray and G. England (Eds.), Stuttering and the Conditioning Therapies. Monterey, Cal.: Monterey Institute for Speech and Hearing.

Lee, B. S., 1951. Artificial stutter. J. Speech Hear. Dis., 16, 53–55.

Lee, I. J. 1941. Language Habits in Human Affairs. New York: Harper & Row.

Luper, H. L., and Mulder, R. L. 1964. Stuttering: Therapy for Children. Englewood Cliffs, N.J.: Prentice-Hall.

Makuen, G. H. 1930/31. Quoted by M. S. Steel in How Dr. G. Hudson Makuen treated stammering. A paper in R. West (Ed.), A Symposium on Stuttering (Stammering). American Society for the Study of Disorders of Speech.

Manning, W. H., and Shrum, W. F. 1973. The concept of control in stuttering therapy: a reappraisal. DCCD Bulletin, 11, 32–34.

Martin, R. 1968. The experimental manipulation of stuttering behavior. In H. Sloane and B. MacAulay (Eds.), Operant Procedures in Remedial Speech and Language Training. Boston: Houghton-Mifflin.

Martin, R., and Haroldson, S. 1969. The effects of two treatment procedures on stuttering. J. Commun. Dis., 2, 115–125.

Martyn, M. M., and Sheehan, J. G. 1968. Onset of stuttering and recovery. Behav. Res. Ther., 6, 295–307.

May, A. 1968. Listenability ratings of stuttering. Unpublished doctoral dissertation, University of California, Los Angeles.

McGuigan, F. J. 1968. Experimental Psychology: a Methodological Approach. Englewood Cliffs, N.J.: Prentice-Hall.

McLelland, J. K., and Cooper, E. B. 1977. Fluency-related behaviors and attitudes of 178 young stutterers. Paper presented at the American Speech and Hearing Association Convention. Chicago.

Mowrer, D. 1975. An instructional program to increase fluent speech of stutterers. J. Fluency Dis., 1, 25–35.

Mowrer, D. 1977. Methods of Modifying Speech Behaviors. Columbus, Ohio: Charles E. Merrill.

Mowrer, O. H. 1953. Psychotherapy: Theory and Research. New York: Ronald Press.

Mowrer, O. H. 1960a. Learning Theory and Behavior. New York: John Wiley & Sons.

Mowrer, O. H. 1960b. Learning Theory and the Symbolic Processes. New York: John Wiley & Sons.

Muma, J. 1971. Syntax of preschool fluent and disfluent speech: a transformational analysis. J. Speech Hear. Res., 14, 428–441.

Murphy, A. (Ed.). 1962. Stuttering: Its Prevention. Memphis, Tenn.: Speech Foundation of America.

Murphy, A. 1970. Stuttering, behavior modification, and the person. In Conditioning in Stuttering Therapy. Memphis, Tenn.: Speech Foundation of America.

Murphy, A. 1974. Feelings and attitudes. In W. Starkweather (Ed.), Therapy for Stutterers. Memphis, Tenn.: Speech Foundation of America.

Murphy, A. 1977. Authenticity and creativity in stuttering theory and therapy. J. Commun. Dis., 10, 25–36.

Murphy, A., and Fitzsimons, R. M. 1960. Stuttering and Personality Dynamics. New York: Ronald Press.

Mysak, E. D. 1960. Servo theory and stuttering. J. Speech Hear. Dis., 25, 188–195.

Mysak, E. D. 1966. Speech Pathology and Feedback Theory. Springfield, Ill.: Charles C Thomas.

Peins, M., McGough, W. E., and Lee, B. S. 1972. Evaluation of a tape-recorded method of stuttering therapy: improvement in a speaking task. J. Speech Hear Res., 15, 364–371.

Perkins, W. 1965. Stuttering: some common denominators. In D. Barbara (Ed.), New Directions in Stuttering. Springfield, Ill.: Charles C Thomas.

Perkins, W. 1967. Modification of stuttering by rate control. Final Report. Vocational Rehabilitation Administration Planning Grant RD-2180-5, University of Southern California, Los Angeles.

Perkins, W. 1970. Physiological studies. In J. Sheehan (Ed.), Stuttering: Research and Therapy. New York: Harper & Row.

Perkins, W. 1973a. Replacement of stuttering with normal speech. I. Rationale. J. Speech Hear. Dis., 38, 283–294.

Perkins, W. 1973b. Replacement of stuttering with normal speech. II. Clinical procedures. J. Speech Hear. Dis., 38, 295–303.

Perkins, W. 1977. Speech Pathology: An Applied Behavioral Science. Rev. ed. St. Louis: C. V. Mosby.

Perkins, W., and Curlee, R. 1969. Clinical impressions of portable masking unit effects in stuttering. J. Speech Hear. Dis., 34, 360–362.

Perkins, W., et al. 1974. Replacement of stuttering with normal speech. III. Clinical effectiveness. J. Speech Hear. Dis., 39, 416–428.

Perkins, W. et al. 1976. Stuttering: discoordination of phonation with articulation and respiration. J. Speech Hear. Res., 19, 509–522.

Prins, D. 1970. Improvement and regression in stutterers following a short-term intensive therapy. J. Speech Hear. Dis., 35, 123–135.

Prins, D. 1976. Stutterers' perceptions of therapy improvement and of post-therapy regression: effects of certain program modifications. J. Speech Hear. Dis., 41, 452–463.

Riley, G. 1972. A stuttering severity instrument for children and adults. J. Speech Hear. Dis., 37, 314–322.

Robbins, S. D. 1930/31. Paper in R. West (Ed.), A Symposium on Stuttering (Stammering). American Society for the Study of Disorders of Speech.

Rogers, C. 1951. Client-centered Therapy. Boston: Houghton-Mifflin.

Rogers, C. 1957. The necessary and sufficient conditions of therapeutic personality change. J. Consult. Psychol., 21, 95–103.

Rosenthal, R. 1966. Experimenter Bias in Behavioral Research. New York: Appleton-Century-Crofts.

Rutherford, D. 1977. Speech and language disorders and minimal brain damage. In J. G. Millichap (Ed.), Learning Disabilities and Related Disorders. Chicago: Year Book Medical Publishers.

Ryan, B. 1964. The construction and evaluation of a program for modifying stuttering behavior. Unpublished doctoral dissertation, University of Pittsburgh.

Ryan, B. 1970. An illustration of operant conditioning therapy for stuttering. In W. Starkweather (Ed.), Conditioning in Stuttering Therapy: Applications and Limitations. Memphis, Tenn.: Speech Foundation of America.

Ryan, B. 1971. Operant procedures applied to stuttering therapy for children. J. Speech Hear. Dis., 36, 264–280.

Ryan, B. 1974. Programmed Therapy for Stuttering in Children and Adults. Springfield, Ill.: Charles C Thomas.

Ryan, B., and Van Kirk, B. 1971. Monterey Fluency Program. Palo Alto: Monterey Learning Systems.

Ryan, B., and Van Kirk, B. 1974a. The establishment, transfer, and maintenance of fluent speech in 50 stutterers using delayed auditory feedback and operant procedures. J. Speech Hear. Dis., 39, 3–10.

Ryan, B., and Van Kirk, B. 1974b. Programmed stuttering therapy for children. Final report. Office of Education Project 0-72-4422, U.S. Department of Health, Education, and Welfare, Washington, D.C.

Sarbin, T. R. 1964. Role-theoretical interpretation of psychological change. In P. Worchel and D. Byrne (Eds.), Personality Change. New York: John Wiley & Sons.

Schuell, H. 1946. Sex differences in relation to stuttering. I. J. Speech Dis., 11, 277–298.

Schwartz, M. F. 1974. The core of the stuttering block. J. Speech Hear. Dis., 39, 169–177.

Schwartz, M. F. 1976. Stuttering Solved. Philadelphia: J. B. Lippincott.

Seligman, M. E. P. 1970. On the generality of the laws of learning. Psychol. Rev., 77, 406–418.

Shames, G. H. 1970. Operant conditioning and therapy for stuttering. In W. Starkweather (Ed.), Conditioning in Stuttering Therapy. Memphis, Tenn.: Speech Foundation of America.

Shames, G. H. 1975. Operant conditioning and stuttering. In J. Eisenson (Ed.), Stuttering: A Second Symposium. New York: Harper & Row.

Shames, G. H., and Egolf, D. 1976. Operant Conditioning and the Management of Stuttering. Englewood Cliffs, N.J.: Prentice-Hall.

Shames, G. H., Egolf, D., and Rhodes, R. 1969. Experimental programs in stuttering therapy. J. Speech Hear. Dis., 34, 30–47.

Shapiro, D., and Surwit, R. 1976. Learned control of physiological function and disease. In H. Leitenberg (Ed.), Handbook of Behavior Modification and Behavior Therapy. Englewood Cliffs, N.J.: Prentice-Hall.

Shaw, C., and Shrum, W. 1972. The effects of response-contingent reward on the connected speech of children who stutter. J. Speech Hear. Res., 37, 75–88.

Shearer, W., and Williams, J. D. 1965. Self-recovery from stuttering. J. Speech Hear. Dis., 30, 288–290.

Sheehan, J. G. 1951. Modification of stuttering through nonreinforcement. J. Abnorm. Soc. Psychol., 46, 51–63.

Sheehan, J. G. 1953. Rorschach changes during psychotherapy in relation to personality of the therapist. Am. Psychol., 8, 434–435.

Sheehan, J. G. 1954a. Rorschach prognosis in psychotherapy and speech therapy. J. Speech Hear. Dis., 19, 217–219.

Sheehan, J. G. 1954b. An integration of psychotherapy and speech therapy through a conflict theory of stuttering. J. Speech Hear. Dis., 19, 474–482.

Sheehan, J. G. 1958a. Projective studies of stuttering. J. Speech Hear. Dis., 23, 18–25.

Sheehan, J. G. 1958b. Conflict theory of stuttering. In J. Eisenson (Ed.) Stuttering: A Symposium. New York: Harper & Row.

Sheehan, J. G. 1968. Stuttering as self-role conflict. In H. Gregory (Ed.), Learning Theory and Stuttering Therapy. Evanston, Ill.: Northwestern University Press.

Sheehan, J. G. (Ed.). 1970a. Stuttering: Research and Therapy. New York: Harper & Row.

Sheehan, J. G. 1970b. Reflections on the behavioral modification of stuttering. In W. Starkweather (Ed.), Stuttering: Behavior Modification. Memphis, Tenn.: Speech Foundation of America.

Sheehan, J. G. 1975. Conflict theory and avoidance-reduction therapy. In J. Eisenson (Ed.), Stuttering: A Second Symposium. New York: Harper & Row.

Sheehan, J. G., Cortese, P., and Hadley, R. 1962. Guilt, shame and tension in graphic projections of stuttering. J. Speech Hear. Dis., 6, 249–254.

Sheehan, J. G., and Costley, M. S. 1977. A reevaluation of the role of heredity in stuttering. J. Speech. Hear. Dis., 42, 47–59.

Sheehan, J. G., Hadley, R., and Gould, E. 1967. Impact of authority on stuttering. J. Abnorm. Psychol., 72, 290–293.

Sheehan, J. G., and Martyn, M. M. 1966. Spontaneous recovery from stuttering. J. Speech Hear. Res., 9, 121–135.

Sheehan, J. G., and Martyn, M. M. 1967. Methodology in studies of recovery from stuttering. J. Speech Hear. Res., 10, 396–400.

Sheehan, J. G., and Martyn, M. M. 1970. Stuttering and its disappearance. J. Speech Hear. Res., 13, 279–287.

Sheehan, J. G., and Martyn, M. M. 1971. Therapy as seen by stutterers. J. Speech Hear. Res., 14, 445–446.

Sheehan, J. G., Martyn, M. M., and Kilburn, K. L. 1968. Speech disorders in retardation. Am. J. Ment. Defic., 73, 251–256.

Sheehan, J. G., and Voas, R. B. 1954. Tension patterns during stuttering in relation to conflict, anxiety-binding, and reinforcement. Speech Monogr. 21, 272–279.

Sheehan, J. G., and Voas, R. B. 1957. Stuttering as conflict: a comparison of therapy techniques involving approach and avoidance. J. Speech Hear. Dis., 22, 714–723.

Sherman, D. 1952. Clinical and experimental use of the Iowa Scale of Severity of moments of stuttering. J. Speech Hear. Dis., 17, 316–320.

Sherman, D. 1955. Reliability and utility of individual ratings of severity of moments of stuttering. J. Speech Hear. Dis., 20, 11–16.

Siegal, G. M. 1970. Punishment, stuttering, and disfluency. J. Speech Hear. Res., 13, 677–714.

Siegal, G. M., and Hanson, B. 1972. The effects of response-contingent neutral stimuli on normal speech disfluency. J. Speech Hear. Res., 15, 123–133.

Skinner, B. F. 1953. Science and Human Behavior. New York: Macmillan.

Speech Foundation of America. 1962. Stuttering: Its Prevention. Memphis, Tenn.: M. Fraser.

Speech Foundation of America. 1964. Treatment of the Young Stutterer in the School. Memphis, Tenn.: M. Fraser.

Speech Foundation of America. 1977. If Your Child Stutters: A Guide for Parents. Memphis, Tenn.: M. Fraser.

Spielberger, C. D. 1966. Anxiety and Behavior. New York: Academic Press.

Staats, A. W. 1977. Fictions in formal analysis' conception of classical conditioning: a case of operantism. Am. Psychol., 32, 231.

Starkweather, C. W. 1973. A behavioral analysis of Van Riperian therapy for stutterers. J. Commun. Dis., 6, 273–291.

Stevens, S. S. 1939. Psychology and the science of science. Psychol. Bull., 36, 221–263.

Stokes, T. F., and Baer, D. M. 1977. An implicit technology of generalization. J. Appl. Behav. Anal., 10, 349–367.

Taylor, M. 1966. An investigation of physiological measures in relation to the moment of stuttering. Unpublished doctoral dissertation, University of Southern California, Los Angeles.

Thomas, L. 1974. The Lives of a Cell. New York: Viking Press.

Travis, L. E. 1936. A Point of View in Speech Correction. Proceedings American Speech Correction Association, 6, 1.

Travis, L. E. 1957. The unspeakable feelings of people with special reference to stuttering. In L. E. Travis (Ed.), Handbook of Speech Pathology, New York: Appleton-Century-Crofts.

Van Kirk, B. 1972. Operant therapy programs for stuttering conducted in a rehabilitation center. Rehab. Lit., 33, 107–108.

Van Riper, C. 1939. Speech Correction: Principles and Methods. Englewood Cliffs, N.J.: Prentice-Hall.

Van Riper, C. 1954. Speech Correction: Principles and Methods. 3rd ed. Englewood Cliffs, N.J.: Prentice-Hall.

Van Riper, C. 1958. Experiments in stuttering therapy. In J. Eisenson (Ed.), Stuttering: A Symposium. New York: Harper & Row.

Van Riper, C. 1963. Speech Correction: Principles and Methods. 4th ed. Englewood Cliffs, N.J.: Prentice-Hall.

Van Riper, C. 1971a. The Nature of Stuttering. Englewood Cliffs, N.J.: Prentice-Hall.

Van Riper, C. 1971b. Symptomatic therapy for stuttering. In L. E. Travis (Ed.), Handbook of Speech Pathology. New York: Appleton-Century-Crofts.

Van Riper, C. 1972. Speech Correction: Principles and Methods. 5th ed. Englewood Cliffs, N.J.: Prentice-Hall.

Van Riper, C. 1973. The Treatment of Stuttering. Englewood Cliffs, N.J.: Prentice-Hall.

Van Riper, C. 1975. The stutterer's clinician. In J. Eisenson (Ed.), Stuttering: A Second Symposium. New York: Harper & Row.

Voelker, C. 1944. A preliminary investigation for a normative study of disfluency: a critical index to the severity of stuttering. Am. J. Orthopsychiatr., 14, 285–294.

Wahler, R., Sperling, K., Thomas, M., Teeter, N., and Luper, H. 1970. The modification of childhood stuttering: some response relationship. J. Exp. Child Psychiatr., 3, 411–428.

Walle, E. L. 1975. To stand and be counted. J. Fluency Dis., 1, 46–48.

Watson, D. L., and Tharp, R. G. 1972. Self-Directed Behavior: Self-Modification for Personal Adjustment. Belmont, Cal.: Wadsworth.

Webster, R. L. 1970. Stuttering: a way to eliminate it and a way to explain it. In R. Ullrich, T. Stachnik, and J. Mabry (Eds.), Control of Human Behavior. Vol. 2. Glenview, Ill.: Scott, Foresman.

Webster, R. L. 1974. A behavioral analysis of stuttering: treatment and theory. In K. Calhoun et al. (Eds.), Innovative Treatment Methods in Psychopathology. New York: John Wiley & Sons.

Webster, R. L. 1975a. A few observations on the manipulation of speech response characteristics in stutterers. In Second Annual Emil Froeschels Conference on the Problem of Stuttering. New York: Pace University Press.

Webster, R. L. 1975b. The Precision Fluency Shaping Program: Speech Reconstruction for Stutterers. Roanoke, Va.: Communication Development Corporation.

Webster, R. L. 1975c. Clinician's Program Guide: The Precision Fluency Shaping Program. Roanoke, Va.: Communications Development Corporation.

Webster, R. L. 1977. Concept and theory in stuttering: an insufficiency of empiricism. In R. W. Rieber (Ed.), The Problems of Stuttering: Theory and Therapy. New York: Elsevier/North-Holland.

Williams, A., and Marks, C. 1972. A comparative analysis of the ITPA and PPVT performances of young stutters and non-stutterers. J. Speech Hear. Res., 11, 622–630.

Williams, D. 1957. A point of view about stuttering. J. Speech Hear. Dis., 22, 390–397.

Williams, D. 1968. Stuttering therapy: an overview. In H. Gregory (Ed.), Learning Theory and Stuttering Therapy. Evanston, Ill.: Northwestern University Press.

Williams, D. 1969. Personal communication to Hugo Gregory.

Williams, D. 1971. Stuttering therapy for children. In L. E. Travis (Ed.), Handbook of Speech Pathology. New York: Appleton-Century-Crofts.

Williams, D. 1978a. Stuttering. In J. F. Curtis (Ed.), Human Communication: Basic Processes and Disorders. New York: Harper & Row.

Williams, D. 1978b. Supplemental case history: stuttering. In F. L. Darley and D. C. Spriestersbach (Eds.), Diagnostic Methods in Speech Pathology. 2nd ed. New York: Harper & Row.

Williams, D. 1978c. The problem of stuttering. In F. L. Darley and D. C. Spriestersbach (Eds.) Diagnostic Methods in Speech Pathology. 2nd ed. New York: Harper & Row.

Williams, D. 1978d. Differential diagnosis of disorders of fluency. In F. L. Darley and D. C. Spriestersbach (Eds.), Diagnostic Methods in Speech Pathology. 2nd ed. New York: Harper & Row.

Williams, D., and Kent, L. 1958. Listener evaluations of speech interruptions. J. Speech Hear. Res., 12, 308–318.

Williams, D., Silverman, F., and Kools, J. 1968. Disfluency behavior of elementary-school stutterers and non-stutterers: the adaptation effect. J. Speech Hear. Res., 11, 622–630.

Williams, D., Silverman, F., and Kools, J. 1969. Disfluency behavior of elementary-school stutterers and non-stutterers: the consistency effect. J. Speech Hear. Res., 12, 301–307.

Wingate, M. 1959. Calling attention to stuttering. J. Speech Hear. Res., 2, 326–335.

Wingate, M. 1962. Evaluation and stuttering. I. Speech characteristics of young children. J. Speech Hear. Dis., 27, 106–115.

Wingate, M. 1964a. A standard definition of stuttering. J. Speech Hear. Dis., 29, 484–489.

Wingate, M. 1964b. Recovery from stuttering. J. Speech Hear. Dis., 29, 312–321.

Wingate, M. 1966. Prosody in stuttering adaptation. J. Speech Hear. Res., 9, 626–629.

Wingate, M. 1967a. Slurvian skill of stutterers. J. Speech Hear. Res., 10, 844–848.

Wingate, M. 1967b. Stuttering and word length. J. Speech Hear. Res., 10, 146–152.

Wingate, M. 1969. Sound and pattern in "artificial" fluency. J. Speech Hear. Res., 12, 677–686.

Wingate, M. 1971. Phonetic ability in stuttering. J. Speech Hear. Res., 14, 189–194.

Wingate, M. 1976. Stuttering: Theory and Treatment. New York: Irvington Publishers. John Wiley & Sons.

Wingate, M. 1978. Disorders of fluency. In P. Skinner and R. L. Shelton (Eds.), Speech, Language and Hearing: Normal Processes and Disorders. Reading, Mass.: Addison-Wesley.

Wischner, G. J. 1969. Stuttering behavior, learning theory and behavior therapy: problems, issues an progress. In B. Gray and G. England (Eds.), Stuttering and the Conditioning Therapies. Monterey, Cal.: Monterey Institute for Speech and Hearing.

Woods, C. L., and Williams, D. 1971. Speech clinicians' conceptions of boys and men who stutter. J. Speech Hear. Dis., 36, 225–334

Woods, C. L., and Williams, D. 1976. Traits attributed to stuttering and normally fluent males. J. Speech Hear. Res., 19, 267–278.

Woolf, G. 1967. The assessment of stuttering as struggle, avoidance and expectancy. Br. J. Dis. Commun., 2, 158–171.

Wyatt, G. 1969. Language Learning and Communication Disorders in Children. New York: The Free Press.

Yairi, E., and Williams, D. 1970. Speech clinicians' stereotypes of elementary-school boys who stutter. J. Commun. Dis., 3, 161–170.

Yalom, I. D. 1975. The Theory and Practice of Group Psychotherapy. Rev. ed. New York: Basic Books.

Young, M. A. 1961. Predicting ratings of severity of stuttering. J. Speech Hear. Dis., Monogr. Suppl. 7, 31–54.

Zwitman, D. H. 1978. The Disfluent Child: A Management Program. Baltimore: University Park Press.

Author Index

Subject Index

Distraction therapy, 105, 180–182,
189, 205, 248, 270
see also Speak more fluently
approach
Dream analysis, 27
Droning, 100, 107
Drug therapies, in stuttering therapy, 59
Duration, prosodic element of, 107
considered in determining stuttering severity, 67, 123

Easy onset, a universal FIG, 79
"Easy Speech," 45, 46
Emphatic responding, 25
Environmental influences
in development of stuttering,
37, 42, 282
in transfer, 56, 61, 286–287
Erickson Scale of Communication
Attitude, 57, 290
Escape behaviors, working with, in
stuttering therapy, 47
Establishment, phase of, in programmed stuttering therapy,
135–136, 149, 157, 273
Expressiveness, as criterion for
measuring normal sounding
speech, 124
External reinforcement, 50
see also Reinforcement
Extinction, of emotional responses,
in stuttering therapy, 16

False fluency, 84, 98, 205
Family, role of, in stuttering therapy, 40, 51–52, 204–205
for preschool-age child, 117–118,
284
in transfer, 153
see also Parent(s), role of
Fear reduction, 249, 251, 255, 256,
272
see also Densensitization
"Feeling of control," 82–84, 242
FIG tree, 79

FIGs, see Fluency-initiating
gestures
Fluency, 32–35
achieving, in stuttering therapy,
2–18, 100–101, 217–221,
247–248, 252, 272, 285
with child, 42, 45
historical overview, 76,
180–182
and issue of relapse, 49–50
and issue of transfer, 152,
153, 217, 226–228, 271
and positive attitude change,
65, 142
programs for, 77, 135–136,
140–141, 212
through the speak more fluently approach, 251
through the stutter more
fluently approach, 251
see also Speak more fluently
approach; Stutter more
fluently approach
controlling, 75–81
see also Fluency-initiating
gestures
as criterion for measurement of
success in therapy, 55, 60,
122, 123, 124, 130, 211, 212,
267
determining, 162
measuring maintenance, 162,
165–166
measuring transfer, 164–165
and effects of specific characteristics of the communicative message on, 37
as goal of stuttering therapy,
82–84, 133, 135, 138–141,
146, 211, 212
maintaining, 65, 85–86, 107,
250, 252
see also Maintenance; Transfer
operational definition, 134, 138
versus stuttering versus normalcy, 98–108
see also Disfluency
Fluency change, resistances to, 86